T0348463

Tuberculosis

Editors

CHARLES L. DALEY
DAVID M. LEWINSOHN

CLINICS IN CHEST MEDICINE

www.chestmed.theclinics.com

December 2019 • Volume 40 • Number 4

ELSEVIER

1600 John F. Kennedy Boulevard • Suite 1800 • Philadelphia, Pennsylvania, 19103-2899

http://www.theclinics.com

CLINICS IN CHEST MEDICINE Volume 40, Number 4
December 2019 ISSN 0272-5231, ISBN-13: 978-0-323-68215-2

Editor: Colleen Dietzler
Developmental Editor: Casey Potter

© **2019 Elsevier Inc. All rights reserved.**

This periodical and the individual contributions contained in it are protected under copyright by Elsevier, and the following terms and conditions apply to their use:

Photocopying
Single photocopies of single articles may be made for personal use as allowed by national copyright laws. Permission of the Publisher and payment of a fee is required for all other photocopying, including multiple or systematic copying, copying for advertising or promotional purposes, resale, and all forms of document delivery. Special rates are available for educational institutions that wish to make photocopies for non-profit educational classroom use. For information on how to seek permission visit www.elsevier.com/permissions or call: (+44) 1865 843830 (UK)/(+1) 215 239 3804 (USA).

Derivative Works
Subscribers may reproduce tables of contents or prepare lists of articles including abstracts for internal circulation within their institutions. Permission of the Publisher is required for resale or distribution outside the institution. Permission of the Publisher is required for all other derivative works, including compilations and translations (please consult www.elsevier.com/permissions).

Electronic Storage or Usage
Permission of the Publisher is required to store or use electronically any material contained in this periodical, including any article or part of an article (please consult www.elsevier.com/permissions). Except as outlined above, no part of this publication may be reproduced, stored in a retrieval system or transmitted in any form or by any means, electronic, mechanical, photocopying, recording or otherwise, without prior written permission of the Publisher.

Notice
No responsibility is assumed by the Publisher for any injury and/or damage to persons or property as a matter of products liability, negligence or otherwise, or from any use or operation of any methods, products, instructions or ideas contained in the material herein. Because of rapid advances in the medical sciences, in particular, independent verification of diagnoses and drug dosages should be made.

Although all advertising material is expected to conform to ethical (medical) standards, inclusion in this publication does not constitute a guarantee or endorsement of the quality or value of such product or of the claims made of it by its manufacturer.

Clinics in Chest Medicine (ISSN 0272-5231) is published quarterly by Elsevier Inc., 360 Park Avenue South, New York, NY 10010-1710. Months of issue are March, June, September, and December. Periodicals postage paid at New York, NY and additional mailing offices. Subscription prices are $377.00 per year (domestic individuals), $726.00 per year (domestic institutions), $100.00 per year (domestic students/residents), $423.00 per year (Canadian individuals), $902.00 per year (Canadian institutions), $484.00 per year (international individuals), $902.00 per year (international institutions), and $230.00 per year (international and Canadian students/residents). International air speed delivery is included in all Clinics subscription prices. All prices are subject to change without notice. **POSTMASTER:** Send address changes to Clinics in Chest Medicine, Elsevier Health Sciences Division, Subscription Customer Service, 3251 Riverport Lane, Maryland Heights, MO 63043. **Customer Service: Telephone: 1-800-654-2452** (U.S. and Canada); **1-314-447-8871** (outside U.S. and Canada). **Fax: 1-314-447-8029. E-mail: journalscustomerservice-usa@elsevier.com (for print support); journalsonlinesupport-usa@elsevier.com (for online support).**

Reprints. For copies of 100 or more of articles in this publication, please contact the Commercial Reprints Department, Elsevier Inc., 360 Park Avenue South, New York, NY 10010-1710. Tel.: 212-633-3874; Fax: 212-633-3820; E-mail: reprints@elsevier.com.

Clinics in Chest Medicine is covered in *MEDLINE/PubMed (Index Medicus), Current Contents/Clinical Medicine, EMBASE/Excerpta Medica, Science Citation Index,* and *ISI/BIOMED.*

Contributors

EDITORS

DAVID M. LEWINSOHN, MD, PhD
Professor and Vice Chair for Research, Department of Medicine, Pulmonary and Critical Care Medicine, Director, OHSU Center for Global Child Health Research, Department of Pediatrics, Oregon Health & Science University, Portland, Oregon, USA

CHARLES L. DALEY, MD
Chief, Division of Mycobacterial and Respiratory Infections, National Jewish Health, Denver, Colorado, USA

AUTHORS

ROBERT W. BELKNAP, MD
Denver Metro Tuberculosis Program, Denver Public Health, Division of Infectious Diseases, Department of Medicine, University of Colorado Anschutz Medical Campus, Aurora, Colorado, USA

PHILIP N. BRITTON, MBBS, PhD
Staff Specialist, Department of Infectious Diseases and Microbiology, The Children's Hospital at Westmead, Clinical Senior Lecturer, Discipline of Child and Adolescent Health, University of Sydney, Sydney, Australia

TERENCE CHORBA, MD, DSc
Division of Tuberculosis Elimination, Centers for Disease Control and Prevention, Atlanta, Georgia, USA

KELLY E. DOOLEY, MD, PhD
Associate Professor of Medicine, Department of Medicine, Center for Tuberculosis Research, Johns Hopkins School of Medicine, Baltimore, Maryland, USA

HELEN FLETCHER, BSc, PhD
Professor, Department of Immunology and Infection, London School of Hygiene and Tropical Medicine, London, United Kingdom

LLOYD N. FRIEDMAN, MD
Clinical Professor of Medicine, Section of Pulmonary, Critical Care, and Sleep Medicine, Yale School of Medicine, New Haven, Connecticut, USA

CHRISTOPHER GILPIN, PhD
Senior Scientist, Global TB Programme, World Health Organization, Geneva, Switzerland

MARK S. GODFREY, MD
Clinical Fellow, Section of Pulmonary, Critical Care, and Sleep Medicine, Yale School of Medicine, New Haven, Connecticut, USA

MICHELLE K. HAAS, MD
Denver Metro Tuberculosis Program, Denver Public Health, Division of Infectious Diseases, Department of Medicine, University of Colorado Anschutz Medical Campus, Aurora, Colorado, USA

MOISES A. HUAMAN, MD, MSc
Assistant Professor of Medicine, Department of Internal Medicine, Division of Infectious Diseases, University of Cincinnati College of Medicine, University of Cincinnati, Hamilton County Public Health Tuberculosis Control Program, Cincinnati, Ohio, USA; Vanderbilt Tuberculosis Center, Vanderbilt University School of Medicine, Nashville, Tennessee, USA

ELISA H. IGNATIUS, MD, MSc
Department of Medicine, Johns Hopkins School of Medicine, Baltimore, Maryland, USA

AMENEH KHATAMI, BHB, MBChB, MD
Clinical Academic, Department of Infectious Diseases and Microbiology, The Children's Hospital at Westmead, Clinical Senior Lecturer, Discipline of Child and Adolescent Health, University of Sydney, Sydney, Australia

ADAM J. LANGER, DVM, MPH
Division of Tuberculosis Elimination, National Center for HIV/AIDS, Viral Hepatitis, STD, and TB Prevention, Centers for Disease Control and Prevention, Atlanta, Georgia, USA

DAVID M. LEWINSOHN, MD, PhD
Professor and Vice Chair for Research, Department of Medicine, Pulmonary and Critical Care Medicine, Director, OHSU Center for Global Child Health Research, Department of Pediatrics, Oregon Health & Science University, Portland, Oregon, USA

DEBORAH A. LEWINSOHN, MD
Oregon Health & Science University, Portland, Oregon, USA

PHILIP LoBUE, MD
Division of Tuberculosis Elimination, National Center for HIV/AIDS, Viral Hepatitis, STD, and TB Prevention, Centers for Disease Control and Prevention, Atlanta, Georgia, USA

BEN J. MARAIS, BMedSc, MBChB, MMed, PhD
Senior Clinical Academic, Department of Infectious Diseases and Microbiology, The Children's Hospital at Westmead, Professor, Discipline of Child and Adolescent Health, Co-Director, Marie Bashir Institute for Infectious Diseases and Biosecurity, University of Sydney, Sydney, Australia

SUNDARI R. MASE, MD, MPH
Medical Officer, Tuberculosis, World Health Organization, Country Office for India, New Delhi, India

FUAD MIRZAYEV, MD, MPH
Medical Officer, Global TB Programme, World Health Organization, Geneva, Switzerland

PAYAM NAHID, MD, MPH
Professor in Residence, Department of Pulmonary, Critical Care, Allergy and Sleep Medicine, UCSF Center for Tuberculosis, University of California, San Francisco, San Francisco, California, USA

EDWARD A. NARDELL, MD
Professor of Medicine, Division of Global Health Equity, Harvard Medical School, Brigham & Women's Hospital, Boston, Massachusetts, USA

THOMAS R. NAVIN, MD
Division of Tuberculosis Elimination, National Center for HIV/AIDS, Viral Hepatitis, STD, and TB Prevention, Centers for Disease Control and Prevention, Atlanta, Georgia, USA

MAX SALFINGER, MD
Professor and Co-Lead DrPH Laboratory Concentration, University of South Florida, College of Public Health, Tampa, Florida, USA

AKOS SOMOSKOVI, MD, PhD, DSc
Head of Respiratory Health, Global Health Technologies, Global Good Fund, Intellectual Ventures Laboratory, Bellevue, Washington, USA

TIMOTHY R. STERLING, MD
Vanderbilt Tuberculosis Center, Professor, Department of Medicine, Division of Infectious Diseases, Vanderbilt University School of Medicine, Vanderbilt University, Nashville, Tennessee, USA

LISA STOCKDALE, BSc, MPH, PhD
Post-Doctoral Researcher, Department of Paediatrics, University of Oxford, NIHR Oxford Biomedical Research Centre and Oxford University Hospitals NHS Foundation Trust, Oxford, United Kingdom

CARLA A. WINSTON, PhD
Division of Tuberculosis Elimination, National Center for HIV/AIDS, Viral Hepatitis, STD, and TB Prevention, Centers for Disease Control and Prevention, Atlanta, Georgia, USA

BETH SHOSHANA ZHA, MD, PhD
Clinical Fellow, Department of Pulmonary, Critical Care, Allergy and Sleep Medicine, UCSF Center for Tuberculosis, University of California, San Francisco, San Francisco, California, USA

Contents

Although considerable progress has been made in reducing US tuberculosis incidence, the goal of eliminating the disease from the United States remains elusive. A continued focus on preventing new tuberculosis infections while also identifying and treating persons with existing tuberculosis infection is needed. Continued vigilance to ensure ongoing control of tuberculosis transmission remains key.

Tuberculosis (TB) host defense depends on cellular immunity, including macrophages and adaptively acquired CD4$^+$ and CD8$^+$ T cells. More recently, roles for new immune components, including neutrophils, innate T cells, and B cells, have been defined, and the understanding of the function of macrophages and adaptively acquired T cells has been advanced. Moreover, the understanding of TB immunology elucidates TB infection and disease as a spectrum. Finally, determinates of TB host defense, such as age and comorbidities, affect clinical expression of TB disease. Herein, the authors comprehensively review TB immunology with an emphasis on new advances.

Biologic drugs have revolutionized the treatment of certain hematologic, autoimmune, and malignant diseases, but they may place patients at risk for reactivation or acquisition of tuberculosis. This risk is highest with the tumor necrosis factor-alpha (TNF-α) inhibitors. Amongst this class of drugs, the monoclonal antibodies (infliximab, adalimumab, golimumab) and antibody fragment (certolizumab) carry an increased risk compared to the soluble receptor fusion molecule, etanercept. Treatment of latent TB is critical to decrease the risk of reactivation. Data continues to emerge regarding tuberculosis risk associated with novel biologics targeting cytokines involved in tuberculosis control.

In 2019, tuberculosis is still a global source of morbidity and mortality. To determine and provide the most effective treatment regimen to patients, the tuberculosis laboratory needs to rapidly but reliably answer 2 main questions: (1) Is Mycobacterium tuberculosis detectable in the patient specimen? and (2) If so, is the strain detected drug susceptible or does it show any form of drug resistance? In cases of drug resistance, health care providers need to have access to minimal inhibitory concentration results and to the type of mutation conferring drug resistance to tailor the most appropriate drug regimen.

The World Health Organization Supranational TB Reference Laboratory Network (SRLN) has served as the backbone for TB drug-resistance surveillance and diagnosis since 1994 and remains a key WHO programme for antimicrobial resistance (AMR) surveillance at the global level. SRLN is a great technical resource for proficiency testing to ensure accuracy of drug-susceptibility testing, scale-up, capacity development in countries and provides unique support to the reliable detection of drug resistance. Technical assistance from individual SRLs has been supported by a variety of mechanisms but funding for the SRLN has become increasingly challenging.

Mycobacterium tuberculosis is a major public health concern and requires prompt treatment. Goals of treatment include curing the individual patient and protecting the community from ongoing tuberculosis transmission. To achieve durable cure, regimens must include multiple agents given concurrently and in a manner to ensure completion of therapy. This article focuses on preferred regimens of drug-susceptible tuberculosis under current guidelines by the American Thoracic Society, Centers for Disease Control and Prevention, and Infectious Diseases Society of America and World Health Organization. In addition, topics including patient centered care, poor treatment outcomes, and adverse effects are also discussed.

The treatment of drug-resistant tuberculosis (TB) is complicated and has evolved significantly in the past decade with the advent of rapid molecular tests and updated evidence-based guidelines of the World Health Organization and other organizations. The latest recommendations incorporate the use of new drugs and regimens that maximize efficacy and minimize toxicity to improve treatment outcomes for patients. This article provides an overview of the latest strategies for clinical and programmatic management of drug-resistant TB.

Children carry a significant tuberculosis disease burden in settings with poor epidemic control and high levels of transmission. Even in high-resource settings, the diagnosis of tuberculosis in children can be challenging, but an accurate diagnosis can be achieved by adopting a systematic approach. This review outlines the general principles of tuberculosis prevention in children, including epidemic control, infection control, contact tracing and preventive therapy, and vaccination; diagnosing pediatric tuberculosis, including specimen collection and microbiological confirmation, highlighting key differences from adults; and tuberculosis treatment in children, including treatment of severe disease that mostly occurs in young children and drug-resistant tuberculosis.

Elisa H. Ignatius and Kelly E. Dooley

Tuberculosis (TB) has now surpassed HIV as the leading infectious cause of death, and treatment success rates are declining. Multidrug-resistant TB, extensively drug-resistant TB, and even totally drug-resistant TB threaten to further destabilize disease control efforts. The second wave in TB drug development, which includes the diarylquinoline, bedaquiline, and the nitroimidazoles delamanid and pretomanid, may offer options for simpler, shorter, and potentially all-oral regimens to treat drug-resistant TB. The "third wave" of TB drug development includes numerous promising compounds, including less toxic versions of older drug classes and candidates with novel mechanisms of action.

Michelle K. Haas and Robert W. Belknap

Diagnosing latent tuberculosis (TB) infection (LTBI) is important globally for TB prevention. LTBI diagnosis requires a positive test for infection and negative evaluation for active disease. Current tests measure an immunologic response and include the tuberculin skin test (TST) and interferon-gamma release assays (IGRAs), T-SPOT.TB and QuantiFERON. The IGRAs are preferred in bacille Calmette-Guérin–vaccinated populations. The TST is still used when cost or logistical advantages over the IGRAs exist. Both TST and IGRAs have low positive predictive values. Tests that differentiate the TB spectrum and better predict future TB risk are needed.

Moises A. Huaman and Timothy R. Sterling

Treatment of latent tuberculosis infection (LTBI) is an important component of TB control and elimination. LTBI treatment regimens include once-weekly isoniazid plus rifapentine for 3 months, daily rifampin for 4 months, daily isoniazid plus rifampin for 3–4 months, and daily isoniazid for 6–9 months. Isoniazid monotherapy is efficacious in preventing TB disease, but the rifampin- and rifapentine-containing regimens are shorter and have similar efficacy, adequate safety, and higher treatment completion rates. Novel vaccine strategies, host immunity-directed therapies and ultrashort antimicrobial regimens for TB prevention, such as daily isoniazid plus rifapentine for 1 month, are under evaluation.

Lisa Stockdale and Helen Fletcher

Exciting clinical results from 2 clinical TB vaccine trials were published in 2018. These, plus promising preclinical candidates form a healthy pipeline of potential vaccines against the leading cause of death from a single infectious agent. The only licensed vaccine, the BCG, continues to be an important tool in protecting against severe forms of TB in children, but has not stopped the diseases causing 1.3 million deaths per year. This review provides an overview of the current TB vaccine pipeline, highlighting recent findings, describes work relating to epidemiologic impact of vaccines, and discusses the future of TB vaccine development.

Edward A. Nardell

Traditional tuberculosis (TB) infection control focuses on the known patient with TB, usually on appropriate treatment. A refocused, intensified TB infection control approach is presented. Combined with active case finding and rapid molecular diagnostics, an approach called FAST is described as a convenient way to call attention to the untreated patient. Natural ventilation is the mainstay of air disinfection in much of the world. Germicidal ultraviolet technology is the most sustainable approach to air disinfection under resource-limited conditions. Testing and treatment of latent TB infection works to prevent reactivation but requires greater risk targeting in both low- and high-risk settings.

CLINICS IN CHEST MEDICINE

SERIES OF RELATED INTEREST

Infectious Disease Clinics
https://www.id.theclinics.com

THE CLINICS ARE AVAILABLE ONLINE!
Access your subscription at:
www.theclinics.com

Preface
Tuberculosis

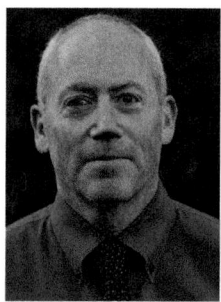

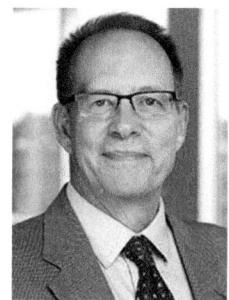

David M. Lewinsohn, MD, PhD   Charles L. Daley, MD
Editors

Caused by *Mycobacterium tuberculosis*, tuberculosis (TB) remains a leading cause of infectious disease morbidity and mortality worldwide. In 2017, there were 10 million cases and 1.6 million deaths. The impact of TB is particularly harsh on vulnerable populations, such as children and those with human immunodeficiency virus, and its importance to global health is highlighted by the inclusion of the goal of ending TB in the Sustainable Development Goals, and by the first United Nations high-level meeting on TB that we held in September 2018.

While TB remains a global health emergency, the diagnosis and management of TB continue to pose challenges as TB is associated with poverty, can be indolent in its clinical presentation, and requires complex and lengthy therapy. Ultimately, the elimination of TB (or eradication) will require improved preventative strategies in those at increased risk to develop TB once infected, or an improved vaccine.

This issue provides a comprehensive overview, encompassing epidemiology, pathogenesis, diagnostics, therapeutics, and recent developments in the prevention of TB. We hope this issue will be of interest to clinicians, scientists, and patients. To the authors, we owe thanks for their excellent contributions. To Casey Potter and the Elsevier staff, and Richard Matthay, we thank you for your support and patience during the long effort to bring this issue to fruition and now publication.

David M. Lewinsohn, MD, PhD
Department of Medicine, Pulmonary and
Critical Care Medicine
OHSU Center for Global Child Health Research
Department of Pediatrics
Oregon Health & Science University
R&D 11, PVAMC, 3710 SW US Veterans Road
Portland, OR 97239, USA

Charles L. Daley, MD
Division of Mycobacterial and
Respiratory Infections
National Jewish Health, Room J204
1400 Jackson Street
Denver, CO 80206, USA

E-mail addresses:
lewinsod@ohsu.edu (D.M. Lewinsohn)
DaleyC@njhealth.org (C.L. Daley)

Epidemiology of Tuberculosis in the United States

Adam J. Langer, DVM, MPH*, Thomas R. Navin, MD, Carla A. Winston, PhD, Philip LoBue, MD

KEYWORDS

- Tuberculosis • Epidemiology • United States • Disease control

KEY POINTS

- Public health efforts have been successful in reducing tuberculosis (TB) morbidity and mortality through an approach largely focused on preventing TB transmission within the United States.
- Future US TB prevention efforts should include a focus on testing for and treating latent tuberculosis infection in order to prevent progression to tuberculosis disease.
- Measures to prevent TB transmission in the United States must be maintained to avoid potential increases in recent transmission that could lead to large outbreaks.

INTRODUCTION

What is now recognized as tuberculosis (TB) has been part of the human experience for all of recorded history, although it was not until the early nineteenth century that the various clinical presentations of the disease were first postulated to be 1 condition and not until later in that century that TB was recognized as an infectious disease caused by *Mycobacterium tuberculosis* complex.[1,2] In addition to the understanding of TB as an infectious disease that was transmissible person to person, researchers applied age-period-cohort methods in the 1930s to demonstrate that the burden of TB in a given cohort at a young age could help to predict the TB burden in that cohort later in life.[3,4] This observation was some of the earliest evidence that TB could remain latent in the body for many years after initial infection before progressing to clinically evident TB disease; this is now commonly known as latent TB infection (LTBI).

Research in the past 10 years to 20 years, however, has drawn into question the classical model of TB as having 2 clinical states: LTBI and active TB disease. Rather, evidence now supports a model where infection with *M tuberculosis* complex (ie, TB infection) is recognized to exist on a clinical spectrum.[5–7] Patients who reside on a part of the spectrum where the cell-mediated immune response to TB infection can be detected through in vivo (ie, tuberculin skin testing [TST]) or in vitro (ie, interferon-gamma release assay [IGRA] testing), but whose degree of tuberculous lesions remain below the limit of detection of available methods (eg, radiography or microbiologic testing) are diagnosed as having LTBI.[5–8] Correspondingly, those persons whose tuberculous disease is severe enough to be detectable are classified as having TB disease.[5–7] However

Disclosure Statements: The authors report no commercial or financial conflicts of interest or outside funding sources. The findings and conclusions in this report are those of the authors and do not necessarily reflect the official position of the Centers for Disease Control and Prevention.
Division of Tuberculosis Elimination, National Center for HIV/AIDS, Viral Hepatitis, STD, and TB Prevention, Centers for Disease Control and Prevention, 1600 Clifton Road Northeast, Mailstop US12-4, Atlanta, GA 30329, USA
* Corresponding author.
E-mail address: ALanger@cdc.gov

Clin Chest Med 40 (2019) 693–702
https://doi.org/10.1016/j.ccm.2019.07.001
0272-5231/19/Published by Elsevier Inc.

flawed a dichotomization might be in terms of the true pathophysiology of TB, it nonetheless can be useful when studying TB epidemiology because it is helpful to think of LTBI as potentially preventable TB disease, even if infected individuals are not now showing any signs of illness or able to transmit the infection to others.

In the United States, TB prevention activities have first focused on early detection and treatment of TB cases, in order to cure the patient and prevent further TB transmission.[9] The second priority is contact investigation around infectious TB cases, to identify other TB disease or LTBI cases and offer treatment to reduce the risk of those individuals progressing to TB disease.[9] Finally, as program resources allow, the third priority is to conduct targeted TB infection testing among high-risk populations to identify persons with remotely acquired LTBI and offer treatment.[9]

US TUBERCULOSIS MORBIDITY, MORTALITY, AND DISABILITY-ADJUSTED LIFE YEARS
Morbidity

Tuberculosis disease
Diagnosis and verification of tuberculosis cases for inclusion in official counts The US government began systematically tracking TB morbidity nationwide in 1953, shortly after the widespread introduction of anti-TB chemotherapy drugs.[10] Definitive diagnosis of TB requires compatible clinical signs and symptoms (eg, persistent cough, unexplained weight loss, and night sweats) in combination with laboratory and diagnostic imaging results consistent with TB.[11] TB disease requires a minimum of 6 months of treatment after diagnosis, and cases often are not detected immediately because of the slow progression of the disease and TB's mimicry of more common illnesses, such as community-acquired pneumonia.[11] This long treatment period makes it is especially important in describing the morbidity of TB to distinguish between incidence (new disease cases observed during a period of interest) and prevalence (all disease cases observed during the period). For TB, the more useful concept is incidence, and TB incidence is commonly described in terms of case counts and incidence rates. The CDC uses US Census Bureau official census and midyear postcensal estimates for population denominator data in the calculation of incidence rates, and rates typically are expressed in CDC TB surveillance data in terms of cases per 100,000 persons in the population of interest during the period of interest.[12] Although both measures are useful, this review focuses on annual incidence rates in order

to account for the effect of changes in the size of the underlying population.

In order for US TB surveillance reporting areas to verify a TB case for surveillance purposes, the case must meet the criteria for 1 of the 3 diagnostic classifications of TB: laboratory confirmation via positive culture or direct testing of a clinical specimen (81%), meeting clinical case criteria in the absence of laboratory confirmation (14%), or expert opinion of a health care provider for cases that do not meet either the laboratory or clinical criteria (5%).[12]

Morbidity trends US TB incidence rates (**Fig. 1**) consistently decreased at annual percent declines from 2.1% to 11.1% from the introduction of systematic national surveillance in 1953 (52.6 cases per 100,000 persons) to 1985 (9.3 cases per 100,000 persons). In 1986, the incidence rate increased (9.5) for the first time over the preceding year (previous recorded increases in 1963 and 1975 were artifacts caused by changes in TB surveillance practices or 1-time immigration events).[10,12] This 1.6% increase in incidence rate could not be explained by either an administrative change in reporting criteria or a 1-time immigration event.[12] Although declines resumed during 1987 to 1988, they were much slower (0.4%–1.1% annual decline in case count and 1.3%–2.0% annual decline in incidence rate).[12] In 1989, a marked increase occurred in incidence rate (3.7%), followed by less dramatic increases during 1990 to 1992 (1.5%–2.3% annual increase in case count and 0.1%–0.9% annual increase in incidence rate).[12] This increase prompted considerable concern, including a Congressional investigation.[10] In 1987, the US Department of Health and Human Services established the Advisory Committee (later Council) for the Elimination of Tuberculosis (ACET) to "provide recommendations for the development of new technology, application of prevention and control methods, and management of state and local tuberculosis programs targeted toward the elimination of tuberculosis as a public health problem."[13] In response, CDC and ACET created a strategic plan for the elimination of TB in the United States, establishing for the first time a national goal of TB elimination (defined as <1 TB case per 1,000,000 population).[13] Major factors that fueled the US TB resurgence were the emergence of human immunodeficiency virus (HIV), the spread of multidrug-resistant (MDR) TB (a problem first noted in 1978), and reductions in resources for US TB control programs.[14–31] A federal task force created the first National Action Plan to Combat Multidrug-Resistant Tuberculosis in 1993.[32] This

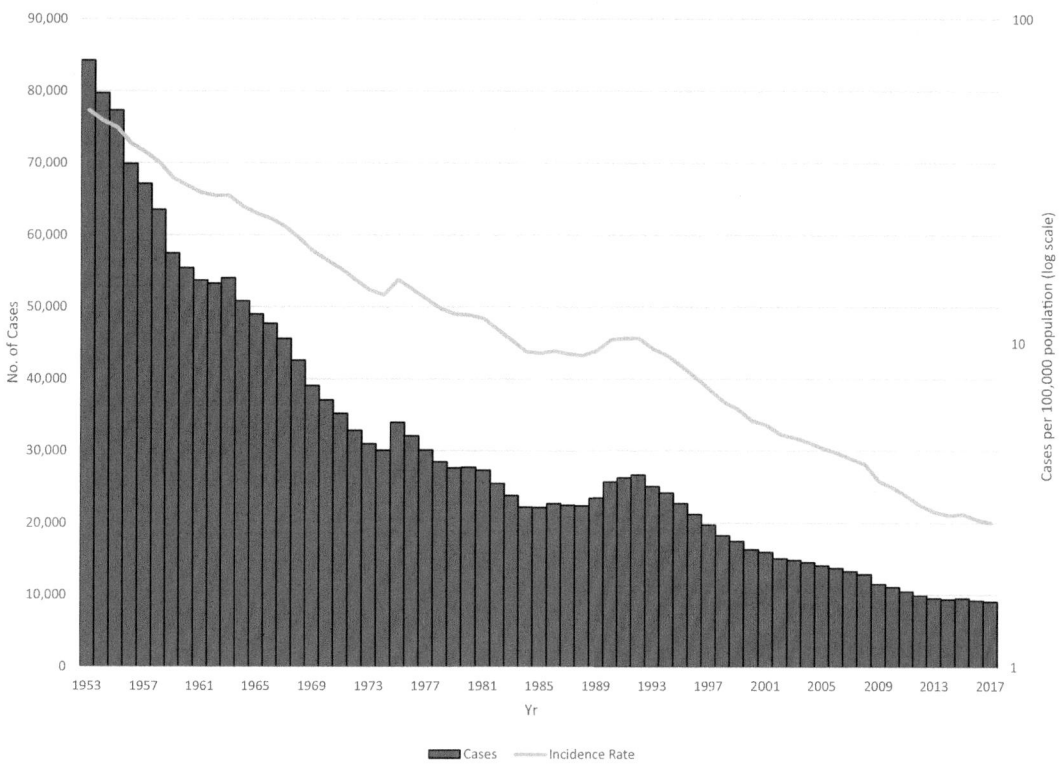

Fig. 1. Tuberculosis cases and incidence rates—United States 1953 to 2017. (*Data from* Centers for Disease Control and Prevention. Reported Tuberculosis in the United States, 2017. Atlanta, GA; 2018. Available at: https://www. cdc.gov/tb/statistics/tbcases.htm.)

initial plan has subsequently been updated and built on with other strategic planning documents, most recently in 2015.[33] As a result of these efforts, primary MDR TB (ie, MDR TB in a patient with no prior history of TB disease) has constituted less than 2% of US TB cases since 1995.[12]

Beginning in 1993, the annual incidence rate began to decline again each year until 2015, when it increased slightly from 2.9 to 3.0 (cases per 100,000 persons) before beginning to decrease again in 2016 (2.9 cases per 100,000 persons) and 2017 (2.8 cases per 100,000 persons).[12] An analysis of incidence rate trends during this period found that there are 3 distinct periods based on average annual percent change (APC) during 1993 to 2012: 1993 to 2000 (APC = −7.3%), 2000 to 2007 (APC = −3.7%), and 2007 to 2012 (APC = −6.7%).[34] The relatively steep 2007 to 2012 decline included an abrupt drop in 2009 from 4.2 to 3.8 (−10%) that raised concerns about potential under-ascertainment of TB cases; however, extensive investigations did not find evidence to support under-detection of TB cases.[35–37] One hypothesis for the abrupt decline was that the contemporaneous US economic recession resulted in changes in migration patterns that influenced the TB incidence rate.[35]

Another potential explanation was the introduction of new technical instructions for overseas panel physicians screening for TB among non–US-born persons who were seeking legal permanent residency in the United States.[38] Since 2012, though, the APC has been only −2.2%.[34] This slowing trend has been observed across geographic and national origin strata, although it is notable that during the entire 1993 to 2017 period, incidence rates among US-born persons declined at a substantially faster pace than rates among non–US-born persons; incidence rates for non–US-born persons during 2013 to 2017 were essentially flat.[34] These data indicate that the percentage of US TB cases occurring among non–US-born persons has been steadily increasing.

Latent tuberculosis infection estimates
Although LTBI has been viewed as an important aspect (and a particular challenge) of TB epidemiology, measuring and reducing LTBI historically have been considered tertiary priorities in the US TB control program.[9] The highest program priority is prompt detection and treatment of TB disease cases in order to prevent further transmission, followed by contact investigation to identify and treat persons recently infected with TB to prevent

progression to TB disease.[9] More recent experience, however, including the results of multiple statistical models, have reinforced the outsized effect of LTBI on the long-term epidemiology of TB disease, particularly in low-incidence countries.[39–41] Unlike TB disease, LTBI is a condition that exists without clinical signs or symptoms. Accordingly, rather than incidence, prevalence is the preferred approach to describing LTBI morbidity. Also, unlike TB disease, because LTBI cases do not come to the attention of the public health system without some form of active case finding, traditional case-based public health surveillance is ill suited to generating LTBI prevalence estimates.

Beginning in 1971, the CDC has conducted periodic TB infection prevalence surveys as part of the National Health and Nutrition Examination Survey (NHANES), which is an annual survey that assesses the health and nutritional status of US residents as part of a continuous program to meet emerging public health needs.[42–44] The 2011 to 2012 NHANES estimated that 4.7% of the civilian, noninstitutionalized US population aged greater than or equal to 6 years were infected with TB, which corresponds to approximately 13.3 million persons.[44] An estimated 5.0% of those infected were male and 4.4% of female, based on TST results, with the highest prevalence of infection among persons 45 years to 64 years of age.[44] Based on TST results, groups with higher LTBI prevalence included non–US-born persons (20.5%), Hispanics (12.3%), and non-Hispanic Asians (22.2%).[44] LTBI prevalence estimates using IGRA resulted in similar patterns as for TST.[44] In all populations, LTBI prevalence estimates did not significantly differ from the NHANES 1999 to 2000 estimates.[43,44]

In addition to supporting periodic NHANES estimates, the CDC continues to explore other innovative approaches to estimating LTBI prevalence. One of these approaches takes advantage of an established, field-validated method using routinely collected US TB surveillance data, linked to molecular genotyping information, to classify TB cases as being attributed to recent transmission (occurring in the preceding 2 years) by using this recent transmission estimate as the basis for back-calculation of the underlying LTBI prevalence.[45–47] Other approaches using mathematical modeling also have been published.[48]

Modeling the future

Given the numerous key determinants of US TB incidence rates, the CDC and its partners have developed several advanced statistical models to explain and predict incidence rate trends.[39–41]

These models include many of the known predictors for TB incidence, and they indicate that without any changes in current US TB control practices, incidence rate declines will continue to slow, with the main contributor to this trend being the prevalence of LTBI in the United States, particularly among non–US-born persons.[39–41]

Mortality and Disability

The United States has made considerable progress in reducing deaths attributed in TB (**Fig. 2**). In 1953, the TB mortality rate was 12.4 deaths per 100,000 persons; however, within 10 years the rate had declined more than 60% to 4.9 in 1963.[12] After another decade, the rate had dropped by a similar degree to 1.8 in 1973, and this trend continued similarly into the early 1980s before slowing during the TB resurgence of the late 1980s.[12] After the end of the resurgence, the mortality rate rapidly declined again until reaching 0.2 in 2003, where it has remained since then.[12] A similar, although slower, trend has occurred with case fatality ratios, declining from 23.4% in 1953 to approximately 5.0% to 6.0% in the past several years.[12] Statistical modeling of TB mortality rates predicts that the mortality rate will remain close to 0.2 until at least 2025 before the pace of decline in mortality begins to accelerate again.[41]

Reliance on vital statistics (death certificate) data for TB mortality estimates has prompted concerns that these estimates might represent persons who died *with* TB (ie, TB was not the actual cause of death) rather than persons who died *from* TB; however, recently published research has found that most (72%) persons who die with TB did have a TB-related death.[49] Delayed diagnosis is the major risk factor for TB mortality; approximately three-fourths of persons who died from TB did so before diagnosis or within a month of treatment initiation.[49] Other risk factors include HIV infection (or not knowing a patient's HIV status), particularly severe forms of TB disease, preexisting comorbidities, use of immunosuppressive medications, MDR, and exclusion of pyrazinamide from the initial treatment regimen (possibly because of concern about hepatotoxicity).[49,50]

In the past 2 decades, public health programs have increasingly understood the importance of long-term effects of disease in patients who survive. The disability-adjusted life year (DALY) is a summary measure combining years of life lost to premature death with time lived in less than perfect health, which the DALY calculation refers to as "disability."[51] **Fig. 3** shows the TB DALY and DALY rate (per 100,000 population) estimates for

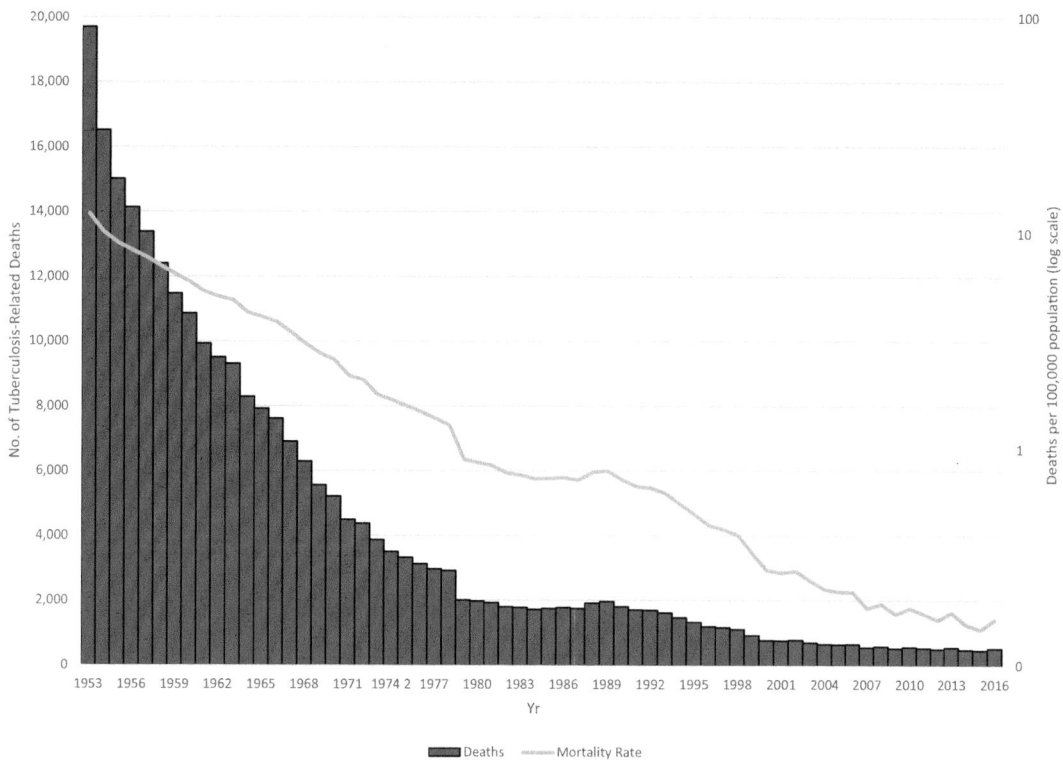

Fig. 2. Tuberculosis deaths and mortality rates—United States 1953 to 2016. (*Data from* Centers for Disease Control and Prevention. Reported tuberculosis in the United States, 2017. Atlanta, GA; 2018.)

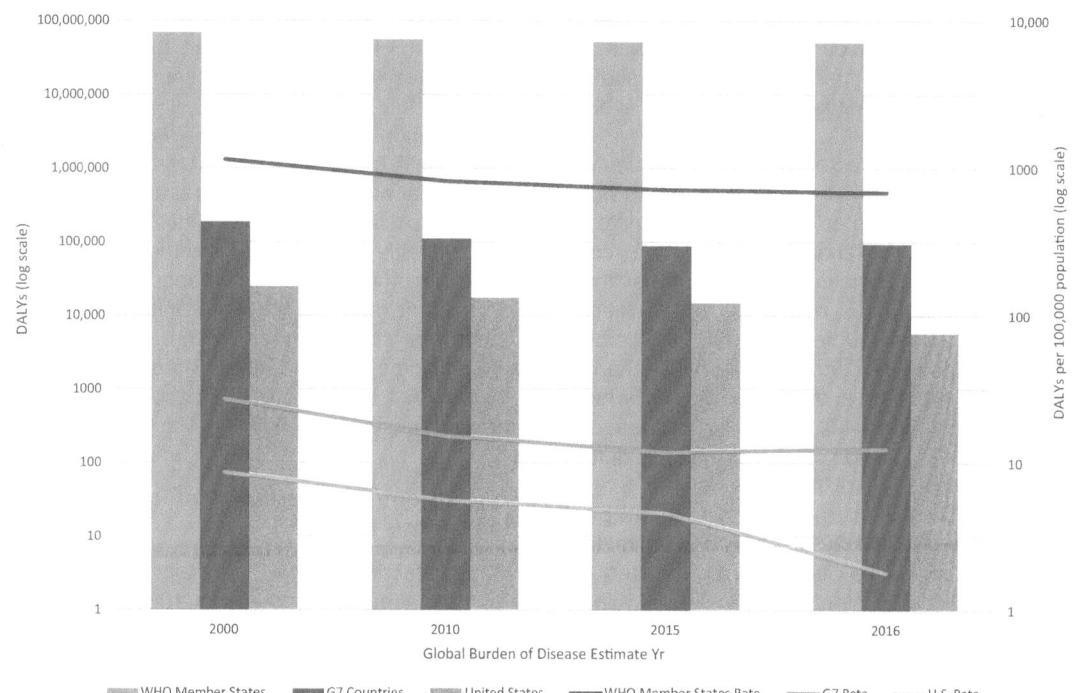

Fig. 3. DALYs lost to tuberculosis and DALYs per 100,000 population—all WHO members states, all G7 countries, and United States, 2000 to 2016. (*Data from* WHO. Global Health Estimates 2016: Disease burden by Cause, Age, Sex, by Country and by Region, 2000-2016. 2018; Available at http://www.who.int/healthinfo/global_burden_disease/estimates/en/index1.html.)

the United States, the Group of Seven (G7) industrialized countries, and for all World Health Organization member states.[51] The US DALY rate is on average greater than 200 times lower than the global rate and approximately 4 times lower than the G7 rate; the US rate also declined by approximately half between 2000 and 2015.[51] This suggests that the United States has been more effective at preventing TB death and disability than the world in general or even the comparably developed economies of the G7 countries; however, it is not clear what factors have led to the US success in this regard.

US TUBERCULOSIS RISK FACTORS
Risk Factors for Acquisition of Tuberculosis Infection

The beginning and end of the TB epidemiologic cycle is transmission of the infection to a new host, and one of the most important goals of public health programs is to prevent uninfected persons from becoming infected. This primary prevention goal is the top priority of the US TB program. Only persons with respiratory forms of TB are considered infectious; however, approximately 80% of all US TB cases reported in 2017 had a respiratory site of disease.[12] More than 70% of 2017 pulmonary TB cases were sputum culture positive, which is an indication of infectiousness.[12] The risk at a population level of becoming infected with TB is directly related to the concentration (case or incidence rate) of infectious TB cases to which that person is exposed.

The strongest risk factor for becoming infected with TB is the country in which a person is born or spends most of his or her life. For example, a person born in sub-Saharan Africa, where most countries report TB incidence rates greater than or equal to 300 cases per 100,000 population, has approximately 100 times the risk on average of being exposed to someone with TB than a person who was born in the United States, where the incidence rate in 2017 was 2.8 cases per 100,000.[12,52] As a nation of immigrants, this difference is particularly striking in the United States when comparing US-born and non–US-born persons. During 2011 to 2012, NHANES estimated the overall prevalence of TB infection (based on a conservative TB infection definition requiring that both TST and IGRA results be positive) in the United States at approximately 2%; however, when stratified by origin of birth, the TB infection prevalence among non–US-born persons using the double-positive definition was approximately 9%, which is considerably higher than the estimate among US-born persons (0.6%).[44] As a

result, non-US birth is the major defining risk factor for greater than 70% of US TB cases, whereas the approximately 30% of cases occurring among US-born persons typically involve 1 or more clinical or social risk factors, such as immunocompromise, homelessness, or substance misuse.[12]

This difference in risk of infection is further demonstrated through the birth cohort effect.[3,4,12] Even when stratifying by origin of birth among US TB disease cases reported during 1996 to 2016 and controlling for age and period effects, all successive birth cohorts had lower age-specific incidence rates than all previous cohorts.[53] This strong birth cohort effect is the consequence of steady reductions over time in the risk of TB exposure for each successive cohort.[53]

The next most important risk factor for acquiring TB infection is documented close contact with a TB patient; the risk of infection increases proportionately to the amount of time spent in close contact with persons who have infectious TB disease.[54] Accordingly, any circumstances that can lead to crowding can increase the risk of TB infection and disease, for example, estimated TB rates among persons experiencing homelessness (36–47 cases per 100,000) and incarceration (8–29 cases per 100,000).[55–57] Two analyses of data from the 1999 to 2000 NHANES cycle identified associations between tobacco smoking or exposure to secondhand tobacco smoke and acquiring TB infection; however, this association has not been identified in subsequent NHANES cycles.[58,59]

Occupation can also increase risk of exposure to TB. Health care workers are at least theoretically at particular risk for TB exposure, although only a small proportion of US TB cases are reported among health care workers, and these individuals often have other risk factors for acquiring TB infection, such as birth outside of the United States.[60] A recent analysis in Canada, which has similar TB epidemiology to the United States, found that occupational exposure to TB (based on workers' compensation claims) was relatively uncommon.[61]

Progression of Tuberculosis Infection to Tuberculosis Disease

HIV coinfection played a major role in the resurgence of TB in the late 1980s and early 1990s.[17,19,21] Systematically assessing the degree of coinfection has been challenging because of low rates of HIV testing of TB patients and incomplete reporting of these data to the CDC; however, efforts to promote testing and treatment of HIV infection have been largely successful.[62] In 1993, only 30% of TB patients were tested for HIV, but approximately half of those tested were HIV positive.[12] In contrast, by 2017 approximately 90% of TB patients had been tested for HIV, and only 5.5% were positive.[12] Even among this small proportion of coinfected patients, it is unclear how many are substantially immunocompromised given the widespread availability of highly effective antiretroviral therapy.

Individuals who misuse alcohol or drugs or who smoke tobacco are also at higher risk of progressing to TB disease, which could be because of a combination of factors, including impaired overall health status.[63–67] Use of tumor necrosis factor α inhibitors for conditions, such as rheumatoid arthritis, is also associated with progression to TB disease.[68] Additional risk factors for progression to TB disease include diabetes mellitus (19.1% of reported TB cases) and other non-HIV immunocompromising conditions, including end-stage renal disease and history of solid organ transplantation (7.5%).[12,69–80]

DISCUSSION

As the US TB control program enters a new decade, a combination of old and new approaches is needed to maintain and accelerate progress toward eliminating TB in the United States. Traditional programmatic priorities focused on early detection of TB cases, prompt treatment of TB cases to prevent further transmission, and early identification and treatment of recently infected persons to reduce the risk of progression to TB disease have been highly successful in reducing TB incidence among US-born persons; however, the decline in TB incidence among the non–US-born has been much slower, largely because US-based efforts to reduce recent transmission are substantially less effective in reducing TB incidence among non–US-born populations who were most likely infected many years before arriving in the United States. Accordingly, more emphasis is needed on testing for and treating LTBI in high-risk populations, such as the non–US-born. Although epidemiologic models have demonstrated that stopping recent transmission in the United States alone will not be sufficient to achieve TB elimination, it is equally clear from the TB resurgence in the late 1980s and early 1990s that control measures aimed at reducing recent transmission must be maintained to prevent a reversal of the substantial gains in TB control achieved during the past 70 years.

Although it cannot be at the expense of transmission control activities, wherever possible TB control programs should increase their investments in testing for and treating LTBI among high-risk populations in order to accelerate progress toward TB elimination in the United States.[81] More sensitive and specific tests are needed for TB infection to ensure that LTBI cases are not missed and persons without LTBI are not treated unnecessarily.[81] Continued progress is also needed on developing LTBI treatment regimens that are less expensive, shorter, and less toxic than current treatments.[81] In addition, development of diagnostic tests that can distinguish which LTBI cases are more likely to progress to TB disease would help to prioritize LTBI cases for treatment.[82] Finally, improvement of overseas TB screening of persons seeking entry into the United States to include more visa types and broaden testing for TB infection beyond children could substantially reduce the burden of TB among non–US-born persons living in the United States.[83]

REFERENCES

1. Dubos RJ, Dubos J. The white plague; tuberculosis, man and society. Boston: Little, Brown; 1952.
2. Koch R. Die atiologic der tuberkulose. Berliner KlinischeWochenschrift 1882;15:221–30.
3. Frost WH. The age selection of mortality from tuberculosis in successive decades. 1939. Am J Epidemiol 1995;141(1):4–9 [discussion: 3].
4. Andvord KF, Wijsmuller G, Blomberg B. What can we learn by following the development of tuberculosis from one generation to another? 1930. Int J Tuberc Lung Dis 2002;6(7):562–8.
5. Dutta NK, Karakousis PC. Latent tuberculosis infection: myths, models, and molecular mechanisms. Microbiol Mol Biol Rev 2014;78(3):343–71.
6. Drain PK, Bajema KL, Dowdy D, et al. Incipient and subclinical tuberculosis: a clinical review of early stages and progression of infection. Clin Microbiol Rev 2018;31(4) [pii:e00021-18].
7. Sousa J, Saraiva M. Paradigm changing evidence that alter tuberculosis perception and detection: focus on latency. Infect Genet Evol 2018;72:78–85.
8. Lewinsohn DM, Leonard MK, LoBue PA, et al. Official American Thoracic Society/Infectious Diseases Society of America/Centers for Disease Control and Prevention Clinical Practice Guidelines: Diagnosis of Tuberculosis in Adults and Children. Clin Infect Dis 2017;64(2):111–5.
9. Centers for Disease Control (CDC). Essential components of a tuberculosis prevention and control program. Recommendations of the Advisory Council for the Elimination of Tuberculosis. MMWR Recomm Rep 1995;44(RR-11):1–16.
10. U.S. Congress Office of Technology Assessment. The continuing challenge of tuberculosis, OTA-H-574. Washington, DC: U.S. Government Printing Office; 1993.

11. Nahid P, Dorman SE, Alipanah N, et al. Official American Thoracic Society/Centers for Disease Control and Prevention/Infectious Diseases Society of America Clinical Practice Guidelines: Treatment of Drug-Susceptible Tuberculosis. Clin Infect Dis 2016; 63(7):e147–95.

12. Centers for Disease Control (CDC). Reported Tuberculosis in the United States, 2017. Atlanta (GA): CDC; 2018.

13. Centers for Disease Control (CDC). A strategic plan for the elimination of tuberculosis in the United States. MMWR Morb Mortal Wkly Rep 1989;38(16): 269–72.

14. Villarino ME, Geiter LJ, Simone PM. The multidrug-resistant tuberculosis challenge to public health efforts to control tuberculosis. Public Health Rep 1992;107(6):616–25.

15. Kent JH. The epidemiology of multidrug-resistant tuberculosis in the United States. Med Clin North Am 1993;77(6):1391–409.

16. Brudney K, Dobkin J. Resurgent tuberculosis in New York City. Human immunodeficiency virus, homelessness, and the decline of tuberculosis control programs. Am Rev Respir Dis 1991;144(4):745–9.

17. Centers for Disease Control (CDC). Nosocomial transmission of multidrug-resistant tuberculosis among HIV-infected persons–Florida and New York, 1988-1991. MMWR Morb Mortal Wkly Rep 1991;40(34):585–91.

18. Reichman LB. The U-shaped curve of concern. Am Rev Respir Dis 1991;144(4):741–2.

19. Beck-Sague C, Dooley SW, Hutton MD, et al. Hospital outbreak of multidrug-resistant Mycobacterium tuberculosis infections. Factors in transmission to staff and HIV-infected patients. JAMA 1992; 268(10):1280–6.

20. Daley CL, Small PM, Schecter GF, et al. An outbreak of tuberculosis with accelerated progression among persons infected with the human immunodeficiency virus. An analysis using restriction-fragment-length polymorphisms. N Engl J Med 1992;326(4):231–5.

21. Dooley SW, Villarino ME, Lawrence M, et al. Nosocomial transmission of tuberculosis in a hospital unit for HIV-infected patients. JAMA 1992;267(19): 2632–4.

22. Edlin BR, Tokars JI, Grieco MH, et al. An outbreak of multidrug-resistant tuberculosis among hospitalized patients with the acquired immunodeficiency syndrome. N Engl J Med 1992;326(23): 1514–21.

23. Pearson ML, Jereb JA, Frieden TR, et al. Nosocomial transmission of multidrug-resistant Mycobacterium tuberculosis. A risk to patients and health care workers. Ann Intern Med 1992;117(3):191–6.

24. Snider DE Jr, Roper WL. The new tuberculosis. N Engl J Med 1992;326(10):703–5.

25. Frieden TR, Sterling T, Pablos-Mendez A, et al. The emergence of drug-resistant tuberculosis in New York City. N Engl J Med 1993;328(8):521–6.

26. Landesman SH. Commentary: tuberculosis in New York City–the consequences and lessons of failure. Am J Public Health 1993;83(5):766–8.

27. Buskin SE, Gale JL, Weiss NS, et al. Tuberculosis risk factors in adults in King County, Washington, 1988 through 1990. Am J Public Health 1994;84(11):1750–6.

28. Cantwell MF, Snider DE Jr, Cauthen GM, et al. Epidemiology of tuberculosis in the United States, 1985 through 1992. JAMA 1994;272(7):535–9.

29. Brown RE, Miller B, Taylor WR, et al. Health-care expenditures for tuberculosis in the United States. Arch Intern Med 1995;155(15):1595–600.

30. Jereb JA, Klevens RM, Privett TD, et al. Tuberculosis in health care workers at a hospital with an outbreak of multidrug-resistant Mycobacterium tuberculosis. Arch Intern Med 1995;155(8):854–9.

31. Centers for Disease Control (CDC). CDC timeline 1940s–1970s. Available at: https://www.cdc.gov/museum/timeline/1940-1970.html. Accessed September 28, 2018.

32. Centers for Disease Control (CDC). National action plan to combat multidrug-resistant tuberculosis. MMWR Recomm Rep 1992;41(RR-11):5–48.

33. National action plan for combating multidrug-resistant tuberculosis. Washington, DC: Executive Office of the President of the United States; 2015. Available at: https://obamawhitehouse.archives.gov/sites/default/files/microsites/ostp/national_action_plan_for_tuberculosis_20151204_final.pdf. Accessed November 3, 2018.

34. Armstrong LR, Winston CA, Stewart B, et al. Changes in tuberculosis epidemiology, United States, 1993–2017. Int J Tuberc Lung Dis 2019 2019;23(7):797–804.

35. Winston CA, Navin TR, Becerra JE, et al. Unexpected decline in tuberculosis cases coincident with economic recession - United States, 2009. BMC Public Health 2011;11:846.

36. Winston CA, Navin TR, Becerra JE, et al. No rebound in tuberculosis in the United States in 2010. Int J Tuberc Lung Dis 2011;15(9):1272.

37. Chen MP, Shang N, Winston CA, et al. A Bayesian analysis of the 2009 decline in tuberculosis morbidity in the United States. Stat Med 2012; 31(27):3278–84.

38. Liu Y, Posey DL, Cetron MS, et al. Effect of a culture-based screening algorithm on tuberculosis incidence in immigrants and refugees bound for the United States: a population-based cross-sectional study. Ann Intern Med 2015;162(6): 420–8.

39. Hill AN, Becerra JE, Castro KG. Modelling tuberculosis trends in the USA. Epidemiol Infect 2012; 140(10):1862–72.

40. Shrestha S, Hill AN, Marks SM, et al. Comparing drivers and dynamics of tuberculosis in California, Florida, New York, and Texas. Am J Respir Crit Care Med 2017;196(8):1050–9.

41. Menzies NA, Cohen T, Hill AN, et al. Prospects for tuberculosis elimination in the United States: results of a transmission dynamic model. Am J Epidemiol 2018;187(9):2011–20.

42. Centers for Disease Control (CDC). About the National Health and Nutrition Examination Survey. Available at: https://www.cdc.gov/nchs/nhanes/about_nhanes.htm. Accessed November 3, 2018.

43. Bennett DE, Courval JM, Onorato I, et al. Prevalence of tuberculosis infection in the United States population: the national health and nutrition examination survey, 1999-2000. Am J Respir Crit Care Med 2008;177(3):348–55.

44. Miramontes R, Hill AN, Woodruff RSY, et al. Tuberculosis infection in the United States: prevalence estimates from the national health and nutrition examination survey, 2011-2012. PLoS One 2015;10(11):e0140881.

45. France AM, Grant J, Kammerer JS, et al. A field-validated approach using surveillance and genotyping data to estimate tuberculosis attributable to recent transmission in the United States. Am J Epidemiol 2015;182(9):799–807.

46. Yuen CM, Kammerer JS, Marks K, et al. Recent transmission of tuberculosis - United States, 2011-2014. PLoS One 2016;11(4):e0153728.

47. Haddad MB, Raz KM, Lash TL, et al. Simple estimates for local prevalence of latent tuberculosis infection, United States, 2011–2015. Emerg Infect Dis 2018;24(10):1930–3.

48. Houben RMGJ, Dodd PJ. The global burden of latent tuberculosis infection: a Re-estimation using mathematical modelling. PLoS Med 2016;13(10):e1002152.

49. Beavers SF, Pascopella L, Davidow AL, et al. Tuberculosis mortality in the United States: epidemiology and prevention opportunities. Ann Am Thorac Soc 2018;15(6):683–92.

50. Hannah HA, Miramontes R, Gandhi NR. Sociodemographic and clinical risk factors associated with tuberculosis mortality in the United States, 2009-2013. Public Health Rep 2017;132(3):366–75.

51. World Health Organization. Global Health estimates 2016: disease burden by cause, age, Sex, by country and by region, 2000-2016. 2018. Available at: http://www.who.int/healthinfo/global_burden_disease/estimates/en/index1.html. Accessed November 3, 2018.

52. World Health Organization. Global tuberculosis report 2018. Geneva (Switzerland): World Health Organization; 2018.

53. Iqbal SA, Winston CA, Bardenheier BH, et al. Age-Period-cohort analyses of tuberculosis incidence rates by nativity, United States, 1996-2016. Am J Public Health 2018;108(S4):S315–20.

54. Wanyeki I, Olson S, Brassard P, et al. Dwellings, crowding, and tuberculosis in Montreal. Social Sci Med 2006;63(2):501–11.

55. Bamrah S, Yelk Woodruff RS, Powell K, et al. Tuberculosis among the homeless, United States, 1994-2010. Int J Tuberc Lung Dis 2013;17(11):1414–9.

56. Lambert LA, Armstrong LR, Lobato MN, et al. Tuberculosis in jails and prisons: United States, 2002-2013. Am J Public Health 2016;106(12):2231–7.

57. Mindra G, Wortham JM, Haddad MB, et al. Tuberculosis among incarcerated hispanic persons in the United States, 1993–2014. J Immigr Minor Health 2017;19(4):982–6.

58. Horne DJ, Campo M, Ortiz JR, et al. Association between smoking and latent tuberculosis in the U.S. Population: an analysis of the national health and nutrition examination survey. PLoS One 2012;7(11):e49050.

59. Lindsay RP, Shin SS, Garfein RS, et al. The Association between active and passive smoking and latent tuberculosis infection in adults and children in the United States: results from NHANES. PLoS One 2014;9(3):e93137.

60. Lambert LA, Pratt RH, Armstrong LR, et al. Tuberculosis among healthcare workers, United States, 1995-2007. Infect Control Hosp Epidemiol 2012;33(11):1126–32.

61. Youakim S. The occupational risk of tuberculosis in a low-prevalence population. Occup Med (Lond) 2016;66(6):466–70.

62. Albalak R, O'Brien RJ, Kammerer JS, et al. Trends in tuberculosis/human immunodeficiency virus comorbidity, United States, 1993-2004. Arch Intern Med 2007;167(22):2443–52.

63. Oeltmann JE, Oren E, Haddad MB, et al. Tuberculosis outbreak in marijuana users, Seattle, Washington, 2004. Emerg Infect Dis 2006;12(7):1156–9.

64. Oeltmann JE, Kammerer JS, Pevzner ES, et al. Tuberculosis and substance abuse in the United States, 1997-2006. Arch Intern Med 2009;169(2):189–97.

65. Volkmann T, Moonan PK, Miramontes R, et al. Tuberculosis and excess alcohol use in the United States, 1997-2012. Int J Tuberc Lung Dis 2015;19(1):111–9.

66. Smith GS, Van Den Feden SK, Baxter R, et al. Cigarette smoking and pulmonary tuberculosis in northern California. J Epidemiol Community Health 2015;69(6):568–73.

67. Davies PDO, Yew WW, Ganguly D, et al. Smoking and tuberculosis: the epidemiological association and immunopathogenesis. Trans R Soc Trop Med Hyg 2006;100(4):291–8.

68. Keane J, Gershon S, Wise RP, et al. Tuberculosis associated with infliximab, a tumor necrosis factor

alpha-neutralizing agent. N Engl J Med 2001; 345(15):1098–104.

69. Epstein DJ, Subramanian AK. Prevention and management of tuberculosis in solid organ transplant recipients. Infect Dis Clin North Am 2018;32(3): 703–18.

70. Gras J, De Castro N, Montlahuc C, et al. Clinical characteristics, risk factors, and outcome of tuberculosis in kidney transplant recipients: a multicentric case-control study in a low-endemic area. Transpl Infect Dis 2018;20(5):e12943.

71. Santoro-Lopes G, Subramanian AK, Molina I, et al. Tuberculosis recommendations for solid organ transplant recipients and donors. Transplantation 2018;102(2S Suppl 2):S60–5.

72. Natori Y, Ferreira VH, Nellimarla S, et al. Incidence, outcomes, and long-term immune response to tuberculosis in organ transplant recipients. Transplantation 2019;103(1):210–5.

73. Gavelli F, Patrucco F. Diabetes and tuberculosis: a closer and closer relationship. Clin Respir J 2018; 12(11):2622–3.

74. Hayashi S, Chandramohan D. Risk of active tuberculosis among people with diabetes mellitus: systematic review and meta-analysis. Trop Med Int Health 2018;23(10):1058–70.

75. Lin SY, Tu HP, Lu PL, et al. Metformin is associated with a lower risk of active tuberculosis in patients with type 2 diabetes. Respirology 2018;23(11):1063–73.

76. Nguyen CH, Pascopella L, Barry PM. Association between diabetes mellitus and mortality among patients with tuberculosis in California, 2010-2014. Int J Tuberc Lung Dis 2018;22(11):1269–76.

77. Siddiqui AN, Hussain S, Siddiqui N, et al. Detrimental association between diabetes and tuberculosis: an unresolved double trouble. Diabetes Metab Syndr 2018;12(6):1101–7.

78. Tegegne BS, Mengesha MM, Teferra AA, et al. Association between diabetes mellitus and multi-drug-resistant tuberculosis: evidence from a systematic review and meta-analysis 11 medical and health sciences 1117 public health and health services. Syst Rev 2018;7(1):161.

79. Moran E, Baharani J, Dedicoat M, et al. Risk factors associated with the development of active tuberculosis among patients with advanced chronic kidney disease. J Infect 2018;77(4):291–5.

80. Okada RC, Barry PM, Skarbinski J, et al. Epidemiology, detection, and management of tuberculosis among end-stage renal disease patients. Infect Control Hosp Epidemiol 2018;39(11): 1367–74.

81. LoBue PA, Mermin JH. Latent tuberculosis infection: the final frontier of tuberculosis elimination in the USA. Lancet Infect Dis 2017;17(10):e327–33.

82. Zak DE, Penn-Nicholson A, Scriba TJ, et al. A blood RNA signature for tuberculosis disease risk: a prospective cohort study. Lancet 2016;387(10035): 2312–22.

83. Maloney SA, Fielding KL, Laserson KF, et al. Assessing the performance of overseas tuberculosis screening programs: a study among US-bound immigrants in Vietnam. Arch Intern Med 2006;166(2): 234–40.

New Concepts in Tuberculosis Host Defense

David M. Lewinsohn, MD, PhD[a], Deborah A. Lewinsohn, MD[b],*

KEYWORDS

- Tuberculosis • Innate immunity • T cells • Adaptive immunity • Trained immunity • Macrophages

KEY POINTS

- New insights into immunometabolism, trained immunity, and neutrophils provide novel targets for host-directed therapies for tuberculosis (TB).
- Donor-unrestricted T cells use highly conserved monomorphic antigen presentation molecules to recognize a diverse repertoire of peptidic and nonpeptidic *Mycobacterium tuberculosis* (Mtb) ligands.
- Recent advances in the understanding of T-cell antigen recognition, memory, and mucosal trafficking have important implications for development of an improved TB vaccine.
- Transcriptomic and cellular immunologic signatures as well as PET-computed tomographic imaging reveal the spectrum of disease caused by Mtb infection.
- Determinates of TB host defense, including young and old age, and comorbidities, such as diabetes and HIV infection, predispose to an increased incidence and severity of TB disease.

INTRODUCTION

It has long been understood that tuberculosis (TB) host defense depends on cellular immunity, including primary containment by macrophages and secondary containment by adaptively acquired CD4[+] and CD8[+] T cells. More recently, roles for new immune components, including neutrophils, innate T cells, and B cells, have been defined, and the understanding of the function of macrophages and adaptively acquired T cells has been advanced. Moreover, the understanding of TB immunology elucidates TB infection and disease as a spectrum rather than dichotomous states. Finally, advances in understanding of the effect of host determinates on TB immunity, such as the spectrum of age and comorbidities, such as human immunodeficiency virus (HIV) infection

and diabetes, elucidate how these factors affect clinical expression of *Mycobacterium tuberculosis* (Mtb) infection and disease. Herein, the authors comprehensively review TB immunology with an emphasis on new advances and describe how recent advances in the understanding of TB defense leads to a more mechanistic understanding of TB infection and clinical expression of disease.

NEW CONCEPTS IN INNATE CELLULAR IMMUNITY
Macrophages

Macrophages serve dual and opposing roles in the pathogenesis of TB in that macrophages are both the predominant host cell and the first line of defense against Mtb infection. Advances in the understanding of the complex interplay between

Disclosure Statement: Oregon Health and Science University (OHSU) and Drs D.M. Lewinsohn and D.A. Lewinsohn have a financial interest in ViTi, a company that is developing biomarkers of TB progression and therefore may have a commercial interest in the contents of this article. This potential individual and institutional conflict of interest has been reviewed and managed by OHSU.
[a] Oregon Health and Science University, 3710 Southwest U.S. Veterans Road, Portland, OR 97239, USA;
[b] Oregon Health and Science University, 707 Southwest Gaines Road, Portland, OR 97239, USA
* Corresponding author.
E-mail address: lewinsde@ohsu.edu

Clin Chest Med 40 (2019) 703–719
https://doi.org/10.1016/j.ccm.2019.07.002
0272-5231/19/© 2019 Elsevier Inc. All rights reserved.

chestmed.theclinics.com

host macrophage and Mtb are relevant to new developments in both TB vaccines and therapeutics. Understanding the mechanisms of Mtb-induced macrophage activation and proinflammatory function provides potential opportunities for host-directed therapeutics (HDT) of multi-drug-resistant and extensively drug-resistant TB. Also, improved understanding of mycobacteria-trained immunity in macrophages (discussed later) may aid in vaccine development.

Immunometabolism and opportunities to improve innate immunity

Mtb infection induces metabolic alterations of infected macrophages, which could be targeted by therapies that enhance the host response to Mtb infection, rather than targeting Mtb itself, defined as HDT (reviewed in Ref.[1]). For example, iron chelation, in addition to depriving Mtb of an essential survival element, may promote the proinflammatory function of activated macrophages. Mtb infection of macrophages directs a shift from oxidative phosphorylation to aerobic glycolysis, which, coupled with interleukin-1β (IL-1β) production, supports proinflammatory functions in monocytes and macrophages and has been shown to decrease intracellular bacterial load in alveolar macrophages.[2] HIF1α regulates both the glycolytic switch and the IL-1β production, which in turn is negatively regulated by prolyl hydroxylase domain (PHD) proteins. As PHD proteins require iron as a cofactor, upregulation of HIF1α activity with iron chelation represents a potential mechanism by which iron chelator therapy could promote macrophage host defense.[1] Another example is the effect of Mtb infection on fatty acid metabolism in macrophages, resulting in the formation of foamy macrophages via TL2-mediated activation and an increase in peroxisome proliferator-activated receptor gamma (PPARγ). In the murine TB model, absence of PPARγ in lung macrophages reduces Mtb growth in vivo,[3] and in human alveolar macrophages, PPARγ upregulated by Mtb suppresses apoptosis via induction of prosurvival Mcl-1, which favors Mtb persistence.[4] In this regard, inhibitors of Mcl-1, which are in preclinical development, may have potential as HDT via promotion of apoptosis.[4] Finally, understanding of the immunometabolism of Mtb-infected macrophages supports micronutrient supplementation to an adjunctive HDT. Human alveolar macrophages metabolize vitamin A to all-trans retinoic acid, which in turn promotes autophagy and reduces intracellular Mtb.[5] Moreover, in human macrophages, interferon-γ (IFN-γ)-mediated activation induces killing of intracellular Mtb via a pathway that depends on the presence of vitamin D (reviewed in Ref.[6]).

Trained immunity

Trained immunity, or heterologous immunity, was first defined by Netea and colleagues[7] as an enhanced, persistent nonspecific T-cell-independent response that can occur following bacterial infection. Trained immunity has been studied widely for Bacillus Calmette–Guérin (BCG) (reviewed in Ref.[8]). For monocytes, and to some extent for natural killer (NK) cells, BCG increases the ability of innate cells to upregulate the expression of proinflammatory cytokines and relevant cell surface molecules and perhaps increase T-cell responses upon secondary stimulus with an unrelated, heterologous stimulus, such as Candida or lipopolysaccharide. This BCG training of monocytes has been demonstrated both in vitro and in vivo in humans and results from the mycobacteria-induced HIF1α and mTOR-mediated switch from oxidative phosphorylation to aerobic glycolysis described earlier, which in turn modulates methylation of histones regulating the expression of the target cytokines and cell surface molecules.[9] Recently, Arts and colleagues[10] demonstrated that BCG can mediate protection from a heterologous infection, in that adults first immunized with BCG followed by yellow fever vaccine 1 month later demonstrated decreased viral load compared with those not receiving BCG. Decreased viremia was correlated with IL-1β upregulation in epigenetically modified monocytes that demonstrated characteristic changes of trained monocytes in vitro. Trained immunity has also been hypothesized to contribute to early protection from Mtb infection[11] as well as from heterologous respiratory and sepsis pathogens after neonatal BCG immunization.

Neutrophils

Studies of TB immunity and TB pathogenesis have focused less on neutrophils than other components of the immune system. However, recent progress in this area has elucidated an important role for neutrophils in promoting TB disease and as potential targets for HDT and as biomarkers of disease severity and treatment response[12,13] (reviewed in Ref.[14]). Both mechanistic studies, using mouse and monkey animal models, and correlative and genetic human studies implicate neutrophils in exacerbating disease pathology and providing a short-term nutrient-rich niche for Mtb growth. Pathogenic Mtb strains, as compared with attenuated mycobacteria, induce necrotic cell death, as opposed to apoptotic cell death of human neutrophils, which in turn is favorable for Mtb growth and tissue destruction.[14] As noted earlier, Mtb infection induces macrophages to produce IL-1β and mediates antimicrobial activity in activated macrophages. However, IL-1β also mediates neutrophil influx via 12/15-lipoxygenase in mice and orthologue, 12-LOX, in humans.[13] Furthermore, IL-1β production and related immunopathology are negatively regulated by IFN-γ-induced nitric oxide (NO) through its negative regulation of the NLRP3 inflammasome.[12] This pathway suggests multiple targets for HDT that could either promote NO generation or inhibit the IL-1β immunopathology pathway. Furthermore, neutrophil signatures, including transcriptional profiles and neutrophil-driven proteins, correlate with TB disease severity and normalize with effective treatment in humans and in this way may warrant further development as TB disease biomarkers (reviewed in Ref.[14]). Finally, study of neutrophils has contributed to the understanding of the complexity of innate immunity and TB. For example, these studies have elucidated that IL-1β has opposing roles in promoting host defense and in exacerbation of host pathology and that NO promotes host defense via downregulation of IL-1β-induced immunopathology and depriving Mtb of a nutrient-rich niche provided by neutrophils.

Innate T Cells

CD8+ and CD4+ T cells can recognize protein antigens through the display of peptides by highly polymorphic major histocompatibility complex (MHC) class I and class II molecules that are in turn recognized by a highly diverse repertoire of T-cell receptors (TCRs). Conceptually, these diverse receptors allow the immune system to distinguish self from non-self proteins. In contrast, donor-unrestricted T (DURT) cells are those that use highly conserved, invariant restriction molecules to detect nonpeptidic antigens, such as lipids, glycolipids, and microbial metabolites.[15] Each of these systems has been shown to present Mtb-derived antigens.[16–18]

CD1-restricted T cells
Humans express 4 CD1 antigen-presenting molecules (CD1a, CD1b, CD1c, CD1d). Although there is some variability, the group 1 CD1 molecules (CD1a, CD1b, and CD1c) are characterized by an unusually hydrophobic binding group, allowing for the presentation of lipid and glycolipid antigens.[19] Interestingly, CD1-presented antigens were first discovered using T cells responsive to Mtb. These mycobacterial antigens include those presented by CD1b (mycolic acid, glucose monomycolate, glycerol monomycolate, and diacylated sulfotrehalose[20–23]), CD1a (mycobacterial lipopeptide), and CD1c (mycoketide).[21,24] Several

these lipid antigens have been chemically synthesized, allowing for the generation of tetramers[25] and the potential development of subunit vaccines targeting these T cells.[26–29]

Human CD1-restricted cells typically demonstrate a T-helper (Th1) phenotype in that they produce IFN-γ and tumor necrosis factor-α (TNF-α)[30] and have cytolytic capacity.[30,31] Interestingly, a recent study that evaluated lung-resident cells in those with either latent tuberculosis infection (LTBI) or having been treated for TB suggested that polyfunctional, CD1-restricted T cells were associated with improved control of Mtb.[32]

HLA-E-restricted T cells
HLA-E classically presents signal sequence peptides from HLA class Ia alleles and as such regulates innate immunity by inhibiting NK-cell activation through ligation to NKG2A/CD94.[33] In addition, mycobacterial peptides and glycopeptides are presented by HLA-E to CD8+ T cells.[17,34,35] Like conventional CD8+ T cells, HLA-E restricted CD8+ T cells are increased in frequency in the blood from TB patients compared with healthy controls.[36] Although the full repertoire of mycobacterial peptides displayed by HLA-E remains incompletely explored, it is clear that peptides derived from a variety of distinct proteins can be displayed.[17,34,35,37,38]

Human HLA-E restricted CD8+ T cells have been shown to have a Th1 effector profile[37] as well as a unique effector profile in that they also produce Th-2 cytokines, such as IL-4, IL-5, and IL-13,[17,36,39] as well as the cytolytic molecules, perforin granzyme and granulysin.[17,39] In addition, these cells appear to have the ability to control intracellular mycobacterial growth.[17,34]

Several lines of evidence would suggest that HLA-E-restricted T cells can contribute to protective immunity. In mice, Qa-1 is the homolog of HLA-E. When challenged with Mtb, Qa-1-deficient mice display increased pathology and microbial burden.[40] In rhesus macaques, vaccination with an attenuated rhesus cytomegalovirus has demonstrated protection against both simian immunodeficiency virus and Mtb.[41,42] Interestingly, in the context of vaccination using Mtb proteins, the vaccine can elicit both classically restricted CD4+ and CD8+ T cells and MHC-II-restricted and MHC-E-restricted CD8+ T cells. In this setting, roughly 4 epitopes can be displayed for each 100 amino acids in the context of MHC-E.[43,44] Together, these studies suggest a contribution of HLA-E-restricted T cells to protective immunity against TB.

γδ T cells

Although T cells expressing the αβ TCR have been extensively studied, those expressing the γδ TCR have been less well studied, despite representing roughly 0.5% to 5% of T cells in the peripheral circulation. In humans, the most abundant TCR expressed is Vδ2 typically paired with Vγ9.[45] These T cells can be activated by "phosphoantigens," small molecules that are produced by mammalian as well as microbial cells. Activation of these antigens is dependent on butyrophilin 3A1 (BTN3A1). BTN3A1 is unusual in that phosphoantigens bind the intracellular domain of BTN3A1, leading to a conformational change on the extracellular domain.[46–48] 6-O-Methylglucose-containing lipopolysaccharides have been identified as phosphoantigens specifically produced by Mtb.[49]

Evidence supporting an association with γδ T cells in the host response to infection with mycobacterial infection can be found in both cattle and humans. In cattle, γδ T cells can be seen in the early stages of infection with Mycobacterium bovis infection.[50] Furthermore, γδ T cells from M bovis-exposed animals preferentially lyse BCG-infected cells at higher efficiency relative to those from naive animals.[51] In humans, γδ T cells can produce both IL-17 and IFN-γ in response to Mtb-infected cells and have been shown to inhibit the growth of intracellular Mtb in vitro.[52–55]

In mice, γδ T cells expand rapidly upon BCG infection, can home to the site of infection (the lung), are cytolytic, and produce IFN-γ.[56] Following challenge with either BCG or Mtb, γδ T-cell-deficient mice have transiently increased bacterial loads and have granulomas that are poorly formed.[57,58] In BCG- or Mtb-infected rhesus macaques, a rapid and robust expansion of γδ T cells was observed.[59] Furthermore, in nonhuman primate (NHP) models, adoptive transfer of γδ T cells reduced the bacterial burden and limited disease to the infected lobe, preventing dissemination.[60]

MR1T cells

MHC-related protein 1 (MR1) is nonpolymorphic and is the most evolutionarily conserved HLA class I-related molecule among mammals.[61,62] MR1 can present small organic molecules derived from the riboflavin biosynthesis pathway of bacteria and fungi.[63,64] Mucosal associated invariant T (MAIT) cells recognize Mtb-infected cells in an MR1-dependent manner and express a semi-invariant TCR.[65,66] However, recent data suggest that MAIT cells are a subset of MR1-restricted T (MR1T) cells displaying a broader repertoire of TCRs. Moreover, this broader TCR repertoire is associated with the ability of MR1T cell clones with distinct TCRs to discriminate between synthetic riboflavin-derived and nonribatyllumazine MR1 ligands.[67–69] Specifically, photolumazines derived from Mycobacterium smegmatis have recently been described as a novel class of MR1 ligands.[70]

Although MR1T cells are often termed "innate," these cells have features of both innate and adaptive immune cells. MR1T cells are present in both the thymus and the peripheral blood and have the capacity to secrete proinflammatory cytokines, such as IFN-γ and TNF-α as well as cytolytic capacity.[71–73] Although MR1T cells can respond to Mtb ligands using the TCR, they can also respond to environmental signals, most notably IL-12, IL-18, and TLR stimulation.[66,67,74–76]

In mice, MAIT cells have been shown to facilitate the control of Klebsiella pneumoniae, M bovis BCG, Francisella tularensis, and Legionella longbeachiae.[77–82] Although mice have MR1T cells, MR1T cell frequency is markedly lower than that seen in humans, and the phenotype of mouse MR1T cells is skewed toward the production of IL-17, which is not typically seen in humans. Therefore, evidence from the mouse model may underestimate the importance of these cells for host defense in humans. Recently, in humans, it was demonstrated that an MR1 polymorphism associated with low messenger RNA expression was also associated with TB meningitis.[83] In addition, a patient with cystic fibrosis with absent MAIT cells was found to have an adverse clinical outcome characterized by severe and recurrent bacterial infection.[84]

Although increasing evidence supports a role for MR1T cells in TB host defense, at present, whether an MR1T cell-targeted vaccination will prove effective remains an open question. One challenge of such a vaccine strategy is that many of the known MR1 ligands are small molecules derived from microbial biosynthesis, for which little is known with regard to vaccine delivery. Moreover, in some cases, these ligands (ie, 5-OP-RU) are highly sensitive to degradation. However, 2 recent reports have demonstrated that in mice, exogenous delivery of MR1 ligands resulted in stable expansion of lung-resident MR1T cells.[78,85] These data might suggest that the expansion of MAIT cells is durable, a key requirement of any vaccination strategy. These data are also concordant with those provided by Howson and colleagues,[86] in which the administration of Salmonella typhi to human volunteers resulted in the clonotypic expansion of MR1T cells.

NEW CONCEPTS IN ADAPTIVE IMMUNITY
T Cells

The essential role for adaptively acquired CD4$^+$ and CD8$^+$ T cells, and the IFN-γ these cells produce, in provision of effective TB immunity, has long been appreciated (reviewed in Ref.[87]). However, recent advances in the understanding of T-cell antigen recognition, memory, and trafficking have important implications for development of an improved TB vaccine and are summarized here.

Definition of immunodominant antigens recognized by T cells

Targeted approaches to delineating the "antigenome" recognized by CD4$^+$ and CD8$^+$ T cells provided an incomplete picture of the Mtb proteins recognized by the human T-cell response (reviewed in Ref.[87]). More recently, however, genome-wide antigen discovery approaches have more completely defined the "antigenome" of immunodominant CD4 and CD8 antigens. Regarding CD4 antigens, to identify immunodominant epitopes and antigens, Lindestam Arlehamn and colleagues[88] used computational prediction methods to predict peptides likely to bind HLA-II and tested these peptides using CD4$^+$ T cells from Mtb-infected adults, and high-throughput assays. Regarding CD8 antigens, the authors comprehensively defined human immunodominant CD8 antigens in TB, using CD8$^+$ T cells from Mtb-infected adults to screen a synthetic peptide library representing 10% of the Mtb genome enriched for predicted immunodominant antigens.[89] These 2 studies shared 2 conclusions. First, certain regions of the Mtb proteome, such as the PE/PPE and ESX-associated proteins, are highly enriched for immunodominant antigens. Second, the profile of immunodominant antigens varied broadly between individuals, even those sharing HLA types. Therefore, although the immunodominant antigens for a particular individual could be readily defined, these profiles were not commonly shared across the population. The results of these studies have important implications for the design of TB vaccines targeting adaptively acquired T cells.

Immune evasion from T-cell recognition

Humans and Mtb have coevolved over thousands of years. Given that CD4$^+$ T cells are essential to host defense to Mtb infection, the hypothesis that Mtb has evolved to evade recognition of CD4$^+$ T cells has been extensively examined (reviewed in Ref.[90]). Mtb infection of specialized antigen-presenting cells (APC) results in decreased expression and altered intracellular trafficking of class II within these APC. In addition,

Mtb uses vesicular transport to divert antigens to the extracellular space and away from the Mtb-infected cell. These data support the hypothesis that these immune evasion mechanisms may contribute to lack of efficacy of vaccines, which nonetheless elicit strong CD4$^+$ T-cell responses.[90]

T cells and Mycobacterium tuberculosis "immune subversion"

By contrast, mutational escape does not seem to be a mechanism by which TB evades T-cell recognition. Studies of Mtb strain diversity comparing regions containing TB epitopes to the rest of the Mtb genome demonstrated that the epitope-containing regions are more conserved, rather than less conserved, as would be expected if T cells were exerting selection pressure for mutational escape from recognition.[91–93] It has been hypothesized that it may be advantageous for Mtb to maintain recognition by T cells because T-cell-mediated destruction creates lung cavities, which facilitate Mtb transmission.[94] The positive correlation between the number of T cells in the lung, cavity size, and transmissibility supports this hypothesis. Nonetheless, it is difficult to reconcile the evidence for immune evasion discussed earlier with this Mtb "immune subversion."

T-cell memory

In the mouse TB model, memory T cells, induced either by vaccination or by infection followed by curative therapy, are essential mediators of protection from subsequent Mtb infectious challenge (reviewed in Ref.[95]). Over the past 20 years, much progress has been made in defining memory T-cell subsets from which effector T cells are derived upon secondary antigen challenge (reviewed in Ref.[95]). These memory T-cell subsets are defined based on their phenotype, function, and tissue distribution. Central memory T cells (TCM) are located in the lymph nodes, spleen, and bone marrow, and effector memory T cells (TEM) are located in peripheral tissues. More recently, additional subsets of memory T cells have been defined, including stem cell-like memory cells (TSCM), located in the spleen and lymph nodes, and resident T cells (TRM), located in the lung. Although there is much controversy in the field, 1 simplified model of memory T-cell development postulates that TCM are derived from naive T cells through a TSCM intermediary, and that TRM are derived from TEM, which in turn are derived from TCM.

Recent studies of all these memory T-cell subsets in the mouse TB model and in humans have elucidated new concepts driving TB vaccine development. In humans, TSCM have been defined in Mtb-specific CD4[+] T cells in adults with LTBI and are induced in adolescents undergoing primary infection and by BCG vaccination in neonates.[96] These TSCM are distinct from naive T cells and are functional, producing proinflammatory cytokines with antigen stimulation and therefore may represent a good target of TB vaccine strategies. In the mouse TB model, BCG induces predominantly TEM relative to TCM and a recombinant BCG, which induces more TCM, protects from Mtb challenge better than BCG, suggesting that induction of predominantly TCM relative to TEM may be advantageous for long-lived vaccine-induced T-cell memory. Finally, in the mouse TB model, Mtb infection and BCG induce TRM in the lung, which depends on the route of delivery. As it follows that having TRM at the site of Mtb infection would be advantageous for an effective TB vaccine, these results have implications for studying vaccine route.

T-cell responses within the context of chronic infection

In the mouse TB model, chronic Mtb infection drives the differentiation of memory T cells to terminally differentiated effector T cells (reviewed in Ref.[95]). Recently, Moguche and colleagues[97] showed in both the mouse TB model and humans with LTBI, that chronic expression of an Mtb antigen results in terminally differentiated CD4[+] T cells displaying the phenotype and function of exhausted T cells. These investigators also demonstrate that an Mtb antigen, which is expressed only early in the course of infection, induces memory T-cell populations, which persist in the chronically infected host but are ineffective owing to the lack of antigen presentation. Therefore, TB vaccine strategies also need to consider vaccine antigen expression over time and how it may shape the repertoire of potent effector T cells over the course of infection.

T-cell trafficking

Studies of T-cell trafficking in the mouse TB model demonstrate differences in the phenotype and function of lung resident CD4[+] T cells, which mediate control of Mtb infection better than those that remain in the pulmonary vasculature (reviewed in Ref.[98]). Protective lung resident CD4[+] T cells express activation markers, such as PD-1 and CD69, do not express the terminal differentiation marker KLRG1, and produce less IFN-γ than intravascular T cells. Moreover, Th1 promoting factors IL-12/23 p40 and T-bet differentially promote the development of these 2 subsets of CD4[+] T cells in the lung.[99] These studies demonstrate the importance of considering tissue location when targeting for

protective immune responses against Mtb infection. Finally, the architecture of the TB granuloma favors the separation of T cells and their targets. Kauffman and colleagues[100] recently showed that in rhesus macaques, T cells remain on the periphery of TB granulomas and are thus spatially removed from the Mtb-infected cells in the center of TB granulomas. Therefore, the ability of TB vaccines to promote the trafficking of T cells to the site of infectious challenge can be an additional important component of vaccine-induced protection.[101,102]

B Cells

Reconsidering tuberculosis immunity dogma

TB immunity dogma dictates that B-cell immunity either plays no role in TB host defense or can even contribute to immunopathology (reviewed in Ref.[103]). This dogma was supported by initial studies of B-cell immunity in the mouse TB model and by observations in humans that demonstrated lack of protection with immune sera, and lack of susceptibility to TB in B-cell-deficient individuals. In addition, because the presence of anti-Mtb antibodies correlates with TB disease, serology has been investigated as possible diagnostic immunodiagnostic of TB disease. As a result, study of protective TB immunity has focused almost exclusively on innate and adaptive cellular immunity. However, in 2013, Tameris and colleagues[104] reported on a phase 2b study of BCG-immunized infants who demonstrated that boost with a modified vaccinia Ankara expressing Ag85A (MVA85A) vaccine failed to augment BCG-induced protection, despite inducing proinflammatory CD4[+] T-cell responses. Since then, the TB vaccine community has been reflecting on what other types of immune components might be required for effective immunity. Hence, a possible role for B-cell immunity in TB host defense has been reconsidered, reinvigorating research in this field (reviewed in Ref.[103]).

Possible role for B-cell immunity in tuberculosis host defense

Although the role of B-cell immunity in TB host defense remains highly controversial, several lines of evidence, most of which is correlative and some of which is mechanistic, support a protective role (reviewed in Ref.[103]). First, observational clinical studies suggest that Mtb-specific antibodies can modulate the severity of disease because high antibody titers are inversely correlated with more severe TB disease. Second, there is evidence for a role of antibody opsonization of Mtb for targeted FcR-mediated phagocytosis. This evidence includes that (1) several whole blood transcription studies in active TB show upregulation of antibody receptors, including phagocyte membrane FcR and intracellular antibody receptor TRIM21; (2) in in vitro studies, human Mtb-specific antibodies augment phagocyte FcR-mediated effector function, resulting in decreased intracellular Mtb survival; (3) FcR mice deficient in FcR are more susceptible to Mtb infection; (4) individuals with LTBI, as compared with individuals with TB disease, have purified protein derivative-specific antibodies with better Fc effector activity, which is associated with differential antibody glycosylation.[105] Moreover, these antibodies enhanced macrophage effector function in killing Mtb in vitro. Finally, correlative evidence supports that Mtb-specific antibodies may have a role in preventing infection in those individuals who remain tuberculin skin test (TST) negative despite that repeated exposures to Mtb have high levels of Mtb-specific antibodies (reviewed in Ref.[103]). These results have led to interest in interrogating, and even targeting, antibody responses in developing new TB vaccines.

IMMUNOLOGIC DEFINITION OF TUBERCULOSIS AS A SPECTRUM OF EXPOSURE TO INFECTION TO DISEASE

Although infection with Mtb has been traditionally defined as either latent or active, recent immunologic advances in conjunction with advanced imaging have made it clear that infection with Mtb reflects a spectrum, ranging from resistance to infection, clearance of infection, persistent infection, subclinical, and clinical TB.[106–108]

Clearance of Infection

Because infection with Mtb is defined by the host T-cell response to mycobacterial antigens, as reflected by a positive TST or interferon gamma release assay (IGRA), rather than direct identification of the microbe, direct evidence for persistent bacterial infection is lacking. Nonetheless, epidemiologic observations would support the hypothesis that following exposure to Mtb, some people are able to resist and/or clear infection. For instance, some individuals exposed to Mtb repeatedly never demonstrate a positive TST or IGRA. In this case, it is possible that Mtb has been eradicated before the generation of an adaptive immune response, a phenomenon termed early clearance. In addition, of those individuals who become infected with Mtb, as defined by a positive TST/IGRA, the majority contain infection without developing active disease, suggesting the development of a protective immune response. In support of this hypothesis, prior infection with Mtb is associated with a diminished risk of TB following subsequent exposure.[109] Finally, those who have reverted from a positive to a negative TST/IGRA have a similar risk of progression to those whose TST/IGRA results are persistently negative.[110]

Predictors for Tuberculosis Progression

Although TB is defined on clinical, radiographic, and microbiologic grounds, increasing evidence suggests that biomarkers can be used to distinguish TB from infection (**Fig. 1**). Practically, infection

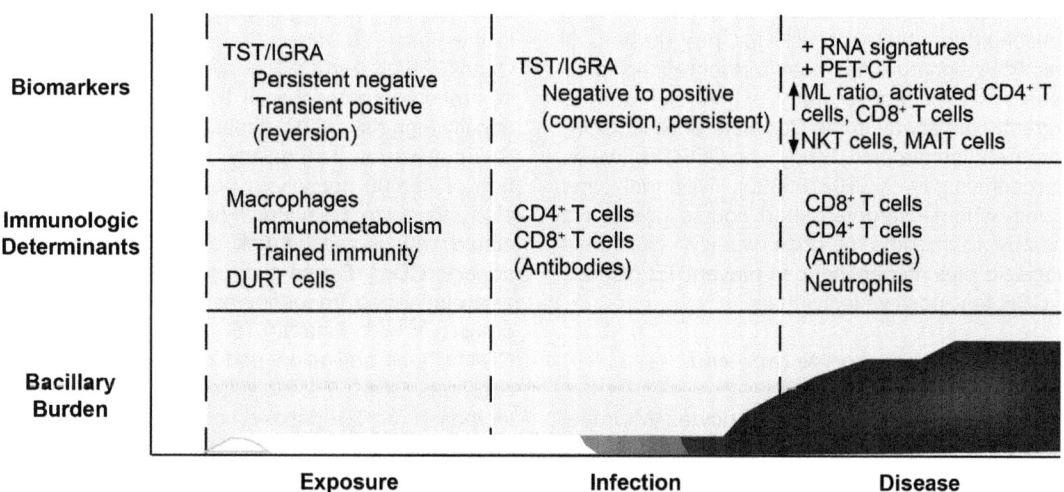

	Exposure	Infection	Disease
Biomarkers	TST/IGRA Persistent negative Transient positive (reversion)	TST/IGRA Negative to positive (conversion, persistent)	+ RNA signatures + PET-CT ↑ML ratio, activated CD4⁺ T cells, CD8⁺ T cells ↓NKT cells, MAIT cells
Immunologic Determinants	Macrophages Immunometabolism Trained immunity DURT cells	CD4⁺ T cells CD8⁺ T cells (Antibodies)	CD8⁺ T cells CD4⁺ T cells (Antibodies) Neutrophils
Bacillary Burden			

Fig. 1. Spectrum of exposure to infection to disease: biomarkers and immunologic determinants of host defense. Infection is distinguished from exposure by the acquisition of an adaptive T-cell response, as reflected by a positive TST or IGRA. Of note, because infection is defined by quantitation of adaptive immunity rather than of Mtb organisms, clearance of infection by innate immunity (*white*) or by adaptive immunity (*light blue*) cannot be distinguished from persistent lifelong infection (*medium blue*). Infection is distinguished from disease by clinical symptoms. However, biomarkers of disease can precede the development of clinical symptoms (*dark blue*).

with Mtb has been classified as either "active," defined clinically, radiologically, and microbiologically, or "latent," as subjects who have evidence of an adaptive T-cell response to Mtb antigens (positive TST/IGRA), but without clinical TB (LTBI). However, recent developments in imaging, transcriptomics, proteomics, and cellular immunology make it clear that there are individuals who would appear to have LTBI, but nonetheless have a biological profile that appears identical to TB. Furthermore, there is mounting evidence that these individuals are at increased risk to develop TB.[108] For example, a recent study of HIV-infected individuals with LTBI found combined PET and computed tomography (CT) to define subjects with subclinical TB. Here, 4 of the 10 individuals were diagnosed with active TB within 6 months, confirming progression from subclinical to active disease.[111] Recent developments in defining biomarkers of progression are summarized here.

Blood transcriptomic signatures of progression
With regard to transcriptomic signatures, type I/II IFN genes have been consistently found to distinguish TB from LTBI.[112–117] In addition, a longitudinal study of adolescents who progressed to TB revealed elevated expression of type I/II IFN responses and complement pathway genes more than a year before TB diagnosis.[118] From these data, a transcriptional signature has been developed that can distinguish adolescents who progressed to TB from nonprogressing, IGRA-positive controls,[119] with a specificity of 82% and sensitivity of 70% within a year of testing.[119] A similar RNA signature could be used to define household contacts at risk for progression.[120] This RNA signature has been further refined to 11 genes.[121] Prospective study of this signature is currently underway in the Correlate of Risk (COR) Targeted Intervention Study, or CORTIS (www.clinicaltrials.gov, NCT02735590). This trial aims to test whether targeted short course preventive therapy (3 months of once weekly, high-dose isoniazid plus rifapentine) can prevent TB disease in COR test-positive individuals.

Myelocyte to lymphocyte ratio and tuberculosis
The ratio of myelocytes to lymphocytes (ML ratio) has consistently proven an indicator of TB.[122,123] A recent study in HIV-infected adults showed a strong association between very high or very low ML ratio and risk of incident TB.[124] An elevated ML ratio was also associated with risk of developing TB in a longitudinal study of contacts of TB patients in Madagascar,[125] and 2 independent studies showed that ML ratios normalized after TB

treatment.[126,127] Finally, transcriptional analyses in the Adolescent Cohort Study found that gene modules representing monocytes and granulocytes increased, whereas T-cell and B-cell gene modules decreased during TB progression.[118]

Donor-unrestricted T cells in latent tuberculosis infection and tuberculosis
DURT cell types have been demonstrated to recognize Mtb-derived products[16,17] and appear to have utility in discerning LTBI from TB. HLA-E restricted CD8+ T cells are increased in frequency in the blood from TB patients compared with healthy controls[36] and can recognize Mtb-derived peptides.[17,34,37] CD1b or CD1c-restricted T cells have been found to be increased in the blood of Mtb-infected individuals compared with healthy controls.[21,23] In contrast, both MR1T cells[65,66,128] and natural killer T (NKT) cells, restricted by CD1d, are reduced in the circulation of individuals with TB compared with healthy controls.[129] Interestingly, in a prospective household contact study, Sutherland and colleagues[130] observed a significantly lower frequency of NKT cells in those who progressed to TB over those who remained asymptomatic.

Adaptive T-cell signatures of progression
Characteristics of antigen-specific CD4+ T-cell responses may be used to distinguish TB disease from LTBI and/or to predict risk of progression to TB disease. In this regard, the quantitative results of IGRAs, which predominantly measure IFN-γ-producing CD4+ T cells, can be used to identify those at risk for progression. Specifically, infants in the phase 2b vaccine trial of MVA85A[104] with QuantiFERON test (QFT) conversions at IFN-γ concentrations greater than 4 IU/mL were at exceptionally high risk of TB disease within 6 months of QFT conversion.[131] Similarly, a longitudinal evaluation of 45,000 household contacts from Norway also showed that elevated IFN-γ values were associated with increased risk of TB.[132] Also, Mtb-specific CD4+ T cells producing IL-2 were found at a diminished frequency as bacterial burden increases.[133,134] Finally, TB is associated with CD4+ T-cell activation and apoptosis.[135,136] For example, CD4+ T cells expressing HLA-DR are increased in TB patients compared with Mtb-infected controls.[136–138] Both in infants in the phase 2b vaccine trial of MVA85A[104,118,139] and in IGRA-positive adolescents from the Adolescent Cohort Study,[118,139] increased HLA-DR expression was associated with progression to TB disease.

Mtb-specific CD8+ T cells can serve as a reflection of in vivo antigen load and disease burden. For example, 2 independent studies report higher frequencies of Mtb-specific CD8$^+$ T cells in smear$^+$ TB than smear$^-$ TB,[134,140] and the presence of Mtb-specific CD8$^+$ T-cell responses distinguishes young children with pulmonary TB from those with pulmonary disease owing to other causes.[141] As further support of their reflection of antigen load, Mtb-specific CD8$^+$ T cells increase during disease progression in NHP[142] and decrease in frequency during TB treatment.[134,143] Finally, the newly introduced QFT assay (QFT-Plus) uses detection of CD8$^+$ T-cell responses to the Mtb-specific antigens ESAT-6 and CFP-10. QFT-Plus uses 2 tubes (TB1 and TB2). TB1 contains long peptides that can only stimulate CD4$^+$ T cells,[144] whereas TB2 contains shorter peptides recognized by both CD4$^+$ and CD8$^+$ T cells.[145] Initial evaluations of QFT-Plus showed high concordance between QFT and QFT-Plus results,[146] with higher TB2-TB1 responses in participants with active TB[147] and increased Mtb exposure,[146,148] which decline during TB treatment.[149] Diagnostic accuracy of QFT-Plus for active TB and treatment response remains to be confirmed.

DETERMINATES OF TUBERCULOSIS HOST DEFENSE
Tuberculosis Immunology in Infants and Young Children

Infants and young children are more likely than older children and adults to develop disease following infection and are more susceptible to severe manifestations of TB, such as disseminated TB and TB meningitis.[150] The most widely administered vaccine worldwide, BCG only provides partial protection from disseminated disease in children,[151] and hence, 1 million children per year develop TB, despite neonatal BCG vaccination.[152] Therefore, an improved infant TB vaccine is urgently needed, and development of a vaccine that is effective in infants requires an improved understanding of both BCG-induced immune responses and of the immunobiology underlying the infant's susceptibility to severe disease. Studies of human infants have not only advanced the understanding of infant TB immunity but also driven approaches in TB vaccine development in general, as illustrated by the results of a recent phase 2b infant vaccine trial, mentioned earlier.[104]

Innate cellular responses in young infants
Studies of activation of monocytes via TLRs, including TLR-1/2 used by Mtb, demonstrate that neonatal monocytes produce less proinflammatory cytokines than do adult monocytes (reviewed in Ref.[153]). In South African infants vaccinated with BCG at birth, BCG in vitro induced diminished expression of proinflammatory cytokines in newborns, which increased over the first 9 months of life.[154] In this same study, TLR-2 ligand induced multiple signaling pathways in 36-week-old infants compared with only one in newborns. Whether these deficiencies in innate cellular responses relevant to Mtb contribute to increased susceptibility of infants and young children to severe disease from TB remains unknown.

Bacillus Calmette–Guérin and trained immunity in infants
Both epidemiologic studies and double-blinded placebo-controlled trials demonstrate that neonatal BCG mediates a TB-independent survival benefit, which is associated with a decreased incidence of pneumonia and sepsis, especially in the first few months of life (reviewed in Ref.[8]). It has been hypothesized that trained immunity, as discussed earlier, is responsible for this BCG-mediated survival advantage. Studies of infants comparing infants immunized at birth versus those with delayed immunization demonstrate the immunologic findings consistent with trained immunity, such as increased proinflammatory cytokine secretion in peripheral blood mononuclear cells or whole blood in response to heterologous stimuli in infants immunized at birth. However, as compared with studies of adults, infants do not demonstrate upregulation of cell surface molecules, and at least 1 study failed to demonstrate BCG-trained increases in cytokine secretion in infants. These inconsistencies leave open the possibility that other innate cells such as MR1T cells that recognize a broad array of pathogens could contribute to this survival benefit.

Innate T cells in infants
MR1T cells are present in cord blood[72] and increase in magnitude over the first year of life.[155] Also, neonatal BCG vaccination is associated with an increase in γδ T cells[156] and with proliferative responses to peptides presented by HLA-E.[34] Future research may determine whether these innate T-cell populations can be harnessed to augment the induction of an adaptive immune response and/or induce a memory population of these T cells.

Adaptive T-cell immunity in infants
Infants and young children are capable of mounting CD4$^+$ Th1 cells within the context of LTBI and TB disease, and CD8$^+$ T cells in TB disease, that are comparable to T-cell responses in older children and adults (reviewed in Ref.[153]). Therefore, deficiency of an adaptive proinflammatory T-cell response is not responsible for the

propensity for severe TB disease in young children. Moreover, the preponderance of published evidence suggests no predominance of CD4$^+$ Th2 cell immunity relative to CD4$^+$ Th1 cell immunity in infants, refuting the often-cited hypothesis that a Th2 cell bias in infants underlies their susceptibility to TB disease.

Regarding BCG-induced immunity in infants, BCG induces robust polyfunctional CD4$^+$ T-cell responses, demonstrating that insufficiency of induction of these proinflammatory T-cell populations is not responsible for the incomplete effectiveness of BCG (reviewed in Ref.[157]). However, as compared with BCG-vaccinated adults, BCG-vaccinated infants demonstrated decreased polyfunctional CD4$^+$ T-cell responses to 2 candidate TB vaccines, AERAS-402 (an adenovirus vector expressing Ag85A, Ag85B, and TB10.4[158]) and MVA85A.[104] This observation suggests that vaccine-induced T-cell immunity is not entirely comparable in infants relative to adults. Moreover, it has been postulated that diminished polyfunctional CD4$^+$ T-cell responses underlie the failure of an MVA85A boost to provide additional efficacy over BCG alone.[104] However, it is not clear if polyfunctional CD4$^+$ T-cell responses represent a correlate of vaccine-induced immunity, as in 2 studies of BCG-vaccinated South African infants.[104,159] The magnitude of polyfunctional CD4$^+$ T cells did not correlate with subsequent risk development of TB.

B-cell immunity in infants

As discussed earlier, there is renewed interest in exploring the role of B-cell immunity in host defense to TB. In this regard, recent studies in infants support a protective role of antibody. First, in the infant trial comparing BCG to BCG boosted with MVA85A, BCG induced Ag85A-specific immunoglobulin G (IgG), which correlated with a decreased risk of developing TB.[139] More recently, Logan and colleagues[160] reported the results of a substudy of this same trial, which showed that a BCG-specific IgG2 response was inversely associated with subsequent Mtb infection, as defined by conversion to a positive QFT. Finally, relevant to the potential protective effects of breastfeeding, mice infected with Mtb inoculated via the intratracheal route demonstrated a reduced bacillary load when the Mtb was coincubated with polyclonal secretory IgA purified from human colostrum.[161]

Tuberculosis Immunology in Elderly Adults

Somewhat similar to infants and young children, elderly adults are more susceptible to TB disease and develop extrapulmonary disease more frequently than younger adults.[162] Comorbid conditions, such as diabetes and chronic obstructive pulmonary disease, both of which are more common with increasing age, likely are partly responsible for this increased susceptibility to TB disease. However, it is also clear that the aging immune system contributes to the susceptibility and expression of TB disease in the elderly. In the mouse TB model, old mice demonstrate better early control of Mtb infection but nonetheless succumb more quickly to primary Mtb infection than adult mice, because of poorer control of Mtb late in infection (reviewed in Ref.[163]). This early Mtb control is mediated by already activated innate immune cells, resulting from "inflammaging" and a population of lung resident memory CD8$^+$ T cells, responding to IL-12 in an antigen-independent manner. The increased susceptibility of old mice to primary Mtb infection is associated with impaired acquisition of an effective CD4$^+$ T-cell response. Additional immune factors thought to contribute to susceptibility of elderly humans to TB include reduced thymic T-cell output and T-cell immune senescence marked by decreased proliferative capacity and effector function and increased immunopathology owing to "inflammaging."[164]

Diabetes

Individuals with diabetes mellitus (DM) demonstrate substantial susceptibility to TB, with an incidence 3 times that of individuals without DM, and DM is associated with more severe pulmonary TB.[165] Moreover, the increasing incidence of DM in countries that already have high burdens of TB has greatly increased the incidence of TB and DM comorbidity. For example, in India, 25% of TB cases also had DM.[166] The effect of DM on TB host defense has been studied both in a DM mouse model and in observational studies of humans with TB comparing those with and without DM.[167,168] Mice with chronic hyperglycemia as the result of streptomycin treatment, which depletes insulin-producing cells, are more susceptible to aerosol infection with Mtb.[168] This increased susceptibility is associated with decreased recruitment of myeloid cells to the lung and delayed migration of dendritic cells to the lymph node and early following infection as well as a delay in acquisition of adaptive immunity. However, this increased susceptibility was also associated with increased inflammation and immunopathology later in infection. Observational studies in humans also demonstrate increased lung immunopathology and an exaggerated proinflammatory response in individuals with DM and TB as compared with nondiabetic individuals with

TB.[167,168] These proinflammatory T-cell responses seen in individuals with TB and DM include more robust Th1 and Th17 CD4$^+$ T-cell responses and diminished regulatory T-cell responses (reviewed in Ref.[167]). Finally, recently Prada-Medina and colleagues[169] defined a cytokine and growth factor signature of individuals with DM and TB that distinguished this cohort from healthy individuals and most individuals with TB alone. Also, neutrophil counts were higher in the TB/DM cohort. Therefore, evidence from both a mouse DM/TB model and observational human studies supports an increased susceptibility to TB owing to impaired innate immunity and delayed acquisition of adaptive immunity and more severe pulmonary disease secondary to an exaggerated pro-inflammatory response.

Human Immunodeficiency Virus

Worldwide, HIV infection is the most important co-morbidity, increasing susceptibility to TB disease with approximately 1 million cases of HIV/TB per year.[152] In addition, susceptibility to TB disease is inversely correlated with CD4 count, and although effective anti-retroviral therapy (ART) reduces the susceptibility to TB, the incidence of TB in HIV-infected individuals on ART remains at higher risk for TB thanks to HIV-uninfected individuals. The effect of HIV infection on host defense to TB HIV/TB has recently been thoroughly reviewed[170] and will only be briefly summarized herein.

HIV comprehensively alters both innate and adaptive immunity in ways favorable for progression of Mtb infection and disease.[170] For example, alveolar macrophages isolated from HIV individuals are dysfunctional in attributes critical to TB host defense, including decreased phagocytosis, APC function, and intracellular killing. Although apoptosis of Mtb-infected macrophages facilitates T-cell priming, Mtb/HIV-infected macrophages are more resistant to apoptosis than Mtb-infected macrophages. HIV infection also depletes DC, which are incompletely restored with ART. Of course, HIV infection depletes CD4$^+$ T-cell numbers, which are depleted not only in the blood but also in the lung. HIV also impairs CD4$^+$ T-cell function in the blood and lung early in infection even before CD4$^+$ T-cell numbers decline. Although ART restores CD4$^+$ T-cell numbers, function of Mtb-specific CD4$^+$ T cells improves but is not fully restored in both blood and lung. CD8$^+$ T cells also demonstrate decreased function in HIV-TB-coinfected individuals. In summary, HIV-mediated depletion and dysfunction of remaining innate and adaptive mediators of TB host defense underlie the increased susceptibility of HIV-infected individuals to TB disease.

SUMMARY

Although it has long been understood that TB host defense is dependent on cellular immunity, recent advances in the understanding of roles for new immune components, including neutrophils, innate T cells, and B cells, have been defined, and the understanding of the function of macrophages and adaptively acquired T cells has been advanced. New insights into immunometabolism, trained immunity, and neutrophils provide novel targets for HDT for TB. DURTs use highly conserved monomorphic antigen presentation molecules to recognize a diverse repertoire of peptidic and non-peptidic Mtb ligands. Recent advances in the understanding of T-cell antigen recognition, memory, and mucosal trafficking have important implications for development of an improved TB vaccine. Transcriptomic and cellular immunologic signatures as well as PET-CT imaging reveal the spectrum of disease caused by Mtb infection. Determinates of TB host defense, including young and old age, and comorbidities, such as diabetes and HIV infection, predispose to an increased incidence and severity of TB disease. Recent advances in the understanding of TB defense leads to a more mechanistic understanding of TB infection and clinical expression of disease.

REFERENCES

1. Phelan JJ, Basdeo SA, Tazoll SC, et al. Modulating iron for metabolic support of TB host defense. Front Immunol 2018;9:2296.
2. Gleeson LE, Sheedy FJ, Palsson-McDermott EM, et al. Cutting edge: *Mycobacterium tuberculosis* induces aerobic glycolysis in human alveolar macrophages that is required for control of intracellular bacillary replication. J Immunol 2016;196(6): 2444–9.
3. Guirado E, Rajaram MV, Chawla A, et al. Deletion of PPARgamma in lung macrophages provides an immunoprotective response against *M. tuberculosis* infection in mice. Tuberculosis (Edinb) 2018;111: 170–7.
4. Arnett E, Weaver AM, Woodyard KC, et al. PPAR-gamma is critical for *Mycobacterium tuberculosis* induction of Mcl-1 and limitation of human macrophage apoptosis. PLoS Pathog 2018;14(6): e1007100.
5. Coleman MM, Basdeo SA, Coleman AM, et al. All-trans retinoic acid augments autophagy during intracellular bacterial infection. Am J Respir Cell Mol Biol 2018;59(5):548–56.

6. Bloom BR, Modlin RL. Mechanisms of defense against intracellular pathogens mediated by human macrophages. Microbiol Spectr 2016;4(3). https://doi.org/10.1128/microbiolspec.MCHD-0006-2015.

7. Netea MG, Quintin J, van der Meer JW. Trained immunity: a memory for innate host defense. Cell Host Microbe 2011;9(5):355–61.

8. Butkeviciute E, Jones CE, Smith SG. Heterologous effects of infant BCG vaccination: potential mechanisms of immunity. Future Microbiol 2018;13: 1193–208.

9. Arts RJW, Carvalho A, La Rocca C, et al. Immunometabolic pathways in BCG-induced trained immunity. Cell Rep 2016;17(10):2562–71.

10. Arts RJW, Moorlag S, Novakovic B, et al. BCG vaccination protects against experimental viral infection in humans through the induction of cytokines associated with trained immunity. Cell Host Microbe 2018;23(1):89–100.e5.

11. Lerm M, Netea MG. Trained immunity: a new avenue for tuberculosis vaccine development. J Intern Med 2016;279(4):337–46.

12. Mishra BB, Rathinam VA, Martens GW, et al. Nitric oxide controls the immunopathology of tuberculosis by inhibiting NLRP3 inflammasome-dependent processing of IL-1beta. Nat Immunol 2013;14(1):52–60.

13. Mishra BB, Lovewell RR, Olive AJ, et al. Nitric oxide prevents a pathogen-permissive granulocytic inflammation during tuberculosis. Nat Microbiol 2017;2:17072.

14. Dallenga T, Schaible UE. Neutrophils in tuberculosis–first line of defence or booster of disease and targets for host-directed therapy? Pathog Dis 2016;74(3) [pii:ftw012].

15. Godfrey DI, Uldrich AP, McCluskey J, et al. The burgeoning family of unconventional T cells. Nat Immunol 2015;16(11):1114–23.

16. De Libero G, Singhal A, Lepore M, et al. Nonclassical T cells and their antigens in tuberculosis. Cold Spring Harb Perspect Med 2014;4(9):a018473.

17. van Meijgaarden KE, Haks MC, Caccamo N, et al. Human CD8+ T-cells recognizing peptides from Mycobacterium tuberculosis (Mtb) presented by HLA-E have an unorthodox Th2-like, multifunctional, Mtb inhibitory phenotype and represent a novel human T-cell subset. PLoS Pathog 2015; 11(3):e1004671.

18. Van Rhijn I, Moody DB. Donor unrestricted T cells: a shared human T cell response. J Immunol 2015; 195(5):1927–32.

19. Van Rhijn I, Ly D, Moody DB. CD1a, CD1b, and CD1c in immunity against mycobacteria. Adv Exp Med Biol 2013;783:181–97.

20. Beckman EM, Porcelli SA, Morita CT, et al. Recognition of a lipid antigen by CD1-restricted alpha beta+ T cells. Nature 1994;372(6507):691–4.

21. Moody DB, Ulrichs T, Muhlecker W, et al. CD1c-mediated T-cell recognition of isoprenoid glycolipids in Mycobacterium tuberculosis infection. Nature 2000;404(6780):884–8.

22. Layre E, Collmann A, Bastian M, et al. Mycolic acids constitute a scaffold for mycobacterial lipid antigens stimulating CD1-restricted T cells. Chem Biol 2009;16(1):82–92.

23. Gilleron M, Stenger S, Mazorra Z, et al. Diacylated sulfoglycolipids are novel mycobacterial antigens stimulating CD1-restricted T cells during infection with Mycobacterium tuberculosis. J Exp Med 2004;199(5):649–59.

24. Moody DB, Reinhold BB, Guy MR, et al. Structural requirements for glycolipid antigen recognition by CD1b-restricted T cells. Science 1997;278(5336): 283–6.

25. Gras S, Van Rhijn I, Shahine A, et al. T cell receptor recognition of CD1b presenting a mycobacterial glycolipid. Nat Commun 2016;7:13257.

26. James CA, Yu KKQ, Gilleron M, et al. CD1b tetramers identify T cells that recognize natural and synthetic diacylated sulfoglycolipids from Mycobacterium tuberculosis. Cell Chem Biol 2018;25(4):392–402.e14.

27. Kasmar AG, van Rhijn I, Cheng TY, et al. CD1b tetramers bind αβ T cell receptors to identify a mycobacterial glycolipid-reactive T cell repertoire in humans. J Exp Med 2011;208(9):1741–7.

28. Kasmar AG, Van Rhijn I, Magalhaes KG, et al. Cutting edge: CD1a tetramers and dextramers identify human lipopeptide-specific T cells ex vivo. J Immunol 2013;191(9):4499–503.

29. Ly D, Kasmar AG, Cheng TY, et al. CD1c tetramers detect ex vivo T cell responses to processed phosphomycoketide antigens. J Exp Med 2013;210(4): 729–41.

30. Rosat JP, Grant EP, Beckman EM, et al. CD1-restricted microbial lipid antigen-specific recognition found in the CD8+ alpha beta T cell pool. J Immunol 1999;162(1):366–71.

31. Stenger S, Hanson DA, Teitelbaum R, et al. An antimicrobial activity of cytolytic T cells mediated by granulysin. Science 1998;282(5386):121–5.

32. Seshadri C, Lin L, Scriba TJ, et al. T cell responses against mycobacterial lipids and proteins are poorly correlated in South African adolescents. J Immunol 2015;195(10):4595–603.

33. Braud VM, Allan DS, O'Callaghan CA, et al. HLA-E binds to natural killer cell receptors CD94/NKG2A, B and C. Nature 1998;391(6669):795–9.

34. Joosten SA, van Meijgaarden KE, van Weeren PC, et al. Mycobacterium tuberculosis peptides presented by HLA-E molecules are targets for human CD8 T-cells with cytotoxic as well as regulatory activity. PLoS Pathog 2010;6(2): e1000782.

35. Harriff MJ, Wolfe LM, Swarbrick G, et al. HLA-E presents glycopeptides from the *Mycobacterium tuberculosis* protein MPT32 to human CD8[+] T cells. Sci Rep 2017;7(1):4622.

36. Caccamo N, Pietra G, Sullivan LC, et al. Human CD8 T lymphocytes recognize *Mycobacterium tuberculosis* antigens presented by HLA-E during active tuberculosis and express type 2 cytokines. Eur J Immunol 2015;45(4):1069–81.

37. Heinzel AS, Grotzke JE, Lines RA, et al. HLA-E-dependent presentation of Mtb-derived antigen to human CD8[+] T cells. J Exp Med 2002;196(11): 1473–81.

38. McMurtrey C, Harriff MJ, Swarbrick GM, et al. T cell recognition of *Mycobacterium tuberculosis* peptides presented by HLA-E derived from infected human cells. PLoS One 2017;12(11):e0188288.

39. Prezzemolo T, van Meijgaarden KE, Franken KL, et al. Detailed characterization of human *Mycobacterium tuberculosis* specific HLA-E restricted CD8[+] T cells. Eur J Immunol 2018;48(2):293–305.

40. Bian Y, Shang S, Siddiqui S, et al. MHC Ib molecule Qa-1 presents *Mycobacterium tuberculosis* peptide antigens to CD8[+] T cells and contributes to protection against infection. PLoS Pathog 2017; 13(5):e1006384.

41. Hansen SG, Piatak M Jr, Ventura AB, et al. Immune clearance of highly pathogenic SIV infection. Nature 2013;502(7469):100–4.

42. Hansen SG, Zak DE, Xu G, et al. Prevention of tuberculosis in rhesus macaques by a cytomegalovirus-based vaccine. Nat Med 2018; 24(2):130–43.

43. Hansen SG, Sacha JB, Hughes CM, et al. Cytomegalovirus vectors violate CD8[+] T cell epitope recognition paradigms. Science 2013;340(6135): 1237874.

44. Hansen SG, Wu HL, Burwitz BJ, et al. Broadly targeted CD8[+] T cell responses restricted by major histocompatibility complex E. Science 2016; 351(6274):714–20.

45. Sherwood AM, Desmarais C, Livingston RJ, et al. Deep sequencing of the human TCRγ and TCRβ repertoires suggests that TCRβ rearranges after αβ and γδ T cell commitment. Sci Transl Med 2011;3(90):90ra61.

46. Vavassori S, Kumar A, Wan GS, et al. Butyrophilin 3A1 binds phosphorylated antigens and stimulates human γδ T cells. Nat Immunol 2013;14(9):908–16.

47. Sandstrom A, Peigne CM, Leger A, et al. The intracellular B30.2 domain of butyrophilin 3A1 binds phosphoantigens to mediate activation of human Vγ9Vδ2 T cells. Immunity 2014;40(4): 490–500.

48. Gu S, Sachleben JR, Boughter CT, et al. Phosphoantigen-induced conformational change of butyrophilin 3A1 (BTN3A1) and its implication on Vγ9Vδ2 T cell activation. Proc Natl Acad Sci U S A 2017;114(35):E7311–20.

49. Xia M, Hesser DC, De P, et al. A subset of protective γ9δ2 T cells is activated by novel mycobacterial glycolipid components. Infect Immun 2016; 84(9):2449–62.

50. McGill JL, Sacco RE, Baldwin CL, et al. The role of gamma delta T cells in immunity to *Mycobacterium bovis* infection in cattle. Vet Immunol Immunopathol 2014;159(3–4):133–43.

51. Rusk RA, Palmer MV, Waters WR, et al. Measuring bovine gammadelta T cell function at the site of Mycobacterium bovis infection. Vet Immunol Immunopathol 2017;193-194:38–49.

52. Peng MY, Wang ZH, Yao CY, et al. Interleukin 17-producing gamma delta T cells increased in patients with active pulmonary tuberculosis. Cell Mol Immunol 2008;5(3):203–8.

53. Spencer CT, Abate G, Blazevic A, et al. Only a subset of phosphoantigen-responsive gamma9delta2 T cells mediate protective tuberculosis immunity. J Immunol 2008;181(7):4471–84.

54. Abate G, Spencer CT, Hamzabegovic F, et al. Mycobacterium-specific γ9δ2 T cells mediate both pathogen-inhibitory and CD40 ligand-dependent antigen presentation effects important for tuberculosis immunity. Infect Immun 2016;84(2):580–9.

55. Spencer CT, Abate G, Sakala IG, et al. Granzyme A produced by γ(9)δ(2) T cells induces human macrophages to inhibit growth of an intracellular pathogen. PLoS Pathog 2013;9(1): e1003119.

56. Dieli F, Ivanyi J, Marsh P, et al. Characterization of lung gamma delta T cells following intranasal infection with *Mycobacterium bovis* bacillus Calmette-Guerin. J Immunol 2003;170(1):463–9.

57. Ladel CH, Blum C, Dreher A, et al. Protective role of gamma/delta T cells and alpha/beta T cells in tuberculosis. Eur J Immunol 1995;25(10): 2877–81.

58. D'Souza CD, Cooper AM, Frank AA, et al. An anti-inflammatory role for gamma delta T lymphocytes in acquired immunity to *Mycobacterium tuberculosis*. J Immunol 1997;158(3):1217–21.

59. Shen Y, Zhou D, Qiu L, et al. Adaptive immune response of Vgamma2Vdelta2+ T cells during mycobacterial infections. Science 2002;295(5563): 2255–8.

60. Qaqish A, Huang D, Chen CY, et al. Adoptive transfer of phosphoantigen-specific γδ T cell subset attenuates *Mycobacterium tuberculosis* infection in nonhuman primates. J Immunol 2017;198(12): 4753–63.

61. Riegert P, Wanner V, Bahram S. Genomics, isoforms, expression, and phylogeny of the MHC class I-related MR1 gene. J Immunol 1998;161(8): 4066–77.

62. Rodgers JR, Cook RG. MHC class Ib molecules bridge innate and acquired immunity. Nat Rev Immunol 2005;5(6):459–71.

63. Corbett AJ, Eckle SB, Birkinshaw RW, et al. T-cell activation by transitory neo-antigens derived from distinct microbial pathways. Nature 2014; 509(7500):361–5.

64. Kjer-Nielsen L, Patel O, Corbett AJ, et al. MR1 presents microbial vitamin B metabolites to MAIT cells. Nature 2012;491(7426):717–23.

65. Le Bourhis L, Martin E, Peguillet I, et al. Antimicrobial activity of mucosal-associated invariant T cells. Nat Immunol 2010;11(8):701–8.

66. Gold MC, Cerri S, Smyk-Pearson S, et al. Human mucosal associated invariant T cells detect bacterially infected cells. PLoS Biol 2010;8(6):e1000407.

67. Gold MC, McLaren JE, Reistetter JA, et al. MR1-restricted MAIT cells display ligand discrimination and pathogen selectivity through distinct T cell receptor usage. J Exp Med 2014;211(8):1601–10.

68. Lepore M, Kalinichenko A, Calogero S, et al. Functionally diverse human T cells recognize non-microbial antigens presented by MR1. eLife 2017; 6 [pii:e24476].

69. Gherardin NA, Keller AN, Woolley RE, et al. Diversity of T cells restricted by the MHC class I-related molecule MR1 facilitates differential antigen recognition. Immunity 2016;44(1):32–45.

70. Harriff MJ, McMurtrey C, Froyd CA, et al. MR1 displays the microbial metabolome driving selective MR1-restricted T cell receptor usage. Sci Immunol 2018;3(25) [pii:eaao2556].

71. Gold MC, Ehlinger HD, Cook MS, et al. Human innate *Mycobacterium tuberculosis*-reactive alphabetaTCR+ thymocytes. PLoS Pathog 2008; 4(2):e39.

72. Gold MC, Eid T, Smyk-Pearson S, et al. Human thymic MR1-restricted MAIT cells are innate pathogen-reactive effectors that adapt following thymic egress. Mucosal Immunol 2013;6(1):35–44.

73. Koay HF, Gherardin NA, Enders A, et al. A three-stage intrathymic development pathway for the mucosal-associated invariant T cell lineage. Nat Immunol 2016;17(11):1300–11.

74. Ussher JE, Bilton M, Attwod E, et al. CD161++ CD8+ T cells, including the MAIT cell subset, are specifically activated by IL-12+IL-18 in a TCR-independent manner. Eur J Immunol 2014;44(1): 195–203.

75. Ussher JE, van Wilgenburg B, Hannaway RF, et al. TLR signaling in human antigen-presenting cells regulates MR1-dependent activation of MAIT cells. Eur J Immunol 2016;46(7):1600–14.

76. Kurioka A, Ussher JE, Cosgrove C, et al. MAIT cells are licensed through granzyme exchange to kill bacterially sensitized targets. Mucosal Immunol 2015;8(2):429–40.

77. Sakala IG, Kjer-Nielsen L, Eickhoff CS, et al. Functional heterogeneity and antimycobacterial effects of mouse mucosal-associated invariant T cells specific for riboflavin metabolites. J Immunol 2015; 195(2):587–601.

78. Wang H, D'Souza C, Lim XY, et al. MAIT cells protect against pulmonary Legionella longbeachae infection. Nat Commun 2018;9(1):3350.

79. Georgel P, Radosavljevic M, Macquin C, et al. The non-conventional MHC class I MR1 molecule controls infection by *Klebsiella pneumoniae* in mice. Mol Immunol 2011;48(5):769–75.

80. Chua WJ, Truscott SM, Eickhoff CS, et al. Polyclonal mucosa-associated invariant T cells have unique innate functions in bacterial infection. Infect Immun 2012;80(9):3256–67.

81. Meierovics A, Yankelevich WJ, Cowley SC. MAIT cells are critical for optimal mucosal immune responses during in vivo pulmonary bacterial infection. Proc Natl Acad Sci U S A 2013;110(33): E3119–28.

82. Meierovics AI, Cowley SC. MAIT cells promote inflammatory monocyte differentiation into dendritic cells during pulmonary intracellular infection. J Exp Med 2016;213(12):2793–809.

83. Seshadri C, Thuong NT, Mai NT, et al. A polymorphism in human MR1 is associated with mRNA expression and susceptibility to tuberculosis. Genes Immun 2017;18(1):8–14.

84. Pincikova T, Paquin-Proulx D, Moll M, et al. Severely impaired control of bacterial infections in a patient with cystic fibrosis defective in mucosal-associated invariant T cells. Chest 2018;153(5): e93–6.

85. Chen Z, Wang H, D'Souza C, et al. Mucosal-associated invariant T-cell activation and accumulation after in vivo infection depends on microbial riboflavin synthesis and co-stimulatory signals. Mucosal Immunol 2017;10(1):58–68.

86. Howson LJ, Napolitani G, Shepherd D, et al. MAIT cell clonal expansion and TCR repertoire shaping in human volunteers challenged with *Salmonella paratyphi A*. Nat Commun 2018;9(1):253.

87. Lindestam Arlehamn CS, Lewinsohn DM, Sette A, et al. Antigens for CD4 and CD8 T cells in tuberculosis. Cold Spring Harb Perspect Med 2014;4(7): a018465.

88. Lindestam Arlehamn CS, Gerasimova A, Mele F, et al. Memory T cells in latent *Mycobacterium tuberculosis* infection are directed against three antigenic islands and largely contained in a CXCR3+CCR6+ Th1 subset. PLoS Pathog 2013; 9(1):e1003130.

89. Lewinsohn DA, Swarbrick GM, Park B, et al. Comprehensive definition of human immunodominant CD8 antigens in tuberculosis. NPJ Vaccines 2017;2 [pii:8].

90. Ernst JD. Mechanisms of *M. tuberculosis* immune evasion as challenges to TB vaccine design. Cell Host Microbe 2018;24(1):34–42.

91. Comas I, Chakravartti J, Small PM, et al. Human T cell epitopes of *Mycobacterium tuberculosis* are evolutionarily hyperconserved. Nat Genet 2010; 42(6):498–503.

92. Copin R, Coscolla M, Seiffert SN, et al. Sequence diversity in the pe_pgrs genes of *Mycobacterium tuberculosis* is independent of human T cell recognition. MBio 2014;5(1):e00960–009613.

93. Coscolla M, Copin R, Sutherland J, et al. *M. tuberculosis* T cell epitope analysis reveals paucity of antigenic variation and identifies rare variable TB antigens. Cell Host Microbe 2015;18(5): 538–48.

94. Gagneux S. Ecology and evolution of *Mycobacterium tuberculosis*. Nat Rev Microbiol 2018;16(4): 202–13.

95. Orme IM, Henao-Tamayo MI. Trying to see the forest through the trees: deciphering the nature of memory immunity to *Mycobacterium tuberculosis*. Front Immunol 2018;9:461.

96. Mpande CAM, Dintwe OB, Musvosvi M, et al. Functional, antigen-specific stem cell memory (TSCM) CD4$^+$ T cells are induced by human *Mycobacterium tuberculosis* infection. Front Immunol 2018;9:324.

97. Moguche AO, Musvosvi M, Penn-Nicholson A, et al. Antigen availability shapes T cell differentiation and function during tuberculosis. Cell Host Microbe 2017;21(6):695–706.e5.

98. Sakai S, Mayer-Barber KD, Barber DL. Defining features of protective CD4 T cell responses to *Mycobacterium tuberculosis*. Curr Opin Immunol 2014;29:137–42.

99. Sallin MA, Sakai S, Kauffman KD, et al. Th1 differentiation drives the accumulation of intravascular, non-protective CD4 T cells during tuberculosis. Cell Rep 2017;18(13):3091–104.

100. Kauffman KD, Sallin MA, Sakai S, et al. Defective positioning in granulomas but not lung-homing limits CD4 T-cell interactions with *Mycobacterium tuberculosi*s-infected macrophages in rhesus macaques. Mucosal Immunol 2018; 11(2):462–73.

101. Bull NC, Stylianou E, Kaveh DA, et al. Enhanced protection conferred by mucosal BCG vaccination associates with presence of antigen-specific lung tissue-resident PD-1$^+$ KLRG1$^-$ CD4$^+$ T cells. Mucosal Immunol 2019;12(2):555–64.

102. Satti I, Meyer J, Harris SA, et al. Safety and immunogenicity of a candidate tuberculosis vaccine MVA85A delivered by aerosol in BCG-vaccinated healthy adults: a phase 1, double-blind, randomised controlled trial. Lancet Infect Dis 2014; 14(10):939–46.

103. Jacobs AJ, Mongkolsapaya J, Screaton GR, et al. Antibodies and tuberculosis. Tuberculosis (Edinb) 2016;101:102–13.

104. Tameris MD, Hatherill M, Landry BS, et al. Safety and efficacy of MVA85A, a new tuberculosis vaccine, in infants previously vaccinated with BCG: a randomised, placebo-controlled phase 2b trial. Lancet 2013;381(9871):1021–8.

105. Lu LL, Chung AW, Rosebrock TR, et al. A functional role for antibodies in tuberculosis. Cell 2016; 167(2):433–43.e14.

106. Drain PK, Bajema KL, Dowdy D, et al. Incipient and subclinical tuberculosis: a clinical review of early stages and progression of infection. Clin Microbiol Rev 2018;31(4) [pii:e00021-18].

107. Meermeier EW, Lewinsohn DM. Early clearance versus control: what is the meaning of a negative tuberculin skin test or interferon-gamma release assay following exposure to Mycobacterium tuberculosis? F1000Res 2018;7 [pii:F1000 Faculty Rev-664].

108. Barry CE 3rd, Boshoff HI, Dartois V, et al. The spectrum of latent tuberculosis: rethinking the biology and intervention strategies. Nat Rev Microbiol 2009;7(12):845–55.

109. Andrews JR, Noubary F, Walensky RP, et al. Risk of progression to active tuberculosis following reinfection with *Mycobacterium tuberculosis*. Clin Infect Dis 2012;54(6):784–91.

110. Simmons JD, Stein CM, Seshadri C, et al. Immunological mechanisms of human resistance to persistent *Mycobacterium tuberculosis* infection. Nat Rev Immunol 2018;18(9):575–89.

111. Esmail H, Lai RP, Lesosky M, et al. Characterization of progressive HIV-associated tuberculosis using 2-deoxy-2-[18F]fluoro-D-glucose positron emission and computed tomography. Nat Med 2016;22(10): 1090–3.

112. Berry MP, Graham CM, McNab FW, et al. An interferon-inducible neutrophil-driven blood transcriptional signature in human tuberculosis. Nature 2010;466(7309):973–7.

113. Bloom CI, Graham CM, Berry MP, et al. Transcriptional blood signatures distinguish pulmonary tuberculosis, pulmonary sarcoidosis, pneumonias and lung cancers. PLoS One 2013;8(8):e70630.

114. Kaforou M, Wright VJ, Oni T, et al. Detection of tuberculosis in HIV-infected and -uninfected African adults using whole blood RNA expression signatures: a case-control study. PLoS Med 2013; 10(10):e1001538.

115. Kaforou M, Wright VJ, Levin M. Host RNA signatures for diagnostics: an example from paediatric tuberculosis in Africa. J Infect 2014;69(Suppl 1):S28–31.

116. Andersen P, Doherty TM, Pai M, et al. The prognosis of latent tuberculosis: can disease be predicted? Trends Mol Med 2007;13(5):175–82.

117. Maertzdorf J, Ota M, Repsilber D, et al. Functional correlations of pathogenesis-driven gene expression signatures in tuberculosis. PLoS One 2011; 6(10):e26938.

118. Scriba TJ, Penn-Nicholson A, Shankar S, et al. Sequential inflammatory processes define human progression from M. tuberculosis infection to tuberculosis disease. PLoS Pathog 2017;13(11): e1006687.

119. Zak DE, Penn-Nicholson A, Scriba TJ, et al. A blood RNA signature for tuberculosis disease risk: a prospective cohort study. Lancet 2016; 387(10035):2312–22.

120. Duffy FJ, Thompson E, Downing K, et al. A serum circulating miRNA signature for short-term risk of progression to active tuberculosis among household contacts. Front Immunol 2018;9:661.

121. Darboe F, Mbandi SK, Thompson EG, et al. Diagnostic performance of an optimized transcriptomic signature of risk of tuberculosis in cryopreserved peripheral blood mononuclear cells. Tuberculosis (Edinb) 2018;108:124–6.

122. Sabin FR, Doan CA. The relation of monocytes and clasmatocytes to early infection in rabbits with bovine tubercle bacilli. J Exp Med 1927;46(4): 627–44.

123. Rogers P. A study of the blood monocytes in children with tuberculosis. N Engl J Med 1928;198: 740–9.

124. Naranbhai V, Hill AV, Abdool Karim SS, et al. Ratio of monocytes to lymphocytes in peripheral blood identifies adults at risk of incident tuberculosis among HIV-infected adults initiating antiretroviral therapy. J Infect Dis 2014;209(4):500–9.

125. Rakotosamimanana N, Richard V, Raharimanga V, et al. Biomarkers for risk of developing active tuberculosis in contacts of TB patients: a prospective cohort study. Eur Respir J 2015;46(4):1095–103.

126. Wang J, Yin Y, Wang X, et al. Ratio of monocytes to lymphocytes in peripheral blood in patients diagnosed with active tuberculosis. Braz J Infect Dis 2015;19(2):125–31.

127. La Manna MP, Orlando V, Dieli F, et al. Quantitative and qualitative profiles of circulating monocytes may help identifying tuberculosis infection and disease stages. PLoS One 2017;12(2):e0171358.

128. Kwon YS, Cho YN, Kim MJ, et al. Mucosal-associated invariant T cells are numerically and functionally deficient in patients with mycobacterial infection and reflect disease activity. Tuberculosis (Edinb) 2015;95(3):267–74.

129. Snyder-Cappione JE, Nixon DF, Loo CP, et al. Individuals with pulmonary tuberculosis have lower levels of circulating CD1d-restricted NKT cells. J Infect Dis 2007;195(9):1361–4.

130. Sutherland JS, Hill PC, Adetifa IM, et al. Identification of probable early-onset biomarkers for tuberculosis disease progression. PLoS One 2011;6(9):e25230.

131. Andrews JR, Nemes E, Tameris M, et al. Serial QuantiFERON testing and tuberculosis disease risk among young children: an observational cohort study. Lancet Respir Med 2017;5(4):282–90.

132. Winje BA, White R, Syre H, et al. Stratification by interferon-γ release assay level predicts risk of incident TB. Thorax 2018 [pii:thoraxjnl-2017-211147].

133. Millington KA, Innes JA, Hackforth S, et al. Dynamic relationship between IFN-gamma and IL-2 profile of Mycobacterium tuberculosis-specific T cells and antigen load. J Immunol 2007;178(8): 5217–26.

134. Day CL, Abrahams DA, Lerumo L, et al. Functional capacity of Mycobacterium tuberculosis-specific T cell responses in humans is associated with mycobacterial load. J Immunol 2011;187(5):2222–32.

135. Day CL, Moshi ND, Abrahams DA, et al. Patients with tuberculosis disease have Mycobacterium tuberculosis-specific CD8 T cells with a pro-apoptotic phenotype and impaired proliferative capacity, which is not restored following treatment. PLoS One 2014;9(4):e94949.

136. Adekambi T, Ibegbu CC, Cagle S, et al. Biomarkers on patient T cells diagnose active tuberculosis and monitor treatment response. J Clin Invest 2015; 125(9):3723.

137. Wilkinson KA, Oni T, Gideon HP, et al. Activation profile of Mycobacterium tuberculosis-specific CD4+ T cells reflects disease activity irrespective of HIV status. Am J Respir Crit Care Med 2016; 193(11):1307–10.

138. Riou C, Berkowitz N, Goliath R, et al. Analysis of the phenotype of Mycobacterium tuberculosis-specific CD4+ T cells to discriminate latent from active tuberculosis in HIV-uninfected and HIV-infected individuals. Front Immunol 2017;8:968.

139. Fletcher HA, Snowden MA, Landry B, et al. T-cell activation is an immune correlate of risk in BCG vaccinated infants. Nat Commun 2016;7: 11290.

140. Rozot V, Vigano S, Mazza-Stalder J, et al. Mycobacterium tuberculosis-specific CD8+ T cells are functionally and phenotypically different between latent infection and active disease. Eur J Immunol 2013;43(6):1568–77.

141. Lancioni C, Nyendak M, Kiguli S, et al. CD8+ T cells provide an immunologic signature of tuberculosis in young children. Am J Respir Crit Care Med 2012;185(2):206–12.

142. Lewinsohn DM, Tydeman IS, Frieder M, et al. High resolution radiographic and fine immunologic definition of TB disease progression in the rhesus macaque. Microbes Infect 2006;8(11):2587–98.

143. Nyendak MR, Park B, Null MD, et al. Mycobacterium tuberculosis specific CD8+ T cells rapidly

decline with antituberculosis treatment. PLoS One 2013;8(12):e81564.

144. Allen NP, Swarbrick G, Cansler M, et al. Characterization of specific CD4 and CD8 T-cell responses in QuantiFERON TB Gold-Plus TB1 and TB2 tubes. Tuberculosis (Edinb) 2018;113:239–41.

145. Petruccioli E, Chiacchio T, Pepponi I, et al. First characterization of the CD4 and CD8 T-cell responses to QuantiFERON-TB plus. J Infect 2016; 73(6):588–97.

146. Pieterman ED, Liqui Lung FG, Verbon A, et al. A multicentre verification study of the QuantiFERON((R))-TB Gold Plus assay. Tuberculosis 2018;108:136–42.

147. Petruccioli E, Vanini V, Chiacchio T, et al. Analytical evaluation of QuantiFERON- plus and QuantiFERON- gold in-tube assays in subjects with or without tuberculosis. Tuberculosis 2017;106:38–43.

148. Barcellini L, Borroni E, Brown J, et al. First evaluation of QuantiFERON-TB Gold Plus performance in contact screening. Eur Respir J 2016;48(5): 1411–9.

149. Kamada A, Amishima M. QuantiFERON-TB((R)) Gold Plus as a potential tuberculosis treatment monitoring tool. Eur Respir J 2017;49(3) [pii: 1601976].

150. Marais BJ, Gie RP, Schaaf HS, et al. Childhood pulmonary tuberculosis: old wisdom and new challenges. Am J Respir Crit Care Med 2006;173(10): 1078–90.

151. Trunz BB, Fine P, Dye C. Effect of BCG vaccination on childhood tuberculous meningitis and miliary tuberculosis worldwide: a meta-analysis and assessment of cost-effectiveness. Lancet 2006; 367(9517):1173–80.

152. World Health Organization. Global tuberculosis report 2018. Geneva (Switzerland): World Health Organization; 2018.

153. Boer MC, Lewinsohn DA, Lancioni CL. Immunobiology of pediatric tuberculosis: lessons learned and implications for an improved TB-vaccine. J Pediatr Infect Dis 2018;13:113–21.

154. Shey MS, Nemes E, Whatney W, et al. Maturation of innate responses to mycobacteria over the first nine months of life. J Immunol 2014;192(10): 4833–43.

155. Ben Youssef G, Tourret M, Salou M, et al. Ontogeny of human mucosal-associated invariant T cells and related T cell subsets. J Exp Med 2018;215(2): 459–79.

156. Zufferey C, Germano S, Dutta B, et al. The contribution of non-conventional T cells and NK cells in the mycobacterial-specific IFNγ response in Bacille Calmette-Guerin (BCG)-immunized infants. PLoS One 2013;8(10):e77334.

157. Lewinsohn DA, Lewinsohn DM, Scriba TJ. Polyfunctional CD4+ T cells as targets for tuberculosis vaccination. Front Immunol 2017;8:1262.

158. Tameris M, Hokey DA, Nduba V, et al. A double-blind, randomised, placebo-controlled, dose-finding trial of the novel tuberculosis vaccine AERAS-402, an adenovirus-vectored fusion protein, in healthy, BCG-vaccinated infants. Vaccine 2015;33(25):2944–54.

159. Kagina BM, Abel B, Scriba TJ, et al. Specific T cell frequency and cytokine expression profile do not correlate with protection against tuberculosis after Bacillus Calmette-Guerin vaccination of newborns. Am J Respir Crit Care Med 2010; 182(8):1073–9.

160. Logan E, Luabeya AKK, Mulenga H, et al. Elevated IgG responses in infants are associated with reduced prevalence of Mycobacterium tuberculosis infection. Front Immunol 2018;9:1529.

161. Alvarez N, Otero O, Camacho F, et al. Passive administration of purified secretory IgA from human colostrum induces protection against Mycobacterium tuberculosis in a murine model of progressive pulmonary infection. BMC Immunol 2013;14(Suppl 1):S3.

162. Rajagopalan S. Tuberculosis in older adults. Clin Geriatr Med 2016;32(3):479–91.

163. Piergallini TJ, Turner J. Tuberculosis in the elderly: why inflammation matters. Exp Gerontol 2018; 105:32–9.

164. Byng-Maddick R, Noursadeghi M. Does tuberculosis threaten our ageing populations? BMC Infect Dis 2016;16:119.

165. Jeon CY, Murray MB. Diabetes mellitus increases the risk of active tuberculosis: a systematic review of 13 observational studies. PLoS Med 2008;5(7): e152.

166. Viswanathan V, Kumpatla S, Aravindalochanan V, et al. Prevalence of diabetes and pre-diabetes and associated risk factors among tuberculosis patients in India. PLoS One 2012;7(7):e41367.

167. Kumar Nathella P, Babu S. Influence of diabetes mellitus on immunity to human tuberculosis. Immunology 2017;152(1):13–24.

168. Martinez N, Kornfeld H. Diabetes and immunity to tuberculosis. Eur J Immunol 2014;44(3): 617–26.

169. Prada-Medina CA, Fukutani KF, Pavan Kumar N, et al. Systems immunology of diabetes-tuberculosis comorbidity reveals signatures of disease complications. Sci Rep 2017;7(1):1999.

170. Du Bruyn E, Wilkinson RJ. The immune interaction between HIV-1 infection and Mycobacterium tuberculosis. Microbiol Spectr 2016;4(6). https://doi.org/10.1128/microbiolspec.TBTB2-0012-2016.

Tuberculosis and Biologic Therapies
Anti-Tumor Necrosis Factor-α and Beyond

Mark S. Godfrey, MD, Lloyd N. Friedman, MD*

KEYWORDS

- Tuberculosis • Biological therapy • Tumor necrosis factor-alpha • Antibodies • Monoclonal
- Opportunistic infection

KEY POINTS

- Tumor necrosis factor-alpha (TNF-α) is integral to the *in vitro* and *in vivo* control of tuberculosis. There is a well-characterized increase in tuberculosis risk for patients with inflammatory disease who are prescribed TNF-α antagonists.
- Screening and treatment of latent tuberculosis infection before TNF-α blockade is effective but remains imperfect in practice because of screening test characteristics, lack of universal adoption, and confounding by immunosuppression.
- Patients treated with TNF-α antagonists remain at risk for tuberculosis throughout treatment, and often present with disseminated or extrapulmonary disease.
- Many biologic drugs that are in increasing clinical use affect T cells or other cytokines peripherally involved in the immune response to tuberculosis, and vigilance for tuberculosis in these patients is advised.

INTRODUCTION

Tumor necrosis factor-alpha (TNF-α) is involved in the pathogenesis of several inflammatory diseases such as rheumatoid arthritis (RA), ankylosing spondylitis, psoriatic arthritis, and inflammatory bowel diseases (IBD), in addition to its role in the host response to infection. This observation led to the first therapeutic trials of TNF-α blockade in patients with RA in 1994, and subsequently these agents have been shown to effectively control symptoms and allow return to function in a variety of inflammatory conditions.[1] Our understanding of the risk of tuberculosis (TB) associated with this therapy has continued to evolve following the seminal report by Keane and colleagues[2] in 2001 on the development of TB in patients receiving the TNF-α antagonist infliximab. The mechanisms and magnitude of risk associated with this class of drugs subsequently has been characterized by numerous *in vitro* and translational studies, and corroborated by 20 years of clinical experience and surveillance through national patient registries. This has resulted in the widespread adoption of recommendations for screening and prophylaxis for latent TB infection (LTBI) before initiation of therapy, and a decrease in TB incidence owing to these drugs. Although the risk associated with TNF-α inhibitors is widely appreciated, there is an increasing number of biologic drugs in use in malignant or inflammatory

Disclosure Statement: The authors have no relationship with a commercial company that has a direct financial interest in subject matter or materials discussed in article or with a company making a competing product.
Section of Pulmonary, Critical Care, and Sleep Medicine, Yale University School of Medicine, 300 Cedar Street, TAC S425, PO Box 208057, New Haven, CT 06520, USA
* Corresponding author.
E-mail address: Lloyd.friedman@yale.edu

0272-5231/19/© 2019 Elsevier Inc. All rights reserved.

conditions. As part of their therapeutic mechanism, these drugs may modulate T cell number, function, or cytokine signaling important for the control of TB infection or the maintenance of granulomas, any of which may place patients at risk for reactivation of latent TB or acquisition of new infection.

This review summarizes what is known about TB risk associated with various classes of biologic drugs and highlights areas where further study is needed. Small molecules, targeted therapies, corticosteroids, and non-biologic disease-modifying antirheumatic drugs (DMARDs) are outside the scope of this review, although it should be noted that they too predispose to an increased risk for TB.[3] We propose practical recommendations for screening, prophylaxis, and management, with a particular focus on patients eligible for or receiving anti-TNF-α biologics.

TUMOR NECROSIS FACTOR-α INHIBITORS: INFLIXIMAB, ADALIMUMAB, GOLIMUMAB, CERTOLIZUMAB PEGOL, AND ETANERCEPT
Tumor Necrosis Factor-α Biology, Available Drugs, and Indications for Use

TNF-α is a cytokine involved in inflammatory and immune responses through its regulation of immune cell proliferation, differentiation, and survival. TNF-α is produced as a membrane-bound homotrimer (mTNF-α) that is cleaved by the membrane metalloproteinase TNF-α converting enzyme to release a soluble form (sTNF-α).[4] mTNF-α and sTNF-α are each biologically active and bind to 2 cell surface receptors: TNFR1 (CD120a) and TNFR2 (CD120b). In addition to acting as a ligand by binding to TNFR1-2, mTNF-α also transmits outside-to-inside (reverse) signals back into the mTNF-α-bearing cells.[5] The immunology of TB and the role of TNF-α in tuberculous control is reviewed in more detail in this issue of *Clinics*, but it is accepted that TNF-α plays a central role in the control of TB infection.[6–9] Both mTNF-α and sTNF-α are important in murine models of TB; TNF-α knockout mice rapidly succumb to TB infection,[10] but restoration of mTNF-α alone can partially restore host defenses, although the mice ultimately succumb to infection.[11] Animal models of TB infection suggest that a failure to control TB during TNF-α blockade is not due to inability to form granulomas, but rather to inability to control intracellular TB growth in macrophages and maintain granulomas.[12,13]

There currently are 5 approved biologic drugs whose therapeutic mechanism of action involves binding and neutralizing TNF-α: 4 monoclonal antibodies (mAbs) and 1 soluble TNF-α receptor (Fig. 1).[14] Infliximab is a chimeric antibody composed of a human immunoglobulin 1 (IgG1) constant region and an antigen-binding murine variable region. Notably, when infliximab is used in RA, it is US Food and Drug Administration (FDA) approved only when co-administered with methotrexate.[15] Adalimumab and golimumab are fully humanized IgG1 antibodies. All 3 mAbs contain an Fc domain that allows them to participate in complement-mediated lysis or cell-mediated cytotoxicity. Certolizumab pegol consists of a human Fab fragment targeting TNF-α, which is conjugated to an approximately 40-kDa polyethylene glycol (PEG) chain. PEGylation of certolizumab leads to an increased half-life, increased solubility, reduced aggregation, and reduced immunogenicity.[16] Etanercept is a soluble TNF-α receptor consisting of a dimer of the extracellular domain of the human TNFR2 fused to an Fc fragment of human IgG1. As such, it is able to bind soluble TNF-α as well as TNF-β (lymphotoxin); TNF-β is itself a cytokine which is important, although not sufficient, for TB control in a murine model.[17]

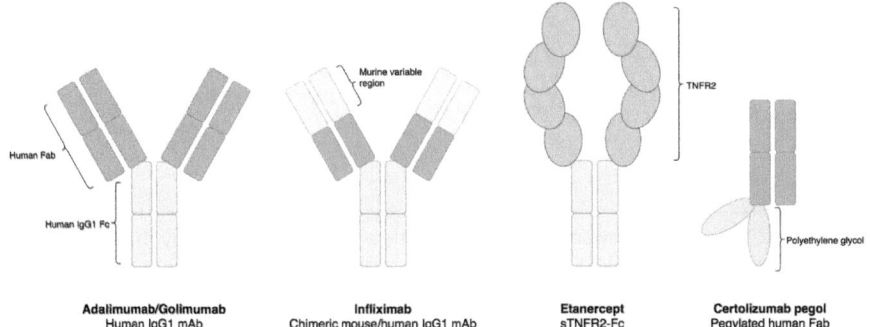

Fig. 1. Structural schematic diagram of the 5 clinically available anti-tumor necrosis factor-α drugs. Fab, fragment, antigen binding; Fc, constant region; mAb, monoclonal antibody; TNFR2, human tumor necrosis factor receptor 2 ("s" indicating soluble).

There may be structural and functional differences between TNF-α antagonists, particularly between the antibodies and soluble receptor constructs, that inform their relationship to clinical TB reactivation.[6] Infliximab and adalimumab inhibit T cell activation and interferon- γ (IFN-γ) production at therapeutic concentrations in healthy human plasma, whereas etanercept does not.[18] Certolizumab is unable to participate in complement-mediated lysis or cell-mediated toxicity because of the absence of an Fc domain. Variability between agents in their pharmacokinetics, binding affinities for TNF-α, and effects on T cell proliferation and apoptosis is reviewed in more detail by Mitoma and colleagues.[4]

Because each TNF-α is a homotrimer with 3 epitopes for antibody binding, and each mAb is bivalent, there is potential for formation of bridging interactions and formation of large immune complexes. Cryo-electron microscope images of adalimumab- and infliximab-TNF-α complexes reveal structures consisting of 1:1, 1:2, 2:2, and 3:2 complexes of antibody:TNF-α, with the dominant form a 598-kDa 3:2 configuration.[19] In contrast, etanercept binds sTNF-α trimers in a 1:1 stoichiometry and does not form stable complexes because 90% of bound cytokine is released after 2 to 3 hours.[20] In addition, infliximab (but not etanercept) seems to bind monomeric sTNF-α, which may slow or even prevent association of monomeric subunits to form bioactive trimeric sTNF-α.[20] Furthermore, etanercept's ability to influence transmembrane TNF-α seems to be weaker than the other agents.[4] The net result of the above interactions is a relative increase in bioavailable sTNF-α and mTNF-α with the use of etanercept compared with the mAb biologics.

Tuberculosis Risk Associated with Different Tumor Necrosis Factor-α Inhibitors

Meta-analyses have been published summarizing the risk of TB associated with TNF-α blockade in thousands of patients with RA or other inflammatory diseases, and have demonstrated a roughly 4-fold increase in TB in those treated with TNF-α antagonists compared with those not exposed to these drugs.[21,22] Several caveats should be noted when interpreting data on the incidence of TB in patients with immune-mediated inflammatory disease, particularly RA. Broadly speaking, many randomized clinical trials of these drugs are conducted in the United States and Western Europe, 2 areas with low TB prevalence. Randomized controlled trials, unless long term, may not have sufficient follow-up to capture all cases and often are underpowered for infrequent adverse events. More contemporary trial protocols involve screening or exclusion of patients with LTBI, which will underestimate risk and dilute hazard ratios when pooled for meta-analyses. In addition, meta-analyses reporting modest increases in risk make use of Yates' correction for continuity when evaluating odds ratios in small studies with zero event rates.[23,24] Such correction can be overly conservative and lead to an underestimation of risk.[25] Furthermore, patients with RA have an increased risk of bacterial infection[26] and TB[21,27,28] compared with the general population regardless of their use of biologic drugs. This may be due to intrinsic defects in cell-mediated immunity,[29] the use of concomitant non-biologic DMARDs or steroids,[3] or structural lung disease such as bronchiectasis.[30]

Therefore, in large part, data are from non-randomized retrospective studies, namely from registries or voluntary public health reporting. Such an approach has intrinsic limitations and likely is an underestimation of actual risk because of detection bias. Alternatively, anti-TNF-α-exposed patients frequently are compared with the background national TB rate, which could lead to an overestimation, and only rarely are compared with a non-TNF-α-exposed population with immune-mediated inflammatory disease as reported by Askling and colleagues.[31] Despite these limitations, it is clear that TNF-α antagonism increases the risk of TB and that the magnitude of this increase is not equal among the different available agents. **Table 1** summarizes the incidence of TB associated with infliximab, adalimumab, and etanercept among selected studies that vary in design from prospective national registries and open-label extension studies to retrospective cohorts, and comprise patients with RA,[3,27,31–40] ankylosing spondylitis,[41] psoriatic arthritis,[42] IBD,[43] or mixed cohorts with multiple TNF-α indications.[44–51] Taken together, it is clear that the incidence of TB is highly dependent on the regional prevalence of TB and that the mAbs infliximab and adalimumab carry a higher risk of TB progression than etanercept.

Data on the incidence of TB with golimumab and certolizumab pegol are limited due to their more recent approval (2009 and 2010, respectively), as well as stringent guidelines for LTBI screening and prophylaxis in their clinical trials. In 1 registry series for golimumab, the incidence was similar to adalimumab, as would be expected given that they are both fully humanized mAbs.[51] Pooled data from 5 phase III trials of golimumab at doses of 100 and 50 mg demonstrated incidence rates of 350 and 170 per 100,000 patient-years in patients who were screened and treated for LTBI.[52] For

Table 1
Summary of selected studies examining the incidence of tuberculosis in patients with inflammatory diseases on anti-TNF-α therapies

Study, Year of Publication	Region	Years of Data	Study Design	Risk Estimate for TB Case Rate per 100,000 Person-Years		
				Infliximab	Adalimumab	Etanercept
Gómez-Reino et al,[33] 2003	Spain	2000–2002	BIOBADASER Registry	1503	—	—
Wallis et al,[44] 2004	USA	1998–2002	FDA AERS	54	—	28
Carmona et al,[34] 2005	Spain	2002–2004	BIOBADASER Registry	32	0	0
Listing et al,[35] 2005	Germany	2001–2003	RABBIT Registry	310	—	0
Askling et al,[31] 2005	Sweden	1999–2004	ARTIS Registry	145	—	80
Brassard et al,[3] 2006	Canada	1998–2003	Pharmaceutical claims database	257[a]		
Sichletidis et al,[45] 2006	Greece	2000–2004	Single center retrospective	449[a]		
Tubach et al,[46] 2009	France	2004–2007	RATIO Registry	188	215	9
Favalli et al,[32] 2009	Italy	1999–2002	LORHEN Registry	375	0	0
		2002–2008		183	191	291
Dixon et al,[36] 2010	UK	2001–2008	BSRBR Registry	136	144	39
Kim et al,[41] 2011	Korea	2002–2009	KTBS Registry	540	490	0
Atzeni et al,[37] 2012	Italy	1999–2012	GISEA Registry	259	113	39
Winthrop et al,[47] 2013	USA	2000–2008	Kaiser Permanente pharmacy database	83	91	17

Study	Country	Period	Database			
Abreu et al,[49] 2013	Portugal	2001–2012	Single center retrospective	1337	792	405
Baddley et al,[50] 2014	USA	1998–2007	Multiple registries	40[a]		
Mok et al,[51] 2014	Hong Kong	2005–2013	Hong Kong Biologics Registry	1680	850	430
Ergun et al,[42] 2015	Turkey	2005–2012	Retrospective study, 4 referral centers	580	130	990
Arkema et al,[27] 2015	Sweden	2002–2011	SRQ Registry	51	47	20
Lim et al,[39] 2017	Taiwan	2000–2015	NHIRD National database	—	1056	889
Hou et al,[43] 2017	USA	2003–2011	National Veterans Affairs administrative data sets	28[a]		
Yonekura et al,[38] 2017	Brazil	2009–2013	BiobadaBrasil Registry	182	443	192
Lee et al,[48] 2017	Korea	2011–2013	HIRA insurance claims database	1234 not treated for LTBI[a] 407 treated for LTBI[a]		
Rutherford et al,[40] 2018	UK	2001–2015	BSRBR Registry	73	83	46

Abbreviations: ARTIS, anti-rheumatic treatment in Sweden; BiobadaBrasil, Brazilian registry of biological therapies in rheumatic diseases; BIOBADASER, Spanish Society of Rheumatology Database on Biologic Products; BSRBR, British Society for Rheumatology Biologics Register; FDA AERS, US Department of Food and Drug Adverse Event Reporting System; GISEA, Gruppo Italiano di Studio sulla early arthritis; HIRA, health insurance review and assessment service; KTBS, Korean tuberculosis surveillance system; LORHEN, Lombardy rheumatology network; LTBI, latent tuberculosis infection; NHIRD, National Health Insurance Research Database; RABBIT, rheumatoid arthritis observation of biologic therapy; RATIO, French research axed on tolerance of biotherapies; SQR, Swedish rheumatology quality.

[a] Indicates studies reporting only a pooled risk among several TNF inhibitors.

Data from BIOBADASER Registry and Favalli et al. are divided before and after 2002 due to implementation of recommendations for the diagnosis and management of latent TB infection in patients receiving TNF antagonists.

certolizumab, national registry data from the United Kingdom have demonstrated an incidence equal to that of infliximab or adalimumab, although with admittedly few total cases.[40] Further analysis of trials and open-label extension studies in RA, in patients who primarily were from endemic regions, demonstrated an incidence of 470 cases per 100,000 patient-years.[53] The incidence was stable throughout the 60 months of follow-up, and 39 of the 44 TB cases occurred in central or Eastern Europe and likely represented new infection. The addition of studies of certolizumab in patients with inflammatory conditions other than RA did not markedly change this overall incidence estimate, but it was noted that the incidence significantly dropped (from 510 to 180 cases per 100,000 patient-years) following more stringent LTBI screening and treatment.[54]

Tuberculosis Associated with Anti- Tumor Necrosis Factor-α Therapy: Time to Onset and Clinical Presentation

TB cases that occur while on anti-TNF-α therapy may result from acquisition of new infection that progresses (primary TB) or from reactivation of latent TB (post-primary TB). The former should be evident as a fixed cumulative case rate dependent on the local TB prevalence, and the latter as cases that cluster shortly after initiation of therapy. **Table 2** summarizes selected studies which presented median time to onset of TB from drug initiation among different TNF-α inhibitors, as well as the sites of TB disease. What is evident is that the median time to onset of TB is shorter with the mAbs infliximab and adalimumab (a median of 3–6 months) compared with greater than 1 year with etanercept. Wallis[55] used mathematical modeling to analyze reported time-to-onset data to reveal the rates of new infection, latent infection, reactivation, and progression to TB in patients on the TNF-α inhibitors infliximab and etanercept. In the groups he studied, with patients on infliximab developing TB at a median of 12 to 21 weeks, he demonstrated that infliximab and etanercept differed markedly with regard to median monthly reactivation rates (20.8% and 1.58%, respectively), but that both seemed to share a high risk for progression from new infection to active disease.

Work in animal models lends further support to the validity of these observational data. Plessner and colleagues[56] investigated the effects of TNF-α inhibition with an anti-TNF-α mAb and soluble TNFR2 (biosimilars analogous to infliximab and etancerept, respectively) in a murine model of primary and chronic TB infection. During acute TB infection, both the mAb and the soluble receptor resulted in rapid mortality. However, when treatment was initiated during an established infection, only mice treated with anti-TNF-α antibody developed overwhelming disease, and the lungs of mice treated with a soluble receptor fusion molecule demonstrated better granuloma formation and decreased mycobacterial burden. Although such animal models can be informative, other host factors in patients make it difficult to translate definitive conclusions on mechanisms of reactivation from such studies. For example, adalimumab at doses higher than used clinically in IBD did not result in 100% TB when administered during acute or latent TB infection in a macaque primate model.[13]

With regard to the site of reactivation (pulmonary versus extrapulmonary) and the rate of disseminated disease, it is also clear from **Table 2** that roughly two-thirds of TB disease in patients receiving anti-TNF-α biologics was extrapulmonary, and half of that (one-third of all TB cases) was disseminated. This seems to be true regardless of the choice of anti-TNF-α drug. There also seems to be a higher than expected TB case-fatality rate; in some series between 12% and 18%,[31,33,36,57] all in areas where the expected case-fatality rate is less than 5%.[58] However, there certainly is confounding data between host factors related to the indication for TNF-α blockade and infection- or TB-specific mortality, and it should be noted that in some series (even those with high rates of disseminated disease) TB-specific mortality was negligible.[46,49,59]

OTHER BIOLOGIC DRUGS WITH INCREASED RISK OR POSSIBLE RISK BASED ON MECHANISM OF ACTION

Many of the biologics discussed in this section (**Table 3**) have no documented increase in TB risk, but these data must be interpreted with the same caveats as were outlined above for TNF-α antagonism. Some of the data do suggest increased risk, but currently there are no specific recommendations for screening or treatment of patients on these drugs. In many cases the only data are from clinical trials conducted in low-prevalence settings, or trials in which LTBI was screened for and treated in anticipation of drug-related immunosuppression, or in which patients with known LTBI were excluded. Some of these drugs have very limited scope or indications for use, or are novel enough that any adverse event reporting in national registries is limited. However, for all of the drugs in this section, we believe that, based on their mechanism of action and what we

Table 2
Summary of selected studies examining the time to onset of tuberculosis in and site of disease in patients with inflammatory diseases on anti-TNF therapies

Study, Year of Publication	Region	Years of Data	Number of TB Cases	TB Deaths	Months to TB Onset (Median)			Site of Disease (n)	
					Infliximab	Adalimumab	Etanercept	Pulmonary	Extrapulmonary (Disseminated)
Keane et al,[2] 2001	USA	1998–2001	70	4 (6%)	3.0	—	—	22[a]	40 (17)
Gómez-Reino et al,[33] 2003	Spain	2000–2002	17	2 (12%)	3.0	—	—	6	11 (5)
Mohan et al,[152] 2004	USA, Europe	1998–2002	25	1 (4%)	—	—	11.5	11[a]	13 (3)
Askling et al,[31] 2005	Sweden	1999–2001	15 (11 infliximab, 4 etanercept)	2 (13%)	7.5	—	4.5	9	6 (2)
Brassard et al,[3] 2006	Canada	1998–2003	51 (19 infliximab, 32 etanercept)	—	4.3	—	19.8	—	—
Sichletidis et al,[45] 2006	Greece	2000–2004	11 (8 infliximab, 3 adalimumab)	0 (0%)	6.0	3.0	—	6	5 (0)
Raval et al,[118] 2007	USA	2001–2006	130	6 (5%)	10	—	—	48[a]	59 (31)
Tubach et al,[46] 2009	France	2004–2007	69 (36 infliximab, 28 adalimumab, 5 etanercept)	1 (1%)	12.0[b]			27	42 (28)
Dixon et al,[36] 2010	UK	2001–2008	40 (12 infliximab, 20 adalimumab, 8 etanercept)	7 (18%)	5.5	18.5	13.4	15	25 (11)
Abreu et al,[49] 2013	Portugal	2001–2012	25 (16 infliximab, 6 adalimumab, 3 etanercept)	0 (0%)	6.0	7.0	89.0	10	15 (9)
Guinard et al,[57] 2016	France	2006–2014	12 (7 infliximab, 4 adalimumab, 1 certolizumab)	2 (17%)	3.8	73.0	—	2	10 (7)
Carpio et al,[59] 2016	Spain	2003–2016	50 (41 infliximab, 9 adalimumab)	1 (2%)	5.2[b]			20	30 (17)
Yonekura et al,[38] 2017	Brazil	2009–2013	5 (1 infliximab, 3 adalimumab, 1 etanercept)	0 (0%)	40	25	31	2	3 (2)

[a] Indicates studies where some patients had an unreported site of primary disease.
[b] Indicates studies reporting only a pooled risk among several TNF inhibitors.

Table 3
Biologic drugs with plausible risk based on mechanism of action, and for which increased vigilance for tuberculosis is recommended by the authors

Biologic Drug	Target Molecule or Pathway
Tofacitinib	JAK1/2/3
Ruxolitinib, oclacitinib, baricitinib, momelitinib	JAK1/2
Decernotinib, peficitinib	JAK3
Filgotinib	JAK1
Fedratinib, lestaurtinib, gandotinib, pacritinib	JAK2
Muromonab-CD3, otelixizumab, teplizumab, visilizumab.	CD3
Anakinra, cabakinumab, gevokizumab, rilonacept	IL-1a and/or IL-1b
Secukinumab, ixekizumab, brodalumab	IL-17A or IL-17RA
Ustekinumab	IL-12/IL-23
Tocilizumab, siltuxumab	IL-6
Nivolumab, pembrolizumab	PD-1
Atezolizumab, durvalumab, avelumab (IRIS-like hypersensitivity)	PD-L1

See accompanying text for references.

understand about the immune response to TB, increased vigilance is reasonable in areas with an intermediate or high prevalence.

Anti-Programmed Cell Death 1

The programmed cell death 1 (PD-1) receptor on T cells plays a vital role in peripheral tolerance, but in the setting of chronic antigen exposure (eg, malignancy or chronic infections) can induce an exhausted or anergic state in T cells.[60] Checkpoint inhibition with mAbs targeting the PD-1 receptor on T cells (pembrolizumab and nivolumab) or its ligand (atezolizumab, durvalumab, or avelumab) allows tumor-specific T cells to return to function, and has been a groundbreaking therapeutic strategy in oncology, which is now standard of care for several malignancies such as melanoma[61] or non-small-cell lung cancer.[62]

CD4 T cells in TB infection display higher levels of PD-1, with the highest levels in smear-positive TB compared with smear-negative TB and LTBI.[63] Functionally, these T cells show blunted proliferation and reduced production of IFN-γ in response to TB antigens, which can be restored with in vitro PD-1 blockade.[64,65] It is intuitive then

that PD-1 blockade should restore T cell function and assist in TB clearance but, surprisingly, PD-1 knockout mice are dramatically susceptible to new TB infection with increased mycobacterial loads, higher levels of interleukin-6 (IL-6) and IL-17, and uniformly fatal necrotizing tuberculous pneumonia compared with wild-type mice.[66,67]

Four cases of TB occurring within a few months of anti-PD-1 therapy in the absence of additional immune suppression were reported recently in Japan[68,69] and China,[70,71] followed by 2 more from a multicenter post-marketing registry in France.[72] In 5 of the 6 cases, onset was within 4 months of initiation of anti-PD-1 therapy, suggesting reactivation of LTBI. It is likely that restoration of effective CD4 T cell function causes a hypersensitivity reaction analogous to the immune-reconstitution inflammatory syndrome (IRIS) seen in patients with HIV, and, indeed, 1 patient in the above cases responded dramatically to steroids.[69] The extraordinary expansion of indications for this class of therapy should make practitioners aware of this potential complication, especially as there may be competing diagnoses for pulmonary or extrapulmonary TB (including progression of lung or extra-thoracic cancer, checkpoint-induced pneumonitis, or other immune-related adverse events).

Janus Kinase Inhibitors

Janus kinases (JAKs) are involved in the intracellular signaling for many cytokines that mediate TNF-α effects (including IFN-γ and IL-12), although not TNF-α per se.[73] The JAK inhibitors in clinical use for various autoimmune conditions include ruxolitinib and baricitinib (JAK1/JAK2 inhibition), tofacitinib and upadacitinib (JAK1/JAK3 inhibition), and filgotinib (selective JAK1 inhibition). Although several case reports of TB reactivation with ruxolitinib are reported,[74,75] the overall risk seems low for the most commonly used JAK inhibitor, tofacitinib.[76] There does not appear to be increased risk in areas of higher TB prevalence for tofacitinib.[39,77,78] Analysis of clinical trials for baricitinib in patients with RA demonstrated TB cases in endemic areas only, and the incidence overall was comparable to the local background rates.[79]

Other T Cell-Directed Biologics

Anti-CD3 drugs (muromonab-CD3, otelixizumab, teplizumab, and visilizumab) can render T cells anergic or induce apoptosis, and are risk factors for TB in solid organ transplant recipients.[80] Anti-CD52 (alemtuzumab) induces severe depletion of peripheral blood lymphocytes (both T and B cells, but a marked reduction in CD4+ T cells), and is used in solid organ transplants, hematopoietic stem cell transplant conditioning, multiple sclerosis, and a variety of hematologic malignancies. Due to its effects on CD4+ T cells, patients are at risk for the same opportunistic infections as in advanced HIV, including TB.[81] In a highly endemic area, TB developed in 7 of 27 patients treated with alemtuzumab, 5 of whom were on alemtuzumab alone (a 1- and 2-year incidence of 31% and 45%, respectively).[82]

Other Cytokine Inhibitors

Tocilizumab is an mAb directed against the soluble receptor for IL-6, and is approved for use in inflammatory arthritis including RA. An incidence of 93 cases per 100,000 patient years was reported in a pooled analysis of tocilizumab in RA clinical trials, although all TB cases were from intermediate-to high-prevalence countries.[83] A Japanese post-marketing registry, in which all patients were screened with chest radiograph and tuberculin skin test (TST) before tocilizumab treatment, suggested that the risk of TB is similar to that observed with anti-TNF-α agents at 130 cases per 100,000 patient-years.[84] This risk can be abrogated with treatment of LTBI before therapy.[85]

Ustekinumab is an mAb directed against IL-12/IL-23 and is approved for psoriasis and Crohn disease. IL-12 is involved in Th1 differentiation and is necessary for effective TB response in a murine model.[86,87] A global registry of psoriasis patients did not find an increased risk for TB,[88] although it should be noted that ustekinumanb trials excluded patients with latent TB, or mandated LTBI testing and treatment before enrollment.[89,90] Biologics directed against the IL-1 pathway (anakinra, canakinumab, gevokizumab, and rilonacept) are used in several inflammatory conditions; IL-1 has been shown to be necessary for control of TB infection in mice.[91,92] Although case reports of TB reactivation exist, pooled data from clinical trials and national biologic registries do not appear to show increased risk.[93,94]

Antibodies directed against IL-17A (secukinumab and ixekizumab) or its receptor (brodalumab) are in use in adults with psoriasis or ankylosing spondylitis. IL-17A knockout mice have higher mycobacterial number and reduced pulmonary granuloma formation after TB infection in comparison with wild-type mice,[95] which may be due to hypoxia-inducible factor 1α-mediated hypoxic changes within granulomata.[96] Genetic polymorphisms in the IL-17 gene have also been associated with increased susceptibility to TB in the Chinese Han population.[97] However, pooled data from phase II and III secukinumab trials did not show any TB cases at 1 year of follow-up,[98] including 107 subjects with LTBI who underwent LTBI treatment concurrent with secukinumab.[99]

BIOLOGIC DRUGS WITH LOW RISK

Rituximab, a mAb directed against CD20, does not appear to have effects on the performance of IFN-γ release assay (IGRA) tests,[100] and does not increase the risk of TB in patients with RA.[81,101,102] These data are likely generalizable to ocrelizumab, a related anti-CD20 mAb. There are no reports of increased TB risk associated with several biologics targeting other lymphoid or myeloid surface antigens, including CD19 (blinatumomab inebilizumab), CD22 (inotuzumab ozogamicin), CD30 (brentuximab vedotin), CD33 (gemtuzumab ozogamicin), CD38 (daratumumab), CD40 (lucatumumab, dacetuzumab), CD319 (elotuzumab), or CCR4 (mogamulizumab).[81,103] A case report of a patient with T cell lymphoma treated with chemotherapy and mogamulizumab who developed disseminated *Mycobacterium chelonae* infection has been described.[104]

Antibodies directed against integrins (natalizumab, vedolizumab, and etrolizumab) disrupt leukocyte adhesion and are in clinical use in patients with multiple sclerosis or Crohn disease. Case reports of active TB among patients on natalizumab exist,[105] but the risk in trial and post-marketing settings seems to be low.[106,107] Eculizumab is a mAb directed against complement component 5, and does not appear to increase the risk of TB.[108] A patient with neuromyelitis optica started eculizumab after completing treatment for pulmonary TB and was maintained on isoniazid without incident.[109]

Several biologics are in use for the treatment of severe, uncontrolled asthma, including anti-IgE (omalizumab), or drugs directed against Th2 cytokines: anti-IL4Ra (dupilumab), anti-IL5 (mepolizumab and reslizumab), anti-IL5R (benralizumab), and anti-IL13 (tralokinumab and lebrikizumab). It is unlikely that these drugs would increase susceptibility to TB given that an increased Th2 response can be detrimental to *in vitro* TB control.[110,111] Consistent with this, there does not appear to be an increased risk of reactivation or de novo TB infection despite the lack of a requirement for LTBI screening in trials or before clinical use.

EVALUATION FOR LATENT TUBERCULOSIS BEFORE INITIATION OF BIOLOGIC THERAPY
Unique Challenges in Patients Who Are Candidates for Biologic Therapy

Testing for LTBI is reviewed separately in this issue of *Clinics*. However, some aspects of LTBI testing have distinctive pitfalls among patients with auto-immune disease, which are reviewed in further detail in Keystone and colleagues.[112] Patients with RA may have impaired cell-mediated immunity and false-negative tuberculin skin testing, regardless of the presence of immunosuppressive medications.[113,114] Furthermore, corticosteroids or methotrexate may decrease TST sensitivity.[115] Notably, patients with psoriasis may develop new psoriatic lesions at the site of minor skin trauma (the Koebner phenomenon), which may be confused with a positive TST.[116]

Tuberculin Skin Testing or Interferon- γ Release Assay Before Biologic Therapy

The performance of TST and the latest-generation IGRAs, predominantly QuantiFERON-Gold In-Tube (QFT; Cellestis, Carnegie, Australia), for LTBI diagnosis was evaluated with data from 157 published articles using a Bayesian latent class analysis, an approach that avoids confounding by varying disease prevalence in a simple pooled meta-analysis.[117] Among immunocompromised adults (HIV/AIDS, solid organ transplantation, stem cell transplantation, immune-mediated inflammatory diseases, end-stage kidney disease, or malignancy), a 5-mm TST cutoff had a sensitivity of 0.71 (95% CI 0.66–0.75) and specificity in non-BCG- and BCG-vaccinated patients of 0.99 (95% CI 0.97–1.00) and 0.93 (95% CI 0.91–0.96), respectively. For QFT, the sensitivity was 0.46 (95% CI 0.43–0.49) and the specificity in non-BCG- and BCG-vaccinated patients was 0.97 (95% CI 0.96–0.98) and 0.92 (95% CI 0.92–0.95), respectively.[117]

Among patients who are screened for LTBI before initiation of TNF-α blockade, early reports raised concern that TST alone was likely inadequate. After the 2001 boxed warning recommending screening for LTBI before infliximab treatment, 34 out of 47 cases (72%) of TB cases reported to the FDA that had available TST results were TST negative (although insufficient data were provided on the actual induration size).[118] Subsequently, combination testing was described by Kleinert and colleagues[119] who evaluated 1529 German patients with both TST and either T-SPOT.TB (TSPOT; Oxford Immunotec, Abingdon, UK) or QFT. There were 161 (10.5%) discordant patients (54 TST–/IGRA+ and 107 TST+/IGRA–), and, from the latter group, 36% were BCG vaccinated. Interestingly, of 71 patients, they reported 27 with TST results of ≥15 mm (38%), none of whom were BCG vaccinated and who had negative IGRA results; no data on prophylaxis or subsequent TB were reported in this group. Whether IGRA testing

or TST have different predictive ability in discriminating who will progress to active TB is controversial, with some studies suggesting the superiority of IGRA testing[115] and more recent data suggesting the superiority of a 15-mm TST compared with QFT.[120]

In a French cohort of 392 patients with a higher background rate of BCG vaccination, a dual IGRA screening strategy was evaluated in patients who were tested with TST followed by both QFT and TSPOT, but only the IGRA result was used to offer prophylaxis.[121] Ninety-one patients had discordance between TST and IGRA at a cutoff of 10 mm, and 122 at a cutoff of 5 mm. Since only the IGRA was used to guide prophylaxis, 50 patients at a 10-mm cutoff or 97 at a 5-mm cutoff who were dual IGRA-negative underwent TNF-α blockade without TB prophylaxis and none developed TB at 1-year follow-up. Contrary to previous studies that demonstrated excellent concordance between QFT and TSPOT,[122] they also had a significant proportion (16.6%) with discordant positive/negative dual-IGRA testing. In an international cohort of golimumab clinical trial patients, high levels of TST/IGRA discordance (kappa 0.22) were demonstrated in those over the age of 65 years, and had previous BCG vaccination, and were resident in Europe or Asia compared with North America as multivariate predictors of discordance.[123] The underlying disease indication (ankylosing spondylitis or psoriatic arthritis compared with RA) was not significant, nor was the use of methotrexate or corticosteroids. In short, discrepancies among IGRA assays and between IGRA and TST may make reliance on any single test unadvisable given the magnitude of the TB risk in this population.

There is evidence that combination testing may decrease the rate of active TB in patients on TNF-α inhibitors. In phase III trials of golimumab for inflammatory arthritis (conducted globally, with 40% of patients from outside North America or Western Europe),[123] patients were screened with TST and IGRA before enrollment and given INH prophylaxis if either test was positive. A meta-analysis of over 2000 such patients showed high levels of TST/IGRA discordance, but no cases of active TB at 1 year among the 317 patients receiving LTBI treatment.[124] A similar "either test positive" prophylaxis strategy in South Korea with a median follow-up of over 2 years demonstrated 4 (0.9%) cases of active TB among 430 treated with TNF-α blockade.[125] Two of the cases occurred within 4 months of treatment initiation, and the other 2 cases likely represented new infection because they occurred after 30 and 42 months of anti-TNF-α therapy. Therefore, using either a positive TST or IGRA as sufficient to treat LTBI before TNF-α blockade may help to reduce TB recurrence in patients on TNF-α therapies, although this has not been proved.

Despite the widespread understanding that such testing before TNF-α blockade is indicated, there remains an unacceptably high rate of noncompliance with screening guidelines. When assessed with anonymous surveys, self-reports of compliance with TB screening guidelines before the initiation of anti-TNF-α therapy among subspecialist prescribing physicians is between 73% and 100%.[126,127] However, retrospective analysis of all patients prescribed anti-TNF-α therapy has demonstrated screening rates between 65%[128] and 72%,[43] although these totals include inadequate and non-guideline-compliant screening (eg, screened with chest radiogaphy alone, or TST alone among patients on prednisone). Unfortunately, even a contemporary report from Japan that reviewed screening of 385 patients in the 2 months before anti-TNF-α prescriptions in a national database found that 10% underwent TST, 44% IGRA, 12% both TST and IGRA, and 34% had no LTBI testing.[129] Although this type of study may underestimate compliance because it will not capture patients who were not re-screened before switching between 2 TNF-α antagonists or patients who were screened but ultimately not prescribed a TNF-α antagonist, it is clear than screening is not universal. These lapses lead directly to cases of TB disease, as shown in a Spanish cohort of anti-TNF-α-treated IBD patients in whom 40% of TB cases did not have adequate baseline screening or were not prescribed prophylaxis when it was indicated.[59]

Surveillance Testing for Latent Tuberculosis Infection While on Biologic Therapy

At present, the Centers for Disease Control and Prevention do not recommend rescreening of individuals during biologic therapy unless they have had a possible TB exposure or ongoing risk factors for TB exposure (ie, visitation to areas with a high prevalence of active TB, residence in correctional facilities, long-term care facilities, or homeless shelters, certain healthcare workers, etc.).[130] Furthermore, treatment with a TNF-α antagonist was shown to decrease the sensitivity of IGRA testing in 1 study, although the IGRA performed better than the TST in patients at risk for infection.[131] Annual rescreening with TST and QFT may identify 12.5% of baseline negative anti-TNF-α patients who convert at least 1 test,[132] a rate that can increase to 29% when screened with TST, QFT, and TSPOT.[133] However, the

significance of test conversion on TNF-α inhibition remains unclear. In a Greek cohort of patients on TNF-α antagonists who were rescreened with TST, QFT, and TSPOT, 60% of patients who converted at least 1 test did not receive INH and none developed active TB.[133] Despite this, because of the severity of TB and the significant frequency of test conversion in patients on biologic drugs, the authors believe the American College of Rheumatology recommendation for annual TB screening (level of evidence C) while on TNF-α inhibitors is reasonable.[134]

Importantly, active TB in patients receiving anti-TNF-α therapy has occurred while receiving treatment for LTBI. This has been described in 2 patients in a clinical trial with certolizumab, as well as in 5 patients in a Colombian cohort (three of whom were on etanercept), although drug resistance information was not available.[53,135] Sichletidis and colleagues[45] described 3 patients treated with anti-TNF-α biologics who developed active TB while properly taking chemoprophylaxis, to which their TB isolate was later found to be susceptible. In the Veterans Affairs data set in the United States, a setting with low TB incidence, reactivation of TB was described in patients who completed treatment for LTBI before starting TNF-α blockade.[43] Advising strict adherence to chemoprophylaxis remains paramount in this population, and periodic symptom assessment should continue during LTBI treatment while on TNF-α antagonists.

Paradoxic Reaction to Biologic Discontinuation

If TB develops while on TNF-α blockade, clinicians should be aware of a paradoxic worsening of TB symptoms in response to TNF-α antagonist discontinuation, which may respond to steroids or resumption of anti-TNF-α therapy. In 2005, there were initial case reports of patients who, on discontinuation of anti-TNF-α therapy in the setting of TB, developed a paradoxic worsening similar to the IRIS seen after initiation of antiretroviral therapy in patient with HIV.[136,137] In such cases, patients experience initial improvement followed by exaggerated inflammatory symptoms such as fever, striking lymphadenopathy, pulmonary infiltrates, or weight loss.[136–141] Typically, the anti-TNF-α IRIS occurs 4 to 20 weeks after discontinuation of the anti-TNF-α drug and while the patient is receiving antituberculous drug therapy, a timing potentially related to the half-life of the TNF-α antagonist. Management has included corticosteroids and, in refractory cases, resumption of the anti-TNF-α biologic.[142–144]

PRACTICAL MANAGEMENT RECOMMENDATIONS
General Principles

Clinical practice guidelines for the screening and treatment of LTBI in medically immunosuppressed patients have been put forth from numerous professional societies and national or international bodies.[145,146] Although there is consensus that patients considered for immunosuppressive therapy, and particularly TNF-α blockade, should be screened for LTBI, there remain areas of difference in the method of screening, interpretation of the TST, and what interventions and at what intervals they should be performed. **Box 1** presents the recommendations of the Centers for Disease Control and Prevention and the British Thoracic Society, both of which developed specific recommendations for individuals receiving TNF-α inhibitors who have either active or latent TB.[147,148] **Box 2** presents the recommendations of the authors, with

acknowledgment that regional practice or recommendations of others may differ.

All patients who are candidates for biologic therapy with anti-TNF-α agents should undergo LTBI screening, and ideally should be screened at the time of diagnosis of an immune or inflammatory condition before starting on any immunosuppressive medications. This avoids confounding of screening tests by concomitant steroids and acknowledges the TB risk intrinsic to some immune-mediated diseases and the risk associated with nonbiologic DMARDs. Screening should consist of a careful history as well as TST, IGRA, and chest radiography. We recommend sequential testing: first a TST and, if negative, an IGRA to take advantage of a possible booster reaction.[149] Either a TST ≥5 mm or a positive IGRA should be considered a positive screen; an indeterminate IGRA should be repeated. Patients should have TST and IGRA testing repeated annually. Increased vigilance should be exercised for patients treated with the drugs shown in **Table 3**.

Box 1
Management of latent tuberculosis infection and active tuberculosis in patients on anti-TNF-α biologics

CDC Recommendations	British Thoracic Society Recommendations
Latent Tuberculosis	Latent Tuberculosis
• Test to exclude TB disease before treatment of LTBI	• Test to exclude TB disease before treatment of LTBI
• Start treatment for LTBI before commencing TNF-α antagonists; the optimal amount of delay is undetermined	• For LTBI with normal CXR, TNF-α antagonist can be given concurrently with LTBI treatment
• Ideally complete LTBI treatment before anti-TNF-α initiation	• For LTBI with abnormal CXR or prior TB not adequately treated, ideally complete LTBI treatment before anti-TNF-α initiation
• Use standard LTBI treatment regimens:	• Use standard LTBI treatment regimens:
Active Tuberculosis	Active Tuberculosis
• Begin treatment of TB disease immediately	• Begin treatment of TB disease immediately
• Use standard active TB treatment regimens	• Use standard active TB treatment regimens
• If active TB disease develops *during TNF-α antagonist therapy*, the TNF-α antagonist should be discontinued at least until the anti-TB regimen has been started and the patient's condition has improved	• For active TB discovered *before initiation* of anti-TNF-α drugs, delay anti-TNF-α treatment for at least 2 mo after starting anti-TB treatment
○ The optimal time for resuming TNF-α antagonist therapy in this setting is undetermined	• If active TB disease *develops during TNF-α antagonist therapy*, the TNF-α antagonist can be continued if clinically indicated
○ Consider postponing TNF-α antagonists until TB treatment completed	

From Centers for Disease Control and Prevention (CDC). Tuberculosis associated with blocking agents against tumor necrosis factor-alpha–California, 2002-2003. MMWR Morb Mortal Wkly Rep. 2004;53(30):683-686 and British Thoracic Society Standards of Care Committee. BTS recommendations for assessing risk and for managing Mycobacterium tuberculosis infection and disease in patients due to start anti-TNF-alpha treatment. Thorax. 2005;60(10):800-805.

Box 2
Practical recommendations for tuberculosis screening and management in patients on anti-TNF-α biologics

Screening and LTBI Treatment

- Screen all patients with interview, CXR, TST and IGRA
- Treat LTBI in a patient with a TST ≥5 mm or positive IGRA with standard LTBI treatment regimens. Repeat indeterminate IGRA tests
- Those with negative testing should be treated if there is a high probability of LTBI (see text)
- Active TB should be excluded in patients with abnormal imaging or history of TB not adequately treated
- Be vigilant for pulmonary, extrapulmonary, and disseminated TB presentations
- Complete LTBI treatment before biologic initiation; if pressing clinical need treat LTBI for at least 1 month before starting biologic
- Patients with old TB or LTBI should be screened monthly for the first 3 months of biologic therapy by symptom assessment ± CXR
- Repeat TST and IGRA testing annually

Management

- If there is a choice among TNF-α antagonists, we favor etanercept in patients with LTBI or old TB
- For active TB on anti-TNF-α biologics, stop the biologic drug until the patient is stable and tolerating the TB treatment
- Resume the biologic after 1 to 2 months of TB treatment, and especially if the patient experiences an IRIS-like reaction

For a positive screen, active TB should be excluded in patients with symptoms, an abnormal chest radiograph, or a past history of TB not adequately treated. In addition, those with a TST less than 5 mm and a negative IGRA should still be treated where circumstances suggest a high probability of LTBI (such as fibrotic lesions on chest imaging, recent exposure, residence in a highly endemic region, or intravenous drug abuse). Ideally, treatment of LTBI should be completed before initiation of anti-TNF-α therapy; newer shorter course regimens such as rifampin for 4 months or isoniazid and rifapentine weekly for 12 weeks can be selected. In some circumstances where there is a pressing clinical need to begin biologic therapy, TNF-α inhibitors can be commenced after the first month of LTBI treatment.

For selection amongst anti-TNF-α agents if there is a choice, we favor etanercept over infliximab, adalimumab, golimumab, or certolizumab in patients with LTBI or a history of treated TB, since the rate of TB is lower. All patients on TNF-α antagonists with a history of treated LTBI or TB should be monitored monthly for reactivation with symptom assessment and chest x-ray for the first 3 months of therapy and with sputum samples if indicated, as treatment of LTBI may not be universally effective in this group. Clinical assessment should include careful screening for extrapulmonary disease, and clinicians should be aware that extrapulmonary TB may mimic a flare-up of the underlying immune or inflammatory condition (eg, intestinal TB in a patient with Crohn disease or tuberculous arthritis in a patient with RA).

If TB develops in a patient on TNF-α blockade, the drug should be held while treating for TB. Following initiation of at least 1 month of antituberculous therapy, the TNF-α antagonist likely can be resumed safely.[148,150] In a cohort of patients with ankylosing spondylitis in South Korea, there was no difference in TB relapse or treatment efficacy between those that resumed anti-TNF-α therapy during TB treatment (at a median of 3.3 months) versus those who waited to complete TB therapy before resuming.[151] If IRIS develops, use corticosteroids and consider resuming the TNF-α antagonist.

SUMMARY

Biologic therapies represent a tremendous advance in our ability to alter the course of inflammatory and neoplastic disease. Despite this, they present unique risks for reactivation of LTBI as well as de novo infection. The longest clinical experience and characterization of risk around the world is for the TNF-α inhibitors, but novel agents whose mechanisms of action present a theoretic risk are increasingly available or have ongoing clinical trials. Awareness of the risks of these agents, particularly in areas of high TB prevalence, is paramount to ensuring their safe use.

REFFRENCES

1. Caporali R, Crepaldi G, Codullo V, et al. 20 years of experience with tumour necrosis factor inhibitors: what have we learned? Rheumatology (Oxford) 2018;57(57 Suppl 7):vii5–10.
2. Keane J, Gershon S, Wise RP, et al. Tuberculosis associated with infliximab, a tumor necrosis factor alpha-neutralizing agent. N Engl J Med 2001; 345(15):1098–104.

3. Brassard P, Kezouh A, Suissa S. Antirheumatic drugs and the risk of tuberculosis. Clin Infect Dis 2006;43(6):717–22.

4. Mitoma H, Horiuchi T, Tsukamoto H, et al. Molecular mechanisms of action of anti-TNF-α agents - comparison among therapeutic TNF-α antagonists. Cytokine 2018;101:56–63.

5. Horiuchi T, Mitoma H, Harashima S, et al. Transmembrane TNF-alpha: structure, function and interaction with anti-TNF agents. Rheumatology (Oxford) 2010;49(7):1215–28.

6. Wallis RS. Tumour necrosis factor antagonists: structure, function, and tuberculosis risks. Lancet Infect Dis 2008;8(10):601–11.

7. O'Garra A, Redford PS, McNab FW, et al. The immune response in tuberculosis. Annu Rev Immunol 2013;31(1):475–527.

8. Xie X, Li F, Chen J-W, et al. Risk of tuberculosis infection in anti-TNF-α biological therapy: from bench to bedside. J Microbiol Immunol Infect 2014;47(4):268–74.

9. Gardam MA, Keystone EC, Menzies R, et al. Anti-tumour necrosis factor agents and tuberculosis risk: mechanisms of action and clinical management. Lancet Infect Dis 2003;3(3):148–55.

10. Flynn JL, Goldstein MM, Chan J, et al. Tumor necrosis factor-alpha is required in the protective immune response against Mycobacterium tuberculosis in mice. Immunity 1995;2(6):561–72.

11. Saunders BM, Tran S, Ruuls S, et al. Transmembrane TNF is sufficient to initiate cell migration and granuloma formation and provide acute, but not long-term, control of Mycobacterium tuberculosis infection. J Immunol 2005;174(8):4852–9.

12. Clay H, Volkman HE, Ramakrishnan L. Tumor necrosis factor signaling mediates resistance to mycobacteria by inhibiting bacterial growth and macrophage death. Immunity 2008;29(2):283–94.

13. Lin PL, Myers A, Smith L, et al. Tumor necrosis factor neutralization results in disseminated disease in acute and latent Mycobacterium tuberculosis infection with normal granuloma structure in a cynomolgus macaque model. Arthritis Rheum 2010; 62(2):340–50.

14. Thalayasingam N, Isaacs JD. Anti-TNF therapy. Best Pract Res Clin Rheumatol 2011;25(4):549–67.

15. Remicade (infliximab) [package insert]. Horsham, PA: Janssen Biotech; 2018.

16. Pasut G. Pegylation of biological molecules and potential benefits: pharmacological properties of certolizumab pegol. BioDrugs 2014;28(Suppl 1): S15–23.

17. Ehlers S, Hölscher C, Scheu S, et al. The lymphotoxin beta receptor is critically involved in controlling infections with the intracellular pathogens Mycobacterium tuberculosis and Listeria monocytogenes. J Immunol 2003;170(10):5210–8.

18. Saliu OY, Sofer C, Stein DS, et al. Tumor-necrosis-factor blockers: differential effects on mycobacterial immunity. J Infect Dis 2006;194(4):486–92.

19. Tran BN, Chan SL, Ng C, et al. Higher order structures of adalimumab, infliximab and their complexes with TNFα revealed by electron microscopy. Protein Sci 2017;26(12):2392–8.

20. Scallon B, Cai A, Solowski N, et al. Binding and functional comparisons of two types of tumor necrosis factor antagonists. J Pharmacol Exp Ther 2002;301(2):418–26.

21. Ai J-W, Zhang S, Ruan Q-L, et al. The risk of tuberculosis in patients with rheumatoid arthritis treated with tumor necrosis factor-α antagonist: a metaanalysis of both randomized controlled trials and registry/cohort studies. J Rheumatol 2015;42(12): 2229–37.

22. Minozzi S, Bonovas S, Lytras T, et al. Risk of infections using anti-TNF agents in rheumatoid arthritis, psoriatic arthritis, and ankylosing spondylitis: a systematic review and meta-analysis. Expert Opin Drug Saf 2016;15(sup1):11–34.

23. Zhang Z, Fan W, Yang G, et al. Risk of tuberculosis in patients treated with TNF-α antagonists: a systematic review and meta-analysis of randomised controlled trials. BMJ Open 2017;7(3):e012567.

24. Higgins J, Green S, editors. The Cochrane handbook for systematic reviews of interventions. Version 5.1.0. The Cochrane Collaboration; 2011. Available at: www.cochrane-handbook.org.

25. Haviland MG. Yates's correction for continuity and the analysis of 2 x 2 contingency tables. Stat Med 1990;9(4):363–7 [discussion: 369–83].

26. Doran MF, Crowson CS, Pond GR, et al. Frequency of infection in patients with rheumatoid arthritis compared with controls: a population-based study. Arthritis Rheum 2002;46(9):2287–93.

27. Arkema EV, Jonsson J, Baecklund E, et al. Are patients with rheumatoid arthritis still at an increased risk of tuberculosis and what is the role of biological treatments? Ann Rheum Dis 2015;74(6):1212–7.

28. Carmona L, Hernández-García C, Vadillo C, et al. Increased risk of tuberculosis in patients with rheumatoid arthritis. J Rheumatol 2003;30(7):1436–9.

29. Wagner UG, Koetz K, Weyand CM, et al. Perturbation of the T cell repertoire in rheumatoid arthritis. Proc Natl Acad Sci U S A 1998;95(24):14447–52.

30. Mori S, Tokuda H, Sakai F, et al. Radiological features and therapeutic responses of pulmonary nontuberculous mycobacterial disease in rheumatoid arthritis patients receiving biological agents: a retrospective multicenter study in Japan. Mod Rheumatol 2012;22(5):727–37.

31. Askling J, Fored CM, Brandt L, et al. Risk and case characteristics of tuberculosis in rheumatoid arthritis associated with tumor necrosis factor

antagonists in Sweden. Arthritis Rheum 2005;52(7):
1986–92.

32. Favalli EG, Desiati F, Atzeni F, et al. Serious infections during anti-TNF-alpha treatment in rheumatoid arthritis patients. Autoimmun Rev 2009;8(3):266–73.

33. Gómez-Reino JJ, Carmona L, Valverde VR, et al, BIOBADASER Group. Treatment of rheumatoid arthritis with tumor necrosis factor inhibitors may predispose to significant increase in tuberculosis risk: a multicenter active-surveillance report. Arthritis Rheum 2003;48(8):2122–7.

34. Carmona L, Gómez-Reino JJ, Rodríguez-Valverde V, et al. Effectiveness of recommendations to prevent reactivation of latent tuberculosis infection in patients treated with tumor necrosis factor antagonists. Arthritis Rheum 2005;52(6):1766–72.

35. Listing J, Strangfeld A, Kary S, et al. Infections in patients with rheumatoid arthritis treated with biologic agents. Arthritis Rheum 2005;52(11):3403–12.

36. Dixon WG, Hyrich KL, Watson KD, et al. Drug-specific risk of tuberculosis in patients with rheumatoid arthritis treated with anti-TNF therapy: results from the British Society for Rheumatology Biologics Register (BSRBR). Ann Rheum Dis 2010;69(3):522–8.

37. Atzeni F, Sarzi-Puttini P, Botsios C, et al. Long-term anti-TNF therapy and the risk of serious infections in a cohort of patients with rheumatoid arthritis: comparison of adalimumab, etanercept and infliximab in the GISEA registry. Autoimmun Rev 2012;12(2):225–9.

38. Yonekura CL, Oliveira RDR, Titton DC, et al. Incidence of tuberculosis among patients with rheumatoid arthritis using TNF blockers in Brazil: data from the Brazilian registry of biological therapies in rheumatic diseases (Registro Brasileiro de Monitoração de Terapias Biológicas - BiobadaBrasil). Rev Bras Reumatol Engl Ed 2017;57(Suppl 2):477–83.

39. Lim CH, Chen H-H, Chen Y-H, et al. The risk of tuberculosis disease in rheumatoid arthritis patients on biologics and targeted therapy: a 15-year real world experience in Taiwan. PLoS One 2017;12(6):e0178035.

40. Rutherford AI, Patarata E, Subesinghe S, et al. Opportunistic infections in rheumatoid arthritis patients exposed to biologic therapy: results from the British Society for Rheumatology Biologics Register for Rheumatoid Arthritis. Rheumatology (Oxford) 2018;57(6):997–1001.

41. Kim E-M, Uhm W-S, Bae S-C, et al. Incidence of tuberculosis among Korean patients with ankylosing spondylitis who are taking tumor necrosis factor blockers. J Rheumatol 2011;38(10):2218–23.

42. Ergun T, Seckin D, Baskan Bulbul E, et al. The risk of tuberculosis in patients with psoriasis treated with anti-tumor necrosis factor agents. Int J Dermatol 2015;54(5):594–9.

43. Hou JK, Kramer JR, Richardson P, et al. Tuberculosis screening and reactivation among a national cohort of patients with inflammatory bowel disease treated with tumor necrosis factor Alpha antagonists. Inflamm Bowel Dis 2017;23(2):254–60.

44. Wallis RS, Broder M, Wong J, et al. Granulomatous infections due to tumor necrosis factor blockade: correction. Clin Infect Dis 2004;39(8):1254–5.

45. Sichletidis L, Settas L, Spyratos D, et al. Tuberculosis in patients receiving anti-TNF agents despite chemoprophylaxis. Int J Tuberc Lung Dis 2006;10(10):1127–32.

46. Tubach F, Salmon D, Ravaud P, et al. Risk of tuberculosis is higher with anti-tumor necrosis factor monoclonal antibody therapy than with soluble tumor necrosis factor receptor therapy: the three-year prospective French Research Axed on Tolerance of Biotherapies registry. Arthritis Rheum 2009;60(7):1884–94.

47. Winthrop KL, Baxter R, Liu L, et al. Mycobacterial diseases and antitumour necrosis factor therapy in USA. Ann Rheum Dis 2013;72(1):37–42.

48. Lee J, Kim E, Jang EJ, et al. Efficacy of treatment for latent tuberculosis in patients undergoing treatment with a tumor necrosis factor Antagonist. Ann Am Thorac Soc 2017;14(5):690–7.

49. Abreu C, Magro F, Santos-Antunes J, et al. Tuberculosis in anti-TNF-α treated patients remains a problem in countries with an intermediate incidence: analysis of 25 patients matched with a control population. J Crohns Colitis 2013;7(10):e486–92.

50. Baddley JW, Winthrop KL, Chen L, et al. Non-viral opportunistic infections in new users of tumour necrosis factor inhibitor therapy: results of the SAfety Assessment of Biologic ThERapy (SABER) study. Ann Rheum Dis 2014;73(11):1942–8.

51. Mok CC, Chan KY, Lee KL, et al, Hong Kong Society of Rheumatology. Factors associated with withdrawal of the anti-TNFα biologics in the treatment of rheumatic diseases: data from the Hong Kong Biologics Registry. Int J Rheum Dis 2014;17(Suppl 3):1–8.

52. Kay J, Fleischmann R, Keystone E, et al. Golimumab 3-year safety update: an analysis of pooled data from the long-term extensions of randomised, double-blind, placebo-controlled trials conducted in patients with rheumatoid arthritis, psoriatic arthritis or ankylosing spondylitis. Ann Rheum Dis 2015;74(3):538–46.

53. Bykerk VP, Cush J, Winthrop K, et al. Update on the safety profile of certolizumab pegol in rheumatoid arthritis: an integrated analysis from clinical trials. Ann Rheum Dis 2015;74(1):96–103.

54. Mariette X, Vencovsky J, Lortholary O, et al. The incidence of tuberculosis in patients treated with certolizumab pegol across indications: impact of baseline skin test results, more stringent screening criteria and geographic region. RMD Open 2015; 1(1):e000044.

55. Wallis RS. Mathematical modeling of the cause of tuberculosis during tumor necrosis factor blockade. Arthritis Rheum 2008;58(4):947–52.

56. Plessner HL, Lin PL, Kohno T, et al. Neutralization of tumor necrosis factor (TNF) by antibody but not TNF receptor fusion molecule exacerbates chronic murine tuberculosis. J Infect Dis 2007; 195(11):1643–50.

57. Guinard E, Bulai Livideanu C, Barthélémy H, et al. Active tuberculosis in psoriasis patients treated with TNF antagonists: a French nationwide retrospective study. J Eur Acad Dermatol Venereol 2016;30(8):1336–41.

58. World Health Organization. Global tuberculosis report 2018. Geneva (Switzerland): World Health Organization; 2018.

59. Carpio D, Jauregui-Amezaga A, de Francisco R, et al. Tuberculosis in anti-tumour necrosis factor-treated inflammatory bowel disease patients after the implementation of preventive measures: compliance with recommendations and safety of retreatment. J Crohns Colitis 2016;10(10): 1186–93.

60. Boussiotis VA. Molecular and biochemical aspects of the PD-1 checkpoint pathway. N Engl J Med 2016;375(18):1767–78.

61. Lugowska I, Teterycz P, Rutkowski P. Immunotherapy of melanoma. Contemp Oncol (Pozn) 2018;22(1A):61–7.

62. Herbst RS, Morgensztern D, Boshoff C. The biology and management of non-small cell lung cancer. Nature 2018;553(7689):446–54.

63. Day CL, Abrahams DA, Bunjun R, et al. PD-1 expression on mycobacterium tuberculosis-specific CD4 T cells is associated with bacterial load in human tuberculosis. Front Immunol 2018; 9:1995.

64. Jurado JO, Alvarez IB, Pasquinelli V, et al. Programmed death (PD)-1:PD-ligand 1/PD-ligand 2 pathway inhibits T cell effector functions during human tuberculosis. J Immunol 2008;181(1): 116–25.

65. Alvarez IB, Pasquinelli V, Jurado JO, et al. Role played by the programmed death-1-programmed death ligand pathway during innate immunity against Mycobacterium tuberculosis. J Infect Dis 2010;202(4):524–32.

66. Lázár-Molnár E, Chen B, Sweeney KA, et al. Programmed death-1 (PD-1)-deficient mice are extraordinarily sensitive to tuberculosis. Proc Natl Acad Sci U S A 2010;107(30):13402–7.

67. Khan N, Vidyarthi A, Amir M, et al. T-cell exhaustion in tuberculosis: pitfalls and prospects. Crit Rev Microbiol 2017;43(2):133–41.

68. Fujita K, Terashima T, Mio T. Anti-PD1 antibody treatment and the development of acute pulmonary tuberculosis. J Thorac Oncol 2016;11(12):2238–40.

69. Takata S, Koh G, Han Y, et al. Paradoxical response in a patient with non-small cell lung cancer who received nivolumab followed by anti-Mycobacterium tuberculosis agents. J Infect Chemother 2019;25(1):54–8.

70. Lee JJX, Chan A, Tang T. Tuberculosis reactivation in a patient receiving anti-programmed death-1 (PD-1) inhibitor for relapsed Hodgkin's lymphoma. Acta Oncol 2016;55(4):519–20.

71. Chu Y-C, Fang K-C, Chen H-C, et al. Pericardial Tamponade caused by a hypersensitivity response to tuberculosis reactivation after anti-PD-1 treatment in a patient with advanced pulmonary adenocarcinoma. J Thorac Oncol 2017;12(8):e111–4.

72. Picchi H, Mateus C, Chouaid C, et al. Infectious complications associated with the use of immune checkpoint inhibitors in oncology: reactivation of tuberculosis after anti PD-1 treatment. Clin Microbiol Infect 2018;24(3):216–8.

73. O'Shea JJ, Kontzias A, Yamaoka K, et al. Janus kinase inhibitors in autoimmune diseases. Ann Rheum Dis 2013;72(Suppl 2):ii111–5.

74. Lussana F, Cattaneo M, Rambaldi A, et al. Ruxolitinib-associated infections: a systematic review and meta-analysis. Am J Hematol 2018;93(3):339–47.

75. Dioverti MV, Abu Saleh OM, Tande AJ. Infectious complications in patients on treatment with Ruxolitinib: case report and review of the literature. Infect Dis (Lond) 2018;50(5):381–7.

76. Cohen SB, Tanaka Y, Mariette X, et al. Long-term safety of tofacitinib for the treatment of rheumatoid arthritis up to 8.5 years: integrated analysis of data from the global clinical trials. Ann Rheum Dis 2017; 76(7):1253–62.

77. Castañeda OM, Romero FJ, Salinas A, et al. Safety of tofacitinib in the treatment of rheumatoid arthritis in Latin America compared with the rest of the world population. J Clin Rheumatol 2017;23(4): 193–9.

78. Lomonte ABV, Radominski SC, Marcolino FMD, et al. Tofacitinib, an oral Janus kinase inhibitor, in patients from Brazil with rheumatoid arthritis: pooled efficacy and safety analyses. Medicine (Baltimore) 2018;97(31):e11609.

79. Smolen JS, Genovese MC, Takeuchi T, et al. Safety profile of Baricitinib in patients with active rheumatoid arthritis with over 2 Years median time in treatment. J Rheumatol 2019;46(1):7–18.

80. Yehia BR, Blumberg EA. Mycobacterium tuberculosis infection in liver transplantation. Liver Transpl 2010;16(10):1129–35.

81. Mikulska M, Lanini S, Gudiol C, et al. ESCMID Study Group for Infections in Compromised Hosts (ESGICH) Consensus Document on the safety of targeted and biological therapies: an infectious diseases perspective (Agents targeting lymphoid cells surface antigens [I]: CD19, CD20 and CD52). Clin Microbiol Infect 2018;24(Suppl 2): S71–82.

82. Au W-Y, Leung AYH, Tse EWC, et al. High incidence of tuberculosis after alemtuzumab treatment in Hong Kong Chinese patients. Leuk Res 2008; 32(4):547–51.

83. Schiff MH, Kremer JM, Jahreis A, et al. Integrated safety in tocilizumab clinical trials. Arthritis Res Ther 2011;13(5):R141.

84. Koike T, Harigai M, Inokuma S, et al. Effectiveness and safety of tocilizumab: postmarketing surveillance of 7901 patients with rheumatoid arthritis in Japan. J Rheumatol 2014;41(1):15–23.

85. Lin C-T, Huang W-N, Hsieh C-W, et al. Safety and effectiveness of tocilizumab in treating patients with rheumatoid arthritis - a three-year study in Taiwan. J Microbiol Immunol Infect 2019;52(1): 141–50.

86. Trinchieri G, Pflanz S, Kastelein RA. The IL-12 family of heterodimeric cytokines: new players in the regulation of T cell responses. Immunity 2003; 19(5):641–4.

87. Cooper AM, Magram J, Ferrante J, et al. Interleukin 12 (IL-12) is crucial to the development of protective immunity in mice intravenously infected with mycobacterium tuberculosis. J Exp Med 1997; 186(1):39–45.

88. Kalb RE, Fiorentino DF, Lebwohl MG, et al. Risk of serious infection with biologic and systemic treatment of psoriasis: results from the psoriasis longitudinal assessment and registry (PSOLAR). JAMA Dermatol 2015;151(9):961–9.

89. Krueger GG, Langley RG, Leonardi C, et al. A human interleukin-12/23 monoclonal antibody for the treatment of psoriasis. N Engl J Med 2007; 356(6):580–92.

90. Leonardi CL, Kimball AB, Papp KA, et al. Efficacy and safety of ustekinumab, a human interleukin-12/23 monoclonal antibody, in patients with psoriasis: 76-week results from a randomised, double-blind, placebo-controlled trial (PHOENIX 1). Lancet 2008;371(9625):1665–74.

91. Bourigault M-l , Segueni N, Rose S, et al. Relative contribution of IL-1α, IL-1β and TNF to the host response to Mycobacterium tuberculosis and attenuated M. bovis BCG. Immun Inflamm Dis 2013;1(1):47–62.

92. Guler R, Parihar SP, Spohn G, et al. Blocking IL-1α but not IL-1β increases susceptibility to chronic Mycobacterium tuberculosis infection in mice. Vaccine 2011;29(6):1339–46.

93. Cantini F, Niccoli L, Goletti D. Tuberculosis risk in patients treated with non-anti-tumor necrosis factor-α (TNF-α) targeted biologics and recently licensed TNF-α inhibitors: data from clinical trials and national registries. J Rheumatol Suppl 2014; 91:56–64.

94. Ridker PM, Everett BM, Thuren T, et al. Antiinflammatory therapy with canakinumab for atherosclerotic disease. N Engl J Med 2017;377(12):1119–31.

95. Okamoto Yoshida Y, Umemura M, Yahagi A, et al. Essential role of IL-17A in the formation of a mycobacterial infection-induced granuloma in the lung. J Immunol 2010;184(8):4414–22.

96. Domingo-Gonzalez R, Das S, Griffiths KL, et al. Interleukin-17 limits hypoxia-inducible factor 1α and development of hypoxic granulomas during tuberculosis. JCI insight 2017;2(19):e92973.

97. Peng R, Yue J, Han M, et al. The IL-17F sequence variant is associated with susceptibility to tuberculosis. Gene 2013;515(1):229–32.

98. Blauvelt A. Safety of secukinumab in the treatment of psoriasis. Expert Opin Drug Saf 2016;15(10): 1413–20.

99. Kammüller M, Tsai TF, Griffiths CEM, et al. Inhibition of IL-17A by secukinumab shows no evidence of increased Mycobacterium tuberculosis infections. Clin Transl Immunol 2017;6(8):e152.

100. Chen Y-M, Chen H-H, Lai K-L, et al. The effects of rituximab therapy on released interferon-γ levels in the QuantiFERON assay among RA patients with different status of Mycobacterium tuberculosis infection. Rheumatology (Oxford) 2013;52(4): 697–704.

101. Alkadi A, Alduaiji N, Alrehaily A. Risk of tuberculosis reactivation with rituximab therapy. Int J Health Sci (Qassim) 2017;11(2):41–4.

102. Buch MH, Smolen JS, Betteridge N, et al. Updated consensus statement on the use of rituximab in patients with rheumatoid arthritis. Ann Rheum Dis 2011;70(6):909–20.

103. Drgona L, Gudiol C, Lanini S, et al. ESCMID Study Group for Infections in Compromised Hosts (ESGICH) Consensus Document on the safety of targeted and biological therapies: an infectious diseases perspective (Agents targeting lymphoid or myeloid cells surface antigens [II]: CD22, CD30, CD33. Clin Microbiol Infect 2018;24(Suppl 2):S83–94.

104. van der Wekken L, Herbrink J, Snijders D, et al. Disseminated Mycobacterium chelonae infection in a patient with T-cell lymphoma. Hematol Oncol Stem Cell Ther 2017;10(2):89–92.

105. Dahdaleh D, Altmann DM, Malik O, et al. Breathlessness, night sweats, and weight loss on natalizumab. Lancet 2012;380(9843):726–7.

106. Boyko AN, Evdoshenko EP, Vorob'eva OV, et al. A prospective, open, non-randomized study on

the safety and efficacy of natalizumab (tisabri) in the Russian population of patients with relapsing-remitting multiple sclerosis. Zh Nevrol Psikhiatr Im S S Korsakova 2015;115(8. Vyp. 2):25–35.

107. Holmén C, Piehl F, Hillert J, et al. A Swedish national post-marketing surveillance study of natalizumab treatment in multiple sclerosis. Mult Scler 2011;17(6):708–19.

108. Winthrop KL, Mariette X, Silva JT, et al. ESCMID Study Group for Infections in Compromised Hosts (ESGICH) Consensus Document on the safety of targeted and biological therapies: an infectious diseases perspective (Soluble immune effector molecules [II]: agents targeting interleukins, immunoglobuli. Clin Microbiol Infect 2018;24(Suppl 2): S21–40.

109. Goncalves MVM, Melo LH, Benedet CM, et al. Eculizumab, neuromyelitis optica, and tuberculosis: we live an era of challenging combinations. CNS Neurosci Ther 2015;21(11):914–5.

110. Rook GAW, Hernández-Pando R, Zumla A. Tuberculosis due to high-dose challenge in partially immune individuals: a problem for vaccination? J Infect Dis 2009;199(5):613–8.

111. Rook GAW. Th2 cytokines in susceptibility to tuberculosis. Curr Mol Med 2007;7(3):327–37.

112. Keystone EC, Papp KA, Wobeser W. Challenges in diagnosing latent tuberculosis infection in patients treated with tumor necrosis factor antagonists. J Rheumatol 2011;38(7):1234–43.

113. Coaccioli S, Di Cato L, Marioli D, et al. Impaired cutaneous cell-mediated immunity in newly diagnosed rheumatoid arthritis. Panminerva Med 2000;42(4):263–6.

114. Ponce de Leon D, Acevedo-Vasquez E, Alvizuri S, et al. Comparison of an interferon-gamma assay with tuberculin skin testing for detection of tuberculosis (TB) infection in patients with rheumatoid arthritis in a TB-endemic population. J Rheumatol 2008;35(5):776–81.

115. Diel R, Loddenkemper R, Nienhaus A. Predictive value of interferon-γ release assays and tuberculin skin testing for progression from latent TB infection to disease state: a meta-analysis. Chest 2012; 142(1):63–75.

116. Sivamani RK, Goodarzi H, Garcia MS, et al. Biologic therapies in the treatment of psoriasis: a comprehensive evidence-based basic science and clinical review and a practical guide to tuberculosis monitoring. Clin Rev Allergy Immunol 2013;44(2):121–40.

117. Doan TN, Eisen DP, Rose MT, et al. Interferon-gamma release assay for the diagnosis of latent tuberculosis infection: a latent-class analysis. PLoS One 2017;12(11):e0188631.

118. Raval A, Akhavan-Toyserkani G, Brinker A, et al. Brief communication: characteristics of spontaneous cases of tuberculosis associated with infliximab. Ann Intern Med 2007;147(10):699–702.

119. Kleinert S, Tony H-P, Krueger K, et al. Screening for latent tuberculosis infection: performance of tuberculin skin test and interferon-γ release assays under real-life conditions. Ann Rheum Dis 2012; 71(11):1791–5.

120. Abubakar I, Drobniewski F, Southern J, et al. Prognostic value of interferon-γ release assays and tuberculin skin test in predicting the development of active tuberculosis (UK PREDICT TB): a prospective cohort study. Lancet Infect Dis 2018; 18(10):1077–87.

121. Mariette X, Baron G, Tubach F, et al. Influence of replacing tuberculin skin test with ex vivo interferon γ release assays on decision to administer prophylactic antituberculosis antibiotics before anti-TNF therapy. Ann Rheum Dis 2012;71(11):1783–90.

122. Bocchino M, Matarese A, Bellofiore B, et al. Performance of two commercial blood IFN-gamma release assays for the detection of Mycobacterium tuberculosis infection in patient candidates for anti-TNF-alpha treatment. Eur J Clin Microbiol Infect Dis 2008;27(10):907–13.

123. Hsia EC, Schluger N, Cush JJ, et al. Interferon-γ release assay versus tuberculin skin test prior to treatment with golimumab, a human anti-tumor necrosis factor antibody, in patients with rheumatoid arthritis, psoriatic arthritis, or ankylosing spondylitis. Arthritis Rheum 2012;64(7):2068–77.

124. Hsia EC, Cush JJ, Matteson EL, et al. Comprehensive tuberculosis screening program in patients with inflammatory arthritides treated with golimumab, a human anti-tumor necrosis factor antibody, in Phase III clinical trials. Arthritis Care Res (Hoboken) 2013;65(2):309–13.

125. Jung YJ, Lee JY, Jo K-W, et al. The "either test positive" strategy for latent tuberculous infection before anti-tumour necrosis factor treatment. Int J Tuberc Lung Dis 2014;18(4):428–34.

126. Smith MY, Attig B, McNamee L, et al. Tuberculosis screening in prescribers of anti-tumor necrosis factor therapy in the European Union. Int J Tuberc Lung Dis 2012;16(9):1168–73.

127. Cantini F, Lubrano E, Marchesoni A, et al. Latent tuberculosis infection detection and active tuberculosis prevention in patients receiving anti-TNF therapy: an Italian nationwide survey. Int J Rheum Dis 2016;19(8):799–805.

128. Vaughn BP, Doherty GA, Gautam S, et al. Screening for tuberculosis and hepatitis B prior to the initiation of anti-tumor necrosis therapy. Inflamm Bowel Dis 2012;18(6):1057–63.

129. Tomio J, Yamana H, Matsui H, et al. Tuberculosis screening prior to anti-tumor necrosis factor therapy among patients with immune-mediated inflammatory diseases in Japan: a longitudinal study

using a large-scale health insurance claims database. Int J Rheum Dis 2017;20(11):1674–83.

130. Centers for Disease Control and Prevention (CDC). Targeted tuberculin testing and treatment of latent tuberculosis infection. American Thoracic Society. MMWR Recomm Rep 2000;49(RR-6):1–51.

131. Matulis G, Jüni P, Villiger PM, et al. Detection of latent tuberculosis in immunosuppressed patients with autoimmune diseases: performance of a Mycobacterium tuberculosis antigen-specific interferon gamma assay. Ann Rheum Dis 2008;67(1): 84–90.

132. Cuomo G, D'Abrosca V, Iacono D, et al. The conversion rate of tuberculosis screening tests during biological therapies in patients with rheumatoid arthritis. Clin Rheumatol 2017;36(2):457–61.

133. Hatzara C, Hadziyannis E, Kandili A, et al. Frequent conversion of tuberculosis screening tests during anti-tumour necrosis factor therapy in patients with rheumatic diseases. Ann Rheum Dis 2015; 74(10):1848–53.

134. Singh JA, Saag KG, Bridges SL, et al. 2015 American College of Rheumatology guideline for the treatment of rheumatoid arthritis. Arthritis Rheumatol 2016;68(1):1–26.

135. Cataño JC, Morales M. Follow-up results of isoniazid chemoprophylaxis during biological therapy in Colombia. Rheumatol Int 2015;35(9):1549–53.

136. Garcia Vidal C, Rodríguez Fernández S, Martínez Lacasa J, et al. Paradoxical response to antituberculous therapy in infliximab-treated patients with disseminated tuberculosis. Clin Infect Dis 2005; 40(5):756–9.

137. Belknap R, Reves R, Burman W. Immune reconstitution to Mycobacterium tuberculosis after discontinuing infliximab. Int J Tuberc Lung Dis 2005; 9(9):1057–8.

138. Hsu DC, Faldetta KF, Pei L, et al. A paradoxical treatment for a paradoxical condition: infliximab use in three cases of mycobacterial IRIS. Clin Infect Dis 2016;62(2):258–61.

139. Gupta M, Jafri K, Sharim R, et al. Immune reconstitution inflammatory syndrome associated with biologic therapy. Curr Allergy Asthma Rep 2015; 15(2):499.

140. Bell LCK, Breen R, Miller RF, et al. Paradoxical reactions and immune reconstitution inflammatory syndrome in tuberculosis. Int J Infect Dis 2015; 32:39–45.

141. Arend SM, Leyten EMS, Franken WPJ, et al. A patient with de novo tuberculosis during anti-tumor necrosis factor-alpha therapy illustrating diagnostic pitfalls and paradoxical response to treatment. Clin Infect Dis 2007;45(11):1470–5.

142. Lwin N, Boyle M, Davis JS. Adalimumab for corticosteroid and infliximab-Resistant immune reconstitution inflammatory syndrome in the setting of TB/HIV Coinfection. Open Forum Infect Dis 2018;5(2): ofy027.

143. Kawamoto H, Takasaki J, Ishii S, et al. Re-administration of abatacept for the control of articular symptoms of rheumatoid arthritis during anti-tuberculous therapy. Respir Med Case Reports 2017;21:147–50.

144. Wallis RS, van Vuuren C, Potgieter S. Adalimumab treatment of life-threatening tuberculosis. Clin Infect Dis 2009;48(10):1429–32.

145. Hasan T, Au E, Chen S, et al. Screening and prevention for latent tuberculosis in immunosuppressed patients at risk for tuberculosis: a systematic review of clinical practice guidelines. BMJ Open 2018;8(9):e022445.

146. Solovic I, Sester M, Gomez-Reino JJ, et al. The risk of tuberculosis related to tumour necrosis factor antagonist therapies: a TBNET consensus statement. Eur Respir J 2010;36(5):1185–206.

147. Centers for Disease Control and Prevention (CDC). Tuberculosis associated with blocking agents against tumor necrosis factor-alpha–California, 2002-2003. MMWR Morb Mortal Wkly Rep 2004; 53(30):683–6.

148. British Thoracic Society Standards of Care Committee. BTS recommendations for assessing risk and for managing Mycobacterium tuberculosis infection and disease in patients due to start anti-TNF-alpha treatment. Thorax 2005;60(10):800–5.

149. van Zyl-Smit RN, Pai M, Peprah K, et al. Within-subject variability and boosting of T-cell interferon-gamma responses after tuberculin skin testing. Am J Respir Crit Care Med 2009;180(1):49–58.

150. Ozguler Y, Hatemi G, Ugurlu S, et al. Re-initiation of biologics after the development of tuberculosis under anti-TNF therapy. Rheumatol Int 2016;36(12): 1719–25.

151. Kim HW, Kwon SR, Jung K-H, et al. Safety of resuming tumor necrosis factor inhibitors in ankylosing spondylitis patients concomitant with the treatment of active tuberculosis: a retrospective nationwide registry of the Korean society of spondyloarthritis research. PLoS One 2016;11(4): e0153816.

152. Mohan AK, Coté TR, Block JA, et al. Tuberculosis following the use of etanercept, a tumor necrosis factor inhibitor. Clin Infect Dis 2004;39(3):295–9.

How Can the Tuberculosis Laboratory Aid in the Patient-Centered Diagnosis and Management of Tuberculosis?

Akos Somoskovi, MD, PhD, DSc[a], Max Salfinger, MD[b],*

KEYWORDS

- Tuberculosis • Minimal inhibitory concentration • Nucleic acid amplification
- Antimicrobial susceptibility testing • Molecular assays • Line probe assays • Drug resistance

KEY POINTS

- The tuberculosis (TB) laboratory needs to employ accurate, timely, and informative methods using molecular assays for detection of TB and antimicrobial susceptibility testing.
- Information on the level of drug resistance using quantitative methods, such as minimal inhibitory concentration assays, is vital to tailor the most appropriate patient-centered drug regimens.
- The type of mutation, if known, could better alert the clinicians and may allow earlier implementation or adjustment of individual and effective treatment options.

INTRODUCTION

Tuberculosis (TB) disease is attributed to a slow-growing acid-fast bacilli (AFB) that requires weeks or even months for a culture to show a positive result. The genus *Mycobacterium* includes more than 200 species and subspecies. Patients with infectious pulmonary TB, which is caused mainly by *M tuberculosis* and to a lesser degree by *M bovis* and *M africanum*, are the main sources of transmission of the disease.

Since the resurgence of TB beginning in the mid-1980s, laboratories have needed better and faster tools for the laboratory diagnosis. In 2018, an American Society for Microbiology work group described contemporary methods for laboratory diagnosis of mycobacterial diseases, for example, updated work-up of specimens, nucleic acid amplification tests (NAATs), AFB smear microscopy, growth detection, identification, and antimicrobial susceptibility testing (AST).[1]

In order to determine and provide the most effective treatment regimen to patients, a clinical TB laboratory needs to rapidly but reliably answer 2 main questions: (1) Is *M tuberculosis* detectable in the patient specimen? and (2) If so, is the strain detected drug susceptible or does it show any form of drug resistance?

APPROPRIATE SPECIMENS

Most specimens received in the mycobacteriology laboratory are from the respiratory tract, since

Disclosure Statement: None of the authors has any relationship with a commercial company that has a direct financial interest in subject matter or materials discussed in article or with a company making a competing product.
[a] Global Health Technologies, Global Good Fund, Intellectual Ventures Laboratory, 3150 139th Avenue Southeast, Building 4, Bellevue, WA 98005, USA; [b] University of South Florida, College of Public Health, 13201 Bruce B. Down Boulevard, MDC56, Tampa, FL 33612-3805, USA
* Corresponding author.
E-mail address: max@health.usf.edu

Clin Chest Med 40 (2019) 741–753
https://doi.org/10.1016/j.ccm.2019.07.004
0272-5231/19/© 2019 Elsevier Inc. All rights reserved.

pulmonary TB is the most common form of TB. A majority of these specimens are sputum, expectorated and induced, along with bronchial aspirates, bronchoalveolar lavage specimens, and tracheal aspirates. Guidelines issued by the American Thoracic Society/Centers for Disease Control and Prevention (CDC)/Infectious Diseases Society of America and National Tuberculosis Controllers Association recommend collection of 3 sputum specimens at 8-hour to 24-hour intervals, with at least 1 being an early-morning specimen to improve the sensitivity of diagnosis.[2] The AFB smear sensitivity of the first specimen is 53.8%, which increases to 64.9% with a second sputum specimen and 65% to 70% with a third.[2] In a study by Leonard and colleagues,[3] the sensitivity of culture among patients with culture-confirmed TB was 91% with 1 sputum specimen, and it increased to 98% with the second and to 100% with the third. The CDC recommends at least 1 of the specimens be a first morning specimen, because the sensitivity is 12% greater than that of a single spot specimen.[3] The amount of sputum collected should be 5 mL to 10 mL. A volume of less than 3 mL compromises the sensitivity of the AFB smear and culture.[2]

It is important that the person collecting specimens be properly trained and be made aware of the appropriate types and volumes of specimens for mycobacterial testing. Knowledge of a laboratory's rejection criteria (eg, pooled sputum, inadequate volume, prolonged transit time) is required. Optimally, specimens should be received in the laboratory within 1 day of collection.[4] When unacceptable specimens are received, the laboratory must let the health care provider know as soon as possible so that a quality specimen may be obtained.

TESTING ALGORITHM

The use of the fluorochrome stain for mycobacterial smears, the use of a liquid-based culture system, and the use of rapid identification methods, such as nucleic acid probe assays, molecular line probe assays (LPAs), and matrix-assisted laser desorption/ionization–time of flight mass spectrometry (MALDI-TOF MS), along with molecular AST directly from clinical specimens or isolates, are optimal for supporting the critical decisions required for effective patient care and management.

The algorithms for testing specimens for mycobacteria are complicated, because several tests and several appropriate algorithms may be used in the clinical laboratory community depending on the patients served and available resources.

Ultimately, any method and algorithm used should ensure that M tuberculosis complex (MTBC) is detected or ruled out as quickly as possible. **Fig. 1** shows a comprehensive diagnostic algorithm for specimens from patients suspected of having TB and from patients for whom suspicion of TB is low but for whom mycobacterial disease needs to be ruled out.[5]

DETECTION OF *MYCOBACTERIUM TUBERCULOSIS* IN CLINICAL SPECIMENS

Use of NAATs to detect the presence of MTBC in specimens from patients suspected of having TB disease has been recommended as a standard of practice by the CDC.[6] By providing rapid detection of the presence of MTBC directly in clinical specimen, NAATs aid in early specific diagnosis of TB and prompt initiation of therapy. NAATs are more sensitive for detection of MTBC than AFB microscopy and more specific because nontuberculous mycobacteria (NTM) may also be detected by AFB microscopy.[6,7]

The 2009 CDC recommendation does not recommend NAATs for all specimens, and it does recommend continued use of culture and AFB microscopy. Overall, it is expected that NAATs can reduce health care costs by helping with decisions about priorities for contact investigations, making decisions about respiratory isolation, and reducing unnecessary TB treatment.

Two commercial NAAT systems have approval or clearance by the US Food and Drug Administration (FDA). One of these (Amplified Mycobacterium tuberculosis Direct, Hologic, San Diego, California) uses transcription-mediated amplification,[8] whereas the other (Xpert MTB/RIF, Cepheid, Sunnyvale, California) uses an automated real-time polymerase chain reaction (PCR) system with molecular beacon probes.[9] In addition, there are commercially available NAAT systems that do not yet have FDA clearance.[10–12] One of these systems is designed to detect mutations associated with resistance to drugs used for treatment of TB, similar to the Xpert MTB/RIF system.[10] The Xpert MTB/RIF is FDA cleared for AFB smear-positive and smear-negative raw sputum and processed sputum sediments. NAATs also are called on to help with decisions about release of patients suspected of having TB disease from airborne infection isolation rooms.[13] Release of a patient from airborne infection isolation historically has been based on multiple consecutive AFB smear-negative sputum specimens. The data presented to the FDA indicated that a single Xpert MTB/RIF assay predicted the absence of AFB smear-positive pulmonary TB, with a negative predictive

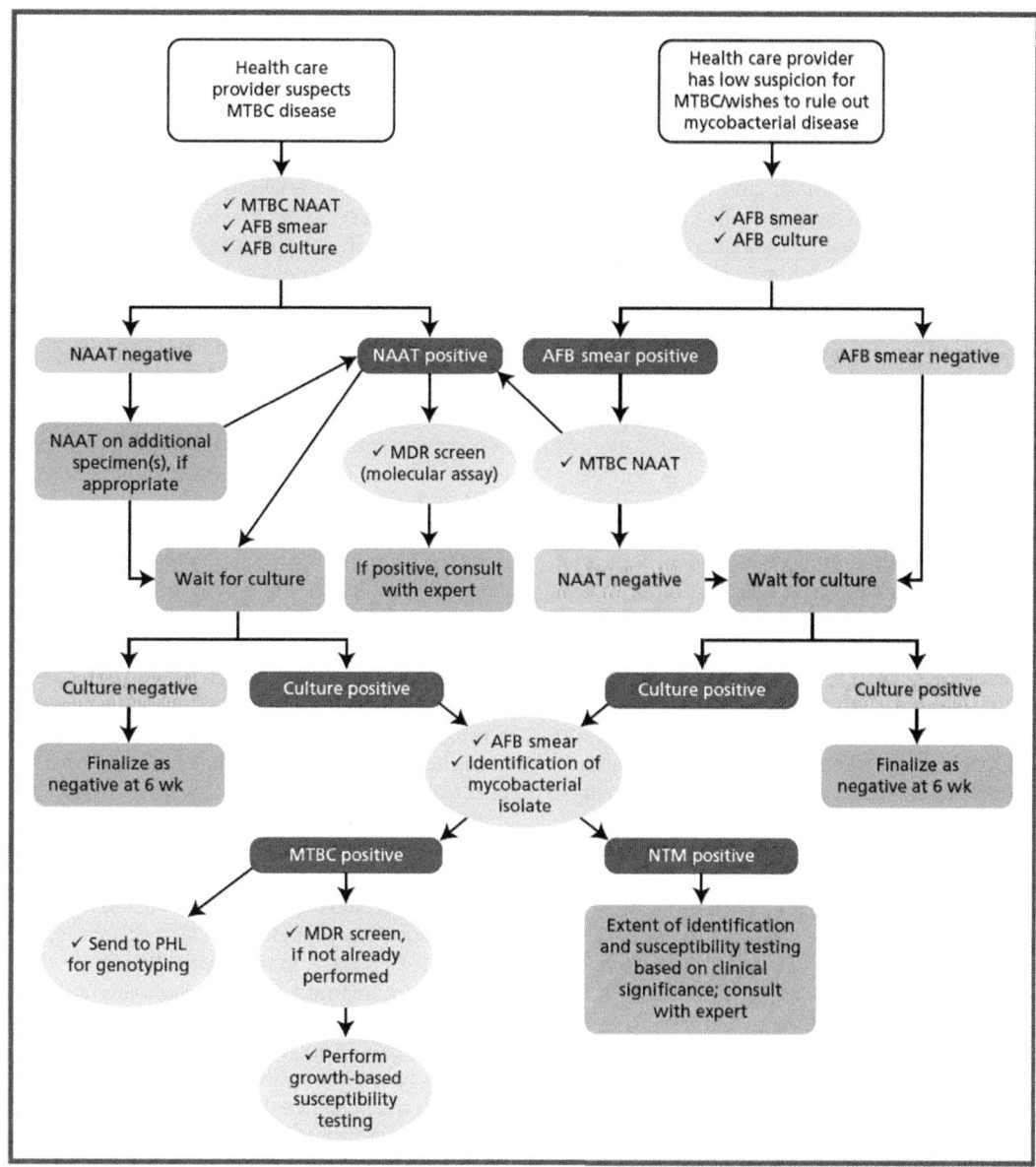

Fig. 1. Schematic of ideal algorithm for mycobacteriology testing in clinical laboratories and public health laboratories (PHLs). (*From* Warshauer DM, Salfinger M, Desmond E, Lin S-Y G. 2019. Chapter 32 *Mycobacterium tuberculosis* complex *In* Carroll, KC and Pfaller MA. (Editors). Manual of Clinical Microbiology. ASM Press. pp. 576-594; with permission.)

value of 99.7%. The newer Xpert MTB/RIF Ultra was reported to have improved sensitivity in a multicenter study.[14] Testing of 2 specimens rather than 1 also is more sensitive for detection of AFB smear-negative but culture-positive TB. The Hologic direct test is FDA cleared for AFB smear-positive and smear-negative processed sediments from sputum, bronchial specimens, and tracheal aspirates. In general, commercially available tests are preferred over laboratory-developed assays because of the standardized protocols and improved quality control and because laboratory-developed NAAT methods have been reported to have highly heterogeneous diagnostic accuracy.[15]

IDENTIFICATION OF ISOLATES

There are 2 commercial MALDI-TOF MS systems available in the United States that are used for rapid identification of culture isolates: the MALDI Biotyper (Bruker Daltonics, Billerica, Massachusetts) and the VITEK MS (bioMérieux, Durham,

North Carolina). The VITEK MS has an FDA-cleared mycobacteria database, and the MALDI Biotyper has a research use–only database for mycobacteria. Laboratories can add spectra to the research use–only database and validate the library as a laboratory-developed test. MALDI-TOF MS requires a large biomass, and, therefore, subculture to solid media and incubation for 1 week to 3 weeks for MTBC may be necessary, resulting in a delay of identification. Studies on the identification of mycobacteria directly from positive liquid media (eg, Mycobacteria Growth Indicator Tube (MGIT) [BD, Sparks, MD] or VersaTREK Myco Media [Thermo Fisher Scientific, Durham, NC]) have shown variable results.

Molecular LPAs provide rapid identification of MTBC directly from clinical specimens and from culture. In LPAs, nucleic acid is extracted from the specimen and then amplified and hybridized onto a nitrocellulose strip with fixed probes that allow the identification of MTBC and other mycobacteria. The patterns on the strips can then be interpreted using a template. There are several manufacturers of LPAs, including Hain Lifescience, Nehren, Germany; Innogenetics, Ghent, Belgium; Nipro Corporation, Osaka, Japan; and Autoimmun Diagnostika, Strassberg, Germany.

The INNO-LiPA Mycobacteria v2 (Innogenetics) can identify MTBC in addition to 15 NTM, and the GenoType Mycobacterium assay (Hain Lifescience) allows identification of MTBC and 13 NTM species. The GenoType MTBC (Hain Lifescience) LPA can differentiate some of the members of the MTBC, including *M tuberculosis*, *M bovis*, *M bovis* bacillus calmette–guérin, *M africanum*, *M microti*, and *M caprae*, from positive cultures.

IMPORTANCE OF ADEQUATE AND INFORMATIVE ANTIMICROBIAL SUSCEPTIBILITY TESTING

Accurate, timely, and informative AST to all first-line, second-line, and newer drugs is essential to develop the best possible treatment approach. Information on the level of drug resistance with the use of quantitative assays, such as limited or full minimal inhibitory concentrations (MICs), in line with the needs of a particular clinical scenario is vital to prevent further transmission of drug-resistant TB. At present, a significant amount of information of molecular assays (such as the type of mutation) is not used or is not available for interpretation, due to the design of current commercial assays. If present or utilized, they could better alert clinicians and may allow earlier implementation or adjustment of more individual and effective treatment options. Routine phenotypic AST approaches usually target only first-line drugs, and second-line AST is performed only when first-line assays identify drug resistance. Judicious use of molecular testing results could possibly trigger testing of both first-line and second-line drugs without delay. Finally, despite the recent revision of treatment of multidrug-resistant (MDR) TB by the World Health Organization (WHO), there are no adequately standardized AST methods for newer drugs, such as bedaquiline or delamanide.[16]

IMPORTANCE OF IDENTIFYING MONORESISTANCE TO KEY DRUGS

Isoniazid (INH) monoresistance can be quite high in certain high-burden settings, such as India, where the rate of INH monoresistance may reach 10%.[17] In cases of isolated phenotypic INH resistance, rapid molecular resistance screening is especially important to adequately orientate clinicians if INH could be continued or should be excluded from the regimen. In the presence of *inhA* mutations, a low level of phenotypic INH mutation can be expected, which usually can be successfully controlled with high-dose INH therapy.[18] With quantitative AST, the isolates of these patients usually show resistance to 0.1 μg/mL and susceptibility at 0.4 μg/mL to INH in the liquid culture-based MGIT system.[19]

When rapid molecular screening confirms the presence of a mutation of the *katG* gene in locus 315, however, the presence of a clinically meaningful and high-level phenotypic resistance (resistance at both 0.1 μg/mL and 0.4 μg/mL INH in the MGIT system) is confirmed. This result clearly indicates that INH treatment is not an option for these patients and should not be continued in the treatment regimen, not even with an increased dose.[20,21] Although molecular testing can be informative for clinicians, exercising caution is needed in therapeutic decisions in cases of detection of a less common and phenotypically not yet well-characterized *katG* mutation (other than locus 315 mutations). This result may be associated with moderate-level phenotypic resistance. The level of phenotypic resistance of a less common *katG* mutation needs to be assessed with quantitative AST, that is, MICs. If patients with INH-resistant TB remain unidentified (eg, screening patients with Xpert MTB/RIF vs LPAs), they are treated with only a single active drug during the continuation phase.

Isolated rifamycin resistance usually is rare. A recent review of the data from various diagnostic settings worldwide, however, supported by 14 WHO supranational laboratories revealed that rifampin (RIF) monoresistance was as high as 11.6% in certain geographic regions.[22] Mukinda and colleagues[23] reported that in the Western Cape of South Africa, RIF monoresistance tripled in 5 years; 12% of these patients were falsely diagnosed and treated for MDR-TB instead of a 12-month regimen with the more effective remaining first-line drugs enhanced with fluoroquinolone (FQ). Rufai and colleagues[17] also reported a high rate of RIF monoresistance (22.2%) in 285 smear-positive MDR-TB suspects in India after AST by LPA. Moreover, a recent drug resistant TB prevalence survey conducted in 2012-14 in South Africa revealed an alarmingly high prevalence of INH mono-resistant TB (not routinely screened for) with a prevalence of RIF-resistant TB that almost doubled, while the overall prevalence of MDR-TB in 2012–14 was similar to that of in 2001–02.[24] These patients should not be lumped together with MDR-TB and treated as such based on the results of an assay that is not informative enough.

Therefore, every effort should be taken to use only such molecular and conventional methods that can reliably differentiate monoresistance to INH and RIF from MDR-TB or extensively drug-resistant (XDR)-TB and also can provide information on the level of drug resistance. Tests that provide only a yes or no answer regarding a drug's susceptibility (mutation present or absent without the type of the mutation that can predict the level of resistance; phenotypic assays using a single critical concertation with susceptible or resistant answer without confirming the level of phenotypic resistance) are not as useful.

GLOBAL ASPECTS: ADVANTAGES AND SHORTCOMINGS OF RECENT NOVEL AND NONCONVENTIONAL DIAGNOSTIC APPROACHES FOR THE RAPID DETECTION AND ANTIMICROBIAL SUSCEPTIBILITY TESTING OF *MYCOBACTERIUM TUBERCULOSIS* COMPLEX

The WHO estimates that approximately 40% of all estimated TB cases and 80% of all estimated MDR TB cases are still missed every year.[25]

The challenges of diagnosing *M tuberculosis* include the need to detect and distinguish latent TB infection (LTBI) (to prevent progression to active TD), active TB disease, drug-resistant TB, and response to treatment. **Table 1** captures major technical gaps in existing diagnostics for the different forms of TB.

The Xpert MTB/RIF assay is a fully automated, cartridge-based, real-time PCR system, which can provide results within 2 hours after specimen collection. This system can detect MTBC with simultaneous prediction of RIF resistance by

Table 1
Major gaps in existing tuberculosis diagnostics

Situation	Gaps
LTBI	1. Biomarkers of progression from LTBI to TB disease 2. Differentiation of those with imminent TB disease from other stages of LTBI
Active TB disease	1. Adequate screening or case detection at POC and POT 2. Increased sensitivity and specificity: paucibacillary (children and immunosuppressed) 3. Non–sputum based, simple, inexpensive
Treatment monitoring	1. Faster and less complex, decentralized 2. Total viability count 3. Persisters/viable bacteria, but not culturable 4. Viability but non–replication dependent
Antimicrobial susceptibility	1. Reliable molecular AST 2. Informative, faster, and less complex phenotypic AST, decentralized 3. Addition of new drugs to assays, monitoring of new regimens
TB bacilli genotype	1. Cheaper and automated systems for whole-genome analysis 2. Directly on clinical specimen 3. Patient management vs surveillance
Specimen referral and reporting	1. Mobilize specimens when patient or diagnostic are not accessible 2. Shorten TAT for reporting to care giver

Abbreviations: POC, point of care; POT, point of treatment; TAT, turnaround time.

From Andama A, Somoskovi A, Mandel B, Bell D, Gutierrez C. Infection, Genetics and Evolution, https://doi.org/10.1016/j.meegid.2018.08.030; with permission.

targeting the *rpoB* gene.[26] The test is best validated for sputum using a simplified and raw sputum-based specimen preparation.

The test presents high sensitivity on AFB smear-positive specimens and acceptable sensitivity on AFB smear-negative specimens, with a good specificity to detect MTBC. The performance for detecting RIF resistance is, however, problematic. There is a lack of detection of certain forms of acquired drug resistance because the system requires the mutated population to be more than 65% or close to 100% to detect a particular mutation; the prediction of RIF resistance in paucibacillary specimens and for a few less common rpoB mutations has resulted in both false-positive and false-negative results.[27] There is no reported information on the type of mutation that may orientate a clinician on the level of phenotypic RIF resistance or presence or absence of potential cross-resistance to rifabutin (RFB).[14,28] Additional parameters that may affect the tests overall performance include HIV prevalence, strain diversity, prevalence of specific RIF resistance-conferring mutations (eg, outside the hot spot region of rpoB targeted by the assay), patient-related diagnostic delays, and default rates.[29]

LPAs were implemented routinely in the late 90s to expedite RIF susceptibility testing of clinical isolates but were endorsed by the WHO for molecular detection of drug resistance for INH and RIF directly from AFB smear-positive patients only in 2008.[30] Three available commercial LPAs are currently used for the rapid detection of MDR-TB: the GenoType MTBDR plus VER 2.0. test (Hain Lifescience), the NTM+MDRTB assay (Nipro Corporation), and the TB Resistance Assay module 1 (AID).[31,32] The WHO recommended for patients with confirmed RIF-resistant TB or MDR-TB that second-line LPA may be used as the initial test, instead of phenotypic culture-based AST, to detect resistance to FQ.[33] The GenoType MTBDR plus VER 2.0. test showed similar performance to the Xpert MTB/RIF on both AFB smear-positive and AFB smear-negative specimens.[34] The MTBDRsl by Hain Lifescience and the TB Resistance Assay module 2 by AID are specifically designed to test for resistance to second-line anti-TB drugs (FQ, aminoglycosides, and cyclic peptides) and which can be used in combination with the GenoType MTBDR plus VER 2.0 or Autoimmun Diagnostika MDR-TB test to identify XDR-TB.[35–37] WHO analysis of systematic reviews and meta-analyses showed that LPAs are highly sensitive (97%) and specific (99%) for the detection of RIF resistance, alone or in combination with INH (sensitivity 90%; specificity 99%), on isolates of M tuberculosis, and on AFB smear-positive sputum specimens.[36] The major advantage of LPAs is that they can be performed directly on AFB smear-positive sputum specimens, giving rapid (approximately 5 hours) AST results without the need for a culture isolate. Based on the LPA performance characteristics for INH and RIF, if screening with the MDR-TB assay does not indicate the presence of resistance-associated mutations, elimination of conventional culture and AST may be considered. For detection of mutations, follow-up can occur with the second-line LPA for rapid culture-based AST for both first-line and second-line drugs together. The disadvantages of LPAs, however, include being labor intensive and requiring highly trained personnel and dedicated laboratory space and equipment.[38] Culture-based AST using microtiter plates, such as the commercially available, quality-controlled, and dry-form Sensititre Mycobacterium tuberculosis MIC Plate by Thermo Scientific (Waltham, Massachusetts), offer a more cost-effective, high-throughput, and relatively fast solution compared with the automated but expensive and complex MGIT system, with a significantly smaller footprint. Recently, this system was further improved by the addition of an Automated Mycobacterial Growth Detection Algorithm (AMyGDA), which excludes manual observation and reading for adequate growth and enables accurate and reproducible prospective growth measurement with an overall faster turnaround time to results.[39]

Whole-genome sequencing (WGS) provides a rapid and comprehensive view of the genotype of M tuberculosis and may offer a clinically meaningful novel path for the detailed diagnosis of drug-resistant TB.[40] The most important questions that still need thorough evaluation and validation to determine if WGS could be an alternative to phenotypic AST are related to (1) the complexity, throughput, and cost of the technology (hardware and software) to perform the tests, to analyze the data, and to provide interpretable information to clinicians; (2) the current discrepancies between genotype and phenotype; (3) the need for large data sets to clarify the role of rare resistance mechanisms and the level of resistance conferred by different mutations; (4) some of the current problems of traditional AST, in particular pyrazinamide (PZA) testing; (5) the clinical impact of different levels of heteroresistance (proportion of wild-type and mutant strains), especially when the assay is directly used on sputum and not isolates; (6) the lack of understanding on phenotypic consequences of mutations and compensatory mutations on drug resistance not only on new drugs but also on several of the old TB drugs; and (7) the lack of understanding of these genetic alterations in different geographic settings with different M tuberculosis lineages or clades.[41]

Despite their limitations concerning their accuracy, turnaround time, and complexity, by combining the use of several different tests for each patient, these novel TB diagnostic technologies have contributed significantly to the progress toward TB elimination in low-burden and high-income settings. Due to the lack of adequate resources, availability, and scalability of these new diagnostic tools, however, the impact in the overall detection and management of TB cases in these settings is so far much more moderate.

PATIENT-CENTERED TREATMENT AND CASE MANAGEMENT

A recent meta-analysis for response to treatment of 6724 MDR-TB patients treated for different forms of drug resistance has highlighted the implications of the oversimplification of present MDR-TB and XDR-TB classification. In the study, overall 62% of patients were successfully treated; in 7% treatment failed or the patients relapsed, 9% died, and 17% defaulted.[42] The analysis revealed that treatment success of patients with only MDR-TB was 64%, with MDR-TB plus aminoglycoside resistance 56%, with MDR-TB plus FQ resistance 48%, and with XDR-TB 40%.

This reality demands better access for TB patients to laboratories that can perform and interpret more detailed molecular and phenotypic AST reliably to detect resistance promptly and provide individualized treatment. Oversimplifying XDR-TB may have a negative impact on strategies to preserve both existing and new treatment regimens. These strategies need timely and individualized treatment optimization to effectively control acquired or to avoid programmatically generated drug resistance.

Even the more recent assays (ie, LPA, Xpert MTB/RIF, and liquid culture with a single screening concentration) for the screening for presumptive drug-resistant cases or the monitoring of treatment are underutilized because the results they generate are reported or interpreted in an oversimplified manner. Typically, these approaches identify strains from patients only as drug susceptible, drug-resistant, MDR-TB, or XDR-TB without trying to predict or determine the phenotypic level of drug resistance, the presence or absence of cross-resistance, and the implications relative to achievable drug concentration.

For example, information on the type of the *rpoB* mutation can be indispensable to rule out cross-resistance to RFB because mutations at codon 516, Phe514PhePhe, and Ser522Leu are usually associated with RFB susceptibility, despite RIF resistance.[43,44] Therefore, if this information is available and properly interpreted, these MDR-TB patients may receive a RIF-based therapy that may offer a much better clinical outcome.[45] A recent study from Bangladesh that was based

on MIC testing of MDR-TB patient isolates showed that 19% of the 62 RIF-resistant isolates in this setting showed susceptibility to RFB.[46] Molecular testing that could have provided a more rapid elucidation in this regard was not available for these patients. In addition, it is clear that some of these less common mutations (rpoB Leu511Pro, Asp 516Tyr, Leu533Pro, His526Leu/Ser, and Ile572Phe), which may reach 22% of all RIF-resistant cases in certain settings,[47,48] are associated with a less than 1.0 μg/mL phenotypic RIF resistance, which is also the definition criterion for MDR-TB. Because phenotypic tests usually only test for this single RIF concentration in the absence of routine quantitative AST (for additional lower concentrations) and molecular resistance screening, these patients often are detected as infected with fully RIF-susceptible strains. Preliminary results indicate that patients with such mutant strains may fail more often under first-line therapy with standard RIF doses.[48]

Ethionamide and prothionamide are drugs that are often used for the treatment of MDR-TB based on their efficacy and low cost. The inclusion of these drugs has to be carefully considered, however, because cross-resistance with INH may be relatively common in the presence of mutations in the *inhA*[21,44] and low-level INH resistance. Therefore, these drugs should not be included in the treatment regimen if rapid molecular prescreening show mutations in this gene or MIC confirms low-level INH resistance. The inclusion of high-dose INH may be beneficial, however, to enhance the standard second-line regimen of these patients. Therefore, future molecular and conventional AST using a quantitative approach must be able to rapidly and adequately identify these particular strains and mutations.

Because discontinuation of FQ has such a significant impact on the outcome of therapy and due to different levels of cross-resistance between aminoglycosides, detection of FQ and aminoglycoside resistance-associated mutations and phenotypic drug resistance to these drugs should not be automatically interpreted as resistance to the entire class of the drug. A more meaningful interpretation of these laboratory results depending on the type of the mutation and the associated different level of phenotypic resistance by conventional AST may enable the continuation of treatment with these key drugs under certain conditions. Laboratory studies indicate that certain mutations associated with *gyrA* and *gyrB* mutations are associated with low or moderate levels of phenotypic drug resistance to FQs.[49] Although this level of resistance already results in MICs for ofloxacin that already are at or above the achievable drug serum concentration, later-generation FQs within the class still may be considered a therapeutic option in the case of certain mutations.[50] The reason is that the associated elevated MIC of these newer FQs may still be below the achievable drug serum concentration.[21] Therefore, it is important to clarify what FQ therapy received by the patient.

Rapid screening for mutations in the *eis, rrs*, and *tlyA* genes can provide similarly valuable information: first, regarding the presence of resistance to the aminoglycoside and polypeptide class of agents, such as kanamycin, amikacin, and viomycin or capreomycin, and, second, on the level of predictable phenotypic resistance that can be confirmed by quantitative AST.[21,44] Mutations in the *eis* are associated with low levels of aminoglycoside resistance, which is much lower than that of the drug serum concentration. Therefore, exclusion of the drug from the regimen may not be necessary, especially if a high-end dose is administered.[21,44] In addition, the type of *rrs* mutations not only can predict aminoglycoside and polypeptide resistance but also may provide information on the absence or presence of cross-resistance within these classes. TB strains with mutation *rrs* A1401 G usually are highly resistant to kanamycin and amikacin, whereas they are susceptible to viomycin or show low levels of resistance to capreomycin, which is still significantly below the achievable drug serum concentration.[51,52] Strains with *rrs* C1402 T mutations usually are associated with high levels of resistance to capreomycin, viomycin, and kanamycin but susceptibility to amikacin, whereas strains with *rrs* G1484 T usually are highly resistant to all aminoglycosides and polypeptides. Mutations in the *tlyA* are good predictors of clinically meaningful polypeptide resistance with intact aminoglycoside susceptibility.

It also is well known that there is no cross-resistance between streptomycin and the other aminoglycoside or polypeptide drugs.[21,44] The reason is that phenotypic streptomycin resistance is usually more associated with different genetic alterations, in the *rpsl* and most commonly in the codons 513-517 of the *rrs* gene, than that of with second-line injectable drugs.[21,44] In cases of clinically significant resistance to kanamycin, amikacin, or capreomycin, the absence of mutations in these loci may suggest phenotypic susceptibility to streptomycin, which, when confirmed by conventional AST, can be extremely valuable in the treatment of XDR-TB. This also was underlined by the observation that streptomycin susceptibility was found to be an important predictor of long-term survival of patients with pre-XDR.[53,54] This information, when well interpreted and complete

with quantitative AST for adequate confirmation of the level of resistance in a particular patient and communicated to the health care provider, may allow continuation of the treatment of the patients with another aminoglycoside. This could save a patient from being labeled as XDR-TB and treated accordingly with a less potent regimen or offered potentially more effective treatment of XDR-TB.

PZA is a key drug of current regimens to treat drug-susceptible TB. Because it has an excellent sterilizing effect on semidormant bacteria, the combination of PZA with RIF was critical to reduce the duration of treatment to 6 months. PZA also plays a central role in evaluation of new drug regimens to shorten the duration of treatment further and to improve the outcome of treatment of drug-resistant TB. Despite its importance in TB therapy, present WHO and International Union Against Tuberculosis and Lung Disease treatment guidelines suggest that because PZA was used in the a failing regimen and AST to this drug may be complicated in many settings, PZA should not be counted in the total of minimum drugs to be selected for MDR-TB treatment.[16,55–57]

The clinical significance of *in vitro* PZA resistance, however, has been highlighted by clinical trials that have shown that an FQ-based MDR-TB regimen increased early culture conversion and treatment completion by 38% versus a similar treatment without PZA.[58] More recent results on the novel 9-month MDR-TB treatment regimen in Bangladesh revealed that bacteriologic treatment failures and relapses were rare except among patients with high-level FQ in the presence of PZA resistance.[18] Often, empiric MDR-TB regimens that include PZA in the initial phase of the treatment suggest discontinuing administration of the drug in the continuation phase if 3-month follow-up cultures are negative. Considering the clinical data discussed previously, this approach also may need reconsideration. Consequently, losing PZA for the treatment of MDR-TB and XDR-TB has a significant clinical impact. Recent investigations indicate that PZA resistance is underestimated and may occur in up to 43% of MDR-TB strains.[59,60] Therefore, rapid and reliable AST testing for PZA is indispensable for TB control. Unfortunately, phenotypic AST for PZA often may be cumbersome or inaccurate due to inconsistencies of the inoculum size, the difficulties to grow TB at the lower pH used in the test, and the fact that PZA has a reduced activity against rapidly growing bacteria.

The primary molecular mechanism behind PZA resistance is mutations in the *pncA* and secondarily in the *rpsA* and *panD*.[61] The drawback of molecular testing for PZA is that genetic alterations in the pncA are found across the more than 500–base pair gene without a genetic hotspot similarly to that of rpoB and RIF. Therefore, patients often present with previously uncharacterized mutations and, in turn, the entire spectrum of pncA, rpsA, and panD alterations, resulting in clinically significant PZA resistance, has not been defined. In addition, polymorphisms in the pncA and rpsA also were found in drug-susceptible strains. In the absence of a systematic assessment of mutations associated with PZA resistance, currently there is no practical and reliable molecular drug resistance prediction tool for PZA, including WGS. To resolve this problem, Yadon and colleagues[61] generated a comprehensive library of pncA mutations using random PCR mutagenesis and screened this catalog of known and more importantly many novel genetic alterations for PZA resistance in vitro and in vivo in mouse experiments. The conclusion of this work was that resistance primarily results from the loss of pncA enzyme activity or protein abundance that can be empirically determined but may not be easily predicated by the sequence analysis. In addition, many substitutions were not associated with resistance to PZA. This thorough mutational and in vivo screening approach shows a good example how to validate the use of potential resistance-associated mutations and their mechanisms.

For decades the TB diagnostic community debated on the need to universal access to AST. It is important not to waste the same amount of time to understand the need to have universal access to quantitative and individualized AST. This is the only reliable way for patients to obtain the treatment that has the most appropriate drug combination and duration. The focus, however, is still on 1-size-fits-all regimens without any meaningful AST guidance and control that inevitably lead to treatment with toxic drugs to which patients are already resistant and prevents the use of affective drugs that could enable adequate treatment outcomes. Unfortunately, similar to the treatment strategies, novel diagnostic methods have also been used in a 1-size-fits-all approach that lumps patients into boxes rather than using information to better understand individual cases and how to optimize treatment according to individuals. This is not a trivial weakness in existing diagnostics; it does not address susceptible cases and allows the continuous regeneration of drug resistance. Previous studies of programmatic selection of ethionamide and PZA-resistant MDR-TB strains in South Africa using inadequately designed and supervised uniform treatment regimens in the absence of using molecular and phenotypic AST clearly underline the importance of the clinical impact of this question.[59] It also is important, however, to use adequate molecular and phenotypic tests that can give full and quantitative information on AST. The need for such an approach was clearly indicated by a recent study from Swaziland that showed that 30% of patients with MDR-TB harbored a mutation outside of the most often examined 81–base pair core region of the rpoB gene, which was missed (and, therefore, reported as susceptible) by commercial molecular assays.[62] The consequence of still not using adequate laboratory tools was dire and again led to the continued and silent programmatic amplification of MDR-TB, which slowly spilled over to South Africa but now with additional bedaquiline resistance after the introduction of this drug in South Africa.[63]

To best use the power that current molecular or phenotypic laboratory tests may provide, these tests should be used in combination and should also have the following basic characteristics:

- Should be able to predict or confirm resistance in a quantitative format (ie, MIC) that can provide clear information if the drug's dose may need to be adjusted or the drug has to be excluded of the regimen
- Should be able to differentiate different forms of monoresistance to key anti-TB drugs
- Should not rely only on hotspots associated with common resistance associated mutations but also preferably on the entire gene and all genes related to the resistance of a particular drug because geographic variations may have an impact on the occurrence of mutations in different genes
- Should be able to provide information on the type of the mutation to exclude misinterpretation of silent mutations, mutations associated with drug-resistant phenotypes, phylogenetic evolution, or compensatory mechanisms of strain fitness
- Should be able to provide information on potential cross-resistance within a particular drug class or between drugs in different classes
- Should be able to monitor the efficacy of treatment
- Should be able to support development of standardized AST of novel drugs

STEPS TO ACCELERATE TUBERCULOSIS ELIMINATION

To achieve improved case detection, follow-up, and management of TB with precision medicine through patient-centered treatment of drug-resistant TB, the following potential approaches should be considered:

1. Improvement of molecular assays to develop a simple, affordable nonsputum (urine, blood, stool, or saliva) biomarker-based (eg, cell free or transrenal DNA), point-of-care and/or point-of-treatment test that can support initiation of anti-TB therapy in patients identified by a referral test. This platform should offer the possibility to rule out MDR-TB or to identify MDR-TB and MDR-TB patients with more XDR, aiding individualized therapeutic decisions and guiding referrals for treatment by predicting different levels of phenotypic resistance and cross-resistances. A recent review suggests that cell-free DNA may be a viable non–sputum-based marker, whereas other recent publications indicate that using oral swab specimens to replace sputum may offer a similar improved detection path for patients with nonproductive cough.[64,65]

2. Individualized case management with focus on the clinical implications of different forms of drug-resistant TB cases by faster, simpler, and more accessible phenotypic detection of the total viable count (including the viable but presently not culturable count that may have significant impact on unsuccessful treatment or relapse). Also, quantitative AST for decentralization can improve individualized case management, follow-up, and monitoring of treatment efficacy with focus on but not limited to treatment failure and different forms of drug-resistant cases. Accepting and repeatedly saying that adequately and informative AST for M tuberculosis is complicated and not possible and continuing to rely on nonquantitative and inaccurate AST is unacceptable. This lack of useful AST testing is clearly associated with repeated programmatic selection of more complex drug-resistant strains and higher mortality.[63,66]

3. Innovative specimen storage and transport systems to preserve specimen integrity or increase testing target yield to further improve access to testing by moving the specimens to the diagnostic sites. The OMNIgene Sputum (DNA Genotek, Ottawa, Canada) transport medium, which allows ambient specimen transportation and storage for both growth detection and molecular testing, and the PrimeStore MTM ambient temperature nucleic acid transport device (Longhorn Vaccines and Diagnostics, Bethesda, Maryland) are good examples of such approaches.[67]

REFERENCES

1. Forbes BA, Hall GS, Miller MB, et al. Practice guidelines for clinical microbiology laboratories: mycobacteria. Clin Microbiol Rev 2018;31(2):1–66.
2. Lewinsohn DM, Leonard MK, LoBue PA, et al. Official American Thoracic Society/infectious diseases Society of America/Centers for disease control and prevention clinical practice guidelines: diagnosis of tuberculosis in adults and children. Clin Infect Dis 2017;64:e1–33.
3. Leonard MK Jr, Kourbatova E, Blumberg HM. Re: how many sputum specimens are necessary to diagnose pulmonary tuberculosis. Am J Infect Control 2006;34:328–9.
4. Centers for Disease Control and Prevention. Tuberculosis laboratory aggregate report. 4th edition. Atlanta (GA): Centers for Disease Control and Prevention; 2017.
5. Warshauer DM, Salfinger M, Desmond E, et al. Mycobacterium tuberculosis complex [Chapter: 32]. In: Carroll KC, Pfaller MA, editors. Manual of clinical microbiology. Washington, DC: ASM Press; 2019. p. 576–94.
6. Centers for Disease Control and Prevention (CDC). Updated guidelines for the use of nucleic acid amplification tests in the diagnosis of tuberculosis. MMWR Morb Mortal Wkly Rep 2009;58:7–10.
7. Peralta G, Barry P, Pascopella L. Use of nucleic acid amplification tests in tuberculosis patients in California, 2010-2013. Open Forum Infect Dis 2016;3:ofw230.
8. Guerra RL, Hooper NM, Baker JF, et al. Use of the amplified Mycobacterium tuberculosis direct test in a public health laboratory: test performance and impact on clinical care. Chest 2007;132:946–51.
9. Luetkemeyer AF, Firnhaber C, Kendall MA, et al, AIDS Clinical Trials Group A5295 and Tuberculosis Trials Consortium Study 34 Teams. Evaluation of Xpert MTB/RIF versus AFB smear and culture to identify pulmonary tuberculosis in patients with suspected tuberculosis from low and higher prevalence settings. Clin Infect Dis 2016;62:1081–8.
10. Hofmann-Thiel S, Molodtsov N, Antonenka U, et al. Evaluation of the Abbott RealTime MTB and RealTime MTB INH/RIF assays for direct detection of Mycobacterium tuberculosis complex and resistance markers in respiratory and extrapulmonary specimens. J Clin Microbiol 2016;54:3022–7.
11. Gray CM, Katamba A, Narang P, et al. Feasibility and operational performance of tuberculosis detection by loop-mediated isothermal amplification platform in decentralized settings: results from a multicenter study. J Clin Microbiol 2016;54:1984–91.
12. Huh HJ, Koh W-J, Song DJ, et al. Evaluation of the Cobas TaqMan MTB test for the detection of Mycobacterium tuberculosis complex according to acid-

fast-bacillus smear grades in respiratory specimens. J Clin Microbiol 2015;53:696–8.

13. Division of Microbiology Devices, Office of In Vitro Diagnostics and Radiological Health, Center for Devices and Radiological Health, Food and Drug Administration. Revised device labeling for the Cepheid Xpert MTB/RIF assay for detecting *Mycobacterium tuberculosis*. MMWR Morb Mortal Wkly Rep 2015;64:193.

14. Chakravorty S, Simmons AM, Rowneki M, et al. The New Xpert MTB/RIF Ultra: improving detection of *Mycobacterium tuberculosis* and resistance to rifampin in an assay suitable for point-of-care testing. MBio 2017;8:e00812–7.

15. Flores LL, Pai M, Colford JM Jr, et al. Inhouse nucleic acid amplification tests for the detection of *Mycobacterium tuberculosis* in sputum specimens: meta-analysis and meta-regression. BMC Microbiol 2005;5:55.

16. World Health Organization. WHO consolidated guidelines on drug-resistant tuberculosis treatment. Geneva (Switzerland): World Health Organization; 2019. License: CC BY-NC-SA 3.0 IGO.

17. Rufai SB, Kumar P, Singh A, et al. Comparison of Xpert MTB/RIF with line probe assay for detection of rifampin-monoresistant *Mycobacterium tuberculosis*. J Clin Microbiol 2014;52:1846–52.

18. Aung KJ, Van Deun A, Declercq E, et al. Successful '9-month Bangladesh regimen' for multidrug-resistant tuberculosis among over 500 consecutive patients. Int J Tuberc Lung Dis 2014;18:1180–7.

19. Cambau E, Viveiros M, Machado D, et al. Revisiting susceptibility testing in MDR-TB by a standardized quantitative phenotypic assessment in a European multicentre study. J Antimicrob Chemother 2015; 70:686–96.

20. Somoskovi A, Parsons LM, Salfinger M. The molecular basis of resistance to isoniazid, rifampin, and pyrazinamide in *Mycobacterium tuberculosis*. Respir Res 2001;2:164–8.

21. Böttger EC. The ins and outs of *Mycobacterium tuberculosis* drug susceptibility testing. Clin Microbiol Infect 2011;17:1128–34.

22. Kurbatova EV, Cavanaugh JS, Shah NS, et al. Rifampicin-resistant *Mycobacterium tuberculosis*: susceptibility to isoniazid and other anti-tuberculosis drugs. Int J Tuberc Lung Dis 2012;16:355–7.

23. Mukinda FK, Theron D, van der Spuy GD, et al. Rise in rifampicin-monoresistant tuberculosis in Western Cape, South Africa. Int J Tuberc Lung Dis 2012;16: 196–202.

24. Ismail NA, Mvusi L, Nanoo A, et al. Prevalence of drug-resistant tuberculosis and imputed burden in South Africa: a national and sub-national cross-sectional survey. Lancet Infect Dis 2018;18(7): 779–87.

25. World Health Organization. The end TB strategy. Geneva (Switzerland): World Health Organization; 2014.

26. World Health Organization. Xpert MTB/RIF implementation manual: technical and operational 'how-to'; practical considerations. Geneva (Switzerland): World Health Organization; 2014.

27. Blakemore R, Story E, Helb D, et al. Evaluation of the analytical performance of the Xpert MTB/RIF assay. J Clin Microbiol 2010;48(7):2495–501.

28. Hanrahan CF, Clouse K, Bassett J, et al. The patient impact of point-of-care vs. laboratory placement of Xpert MTB/RIF. Int J Tuberc Lung Dis 2015;19(7): 811–6.

29. Van Rie A, Page-Shipp L, Scott L, et al. Xpert ® MTB/RIF for point-of- care diagnosis of TB in high-HIV burden , resource-limited countries : hype or hope ? Expert Rev Mol Diagn 2010;10(7):937–46.

30. World Health Organization. Molecular line probe assays for rapid screening of patients at risk of multidrug-resistant tuberculosis. Geneva (Switzerland): World Health Organization; 2008.

31. Pai M, Minion J, Sohn H, et al. Novel and improved technologies for tuberculosis diagnosis: progress and challenges. Clin Chest Med 2009;30(4):701–16.

32. Ritter C, Lucke K, Sirgel FA, et al. Evaluation of the AID TB resistance line probe assay for rapid detection of genetic alterations associated with drug resistance in *Mycobacterium tuberculosis* strains. J Clin Microbiol 2014;52(3):940–6.

33. World Health Organization. The use of molecular line probe assays for the detection of mutations associated with resistance to fluoroquinolones (FQs) and second-line injectable drugs (SLIDs). Geneva (Switzerland): Policy Guidance; 2016. ISBN 978 92 4 150154 5.

34. Barnard M, Gey van Pittius NC, van Helden PD, et al. The diagnostic performance of the GenoType MTBDRplus version 2 line probe assay is equivalent to that of the Xpert MTB/RIF assay. J Clin Microbiol 2012;50(11):3712–6.

35. Kiet VS, Lan NTN, An DD, et al. Evaluation of the MTBDRsl test for detection of second-line-drug resistance in *Mycobacterium tuberculosis*. J Clin Microbiol 2010;48(8):2934–9.

36. Hillemann D, Rüsch-Gerdes S, Richter E. Feasibility of the GenoType MTBDRsl assay for fluoroquinolone, amikacin-capreomycin, and ethambutol resistance testing of *Mycobacterium tuberculosis* strains and clinical specimens. J Clin Microbiol 2009;47(6):1767–72.

37. Brossier F, Veziris N, Aubry A, et al. Detection by GenoType MTBDRsl test of complex mechanisms of resistance to second-line drugs and ethambutol in multidrug-resistant *Mycobacterium tuberculosis* complex isolates. J Clin Microbiol 2010;48(5): 1683–9.

38. Nicol M. New developments in the laboratory diagnosis of tuberculosis. CME 2010;28(6):246–50. Available at: https://www.ajol.info/index.php/cme/article/download/71268/60220.

39. Fowler PW, Gibertoni Cruz AL, Hoosdally SJ, et al. Automated detection of bacterial growth on 96-well plates for high-throughput drug susceptibility testing of Mycobacterium tuberculosis. Microbiology 2018; 164(12):1522–30.

40. Cabibbe AM, Walker TM, Niemann S, et al. Whole genome sequencing of Mycobacterium tuberculosis. Eur Respir J 2018;52(5) [pii:1801163].

41. Salfinger M, Somoskovi A. More on treatment outcomes in multidrug-resistant tuberculosis. N Engl J Med 2016;375(26):2609.

42. Falzon D, Gandhi N, Migliori GB, et al, Collaborative Group for Meta-Analysis of Individual Patient Data in MDR-TB. Resistance to fluoroquinolones and second-line injectable drugs: impact on multidrug-resistant TB outcomes. Eur Respir J 2013;42(1): 156–68.

43. Zhang Y, Yew W-W. Mechanisms of drug resistance in Mycobacterium tuberculosis: update 2015. Int J Tuberc Lung Dis 2015;19:1276–89.

44. Somoskovi A, Salfinger M. The race is on to shorten the turnaround time for diagnosis of multidrug-resistant tuberculosis. J Clin Microbiol 2015;53(12): 3715–8.

45. Jo KW, Ji W, Hong Y, et al. The efficacy of rifabutin for rifabutin-susceptible, multidrug-resistant tuberculosis. Respir Med 2013;107:292–7.

46. Heysell SK, Ahmed S, Ferdous SS, et al. Quantitative drug-susceptibility in patients treated for multidrug-resistant tuberculosis in Bangladesh: implications for regimen choice. PLoS One 2015;10(2): e0116795.

47. Somoskovi A, Dormandy J, Mitsani D, et al. Use of smear-positive samples to assess the PCR-based genotype MTBDR assay for rapid, direct detection of the Mycobacterium tuberculosis complex as well as its resistance to isoniazid and rifampin. J Clin Microbiol 2006;44:4459–63.

48. Van Deun A, Aung KJ, Hossain A, et al. Disputed rpoB mutations can frequently cause important rifampicin resistance among new tuberculosis patients. Int J Tuberc Lung Dis 2015;19:185–90.

49. Sirgel FA, Warren RM, Streicher EM, et al. gyrA mutations and phenotypic susceptibility levels to ofloxacin and moxifloxacin in clinical isolates of Mycobacterium tuberculosis. J Antimicrob Chemother 2012;67:1088–93.

50. Yew WW, Nuermberger E. High-dose fluoroquinolones in short-course regimens for treatment of MDR-TB: the way forward? Int J Tuberc Lung Dis 2013;7:853–4.

51. Maus CE, Plikaytis BB, Shinnick TM. Molecular analysis of cross-resistance to capreomycin, kanamycin, amikacin, and viomycin in Mycobacterium tuberculosis. Antimicrob Agents Chemother 2005;49: 3192–7.

52. Sirgel FA, Tait M, Warren RM, et al. Mutations in the rrs A1401G gene and phenotypic resistance to amikacin and capreomycin in Mycobacterium tuberculosis. Microb Drug Resist 2012;18:193–7.

53. Hwang SS, Kim HR, Kim HJ, et al. Impact of resistance to first-line and injectable drugs on treatment outcomes in MDR-TB. Eur Respir J 2009;33:581–5.

54. Kim DH, Kim HJ, Park SK, et al. Treatment outcomes and survival based on drug resistance patterns in multidrug-resistant tuberculosis. Am J Respir Crit Care Med 2010;182:113–9.

55. World Health Organization. Guidelines for treatment of tuberculosis. 4th edition. Geneva (Switzerland): World Health Organization; 2010 (WHO/HTM/TB/2009.420).

56. World Health Organization. Guidelines for the programmatic management of drug-resistant tuberculosis. Geneva (Switzerland): World Health Organization; 2011. Update (WHO/HTM/TB/2011.6).

57. Caminero JA, editor. Guidelines for clinical and operational management of drug-resistant tuberculosis. Paris: International Union Against Tuberculosis and Lung Disease; 2013.

58. Chang KC, Leung CC, Yew WW, et al. Pyrazinamide may improve fluoroquinolone-based treatment of multidrug-resistant tuberculosis. Antimicrob Agents Chemother 2012;56:5465–75.

59. Müller B, Chihota VN, Pillay M, et al. Programmatically selected multidrug-resistant strains drive the emergence of extensively drug-resistant tuberculosis in South Africa. PLoS One 2013;8(8):e70919.

60. Stoffels K, Mathys V, Fauville-Dufaux M, et al. Systematic analysis of pyrazinamide-resistant spontaneous mutants and clinical isolates of Mycobacterium tuberculosis. Antimicrob Agents Chemother 2012;56: 5186–93.

61. Yadon AN, Maharaj K, Adamson JH, et al. A comprehensive characterization of pncA polymorphisms that confer resistance to pyrazinamide. Nat Commun 2017;8(1):588.

62. Sanchez-Padilla E, Merker M, Beckert P, et al. Detection of drug-resistant tuberculosis by Xpert MTB/RIF in Swaziland. N Engl J Med 2015;372: 1181–2.

63. Makhado NA, Matabane E, Faccin M, et al. Outbreak of multidrug-resistant tuberculosis in South Africa undetected by WHO-endorsed commercial tests: an observational study. Lancet Infect Dis 2018;18(12):1350–9.

64. Fernández-Carballo BL, Broger T, Wyss R, et al. Toward the development of a circulating free DNA-based in vitro diagnostic test for infectious diseases: a review of evidence for tuberculosis. J Clin Microbiol 2019;57(4) [pii:e01234-18].

65. Luabeya AK, Wood RC, Shenje J, et al. Noninvasive detection of tuberculosis by oral swab analysis. J Clin Microbiol 2019;57(3) [pii:e01847-18].
66. Zürcher K, Ballif M, Fenner L, et al. International epidemiology databases to Evaluate AIDS (IeDEA) consortium. Drug susceptibility testing and mortality in patients treated for tuberculosis in high-burden countries: a multicentre cohort study. Lancet Infect Dis 2019;19(3): 298–307.
67. Reeve BWP, McFall SM, Song R, et al. Commercial products to preserve specimens for tuberculosis diagnosis: a systematic review. Int J Tuberc Lung Dis 2018;22(7):741–53.

Tuberculosis Supranational Reference Laboratories: A Global Approach

Christopher Gilpin, PhD, Fuad Mirzayev, MD, MPH*

KEYWORDS

- Tuberculosis • WHO TB supranational reference laboratory • Drug susceptibility testing
- Quality assurance

KEY POINTS

- The Word health Organization tuberculosis Supranational Reference Laboratories Network has supported the Global Project on Anti-Tuberculosis Drug Resistance Surveillance, the oldest and largest initiative on the surveillance of antimicrobial resistance.
- By 2018, the Supranational Reference Laboratories Network had expanded from initial 14 to 32 Supranational Reference Laboratories, and 4 National Centers of Excellence.
- Individual laboratories and the network are a great technical resource for laboratory scale-up and capacity development in countries, providing support to the reliable detection of anti-tuberculosis drug resistance.
- Technical assistance from individual laboratories has been supported by a variety of mechanisms, but funding has become increasingly challenging in recent years.

INTRODUCTION

Tuberculosis (TB) is one of the top 10 causes of death and the single leading infectious cause of mortality worldwide.[1] Ending the TB epidemic is one of the targets of the Sustainable Development Goals that requires intensive action by all countries, especially those with a high TB burden. According to the World Health Organization (WHO) Global Tuberculosis Report, in 2017 more than 10 million persons developed the disease resulting in an estimated 1.6 million deaths, including among 300,000 persons living with human immunodeficiency virus. Multidrug-resistant (MDR) TB remains a major public health concern in many countries with an estimated 558,000 new cases of rifampicin-resistant (RR) TB in 2017. Of these cases, almost one-half were estimated to be from 3 countries, namely, China, India, and the Russian Federation. Globally, MDR/RR-TB accounts for 3.5% of new TB cases and 18% of previously treated persons. The lack of diagnostic capacity is a crucial barrier preventing an effective response to the challenges of TB and MDR/RR-TB, with only slightly more than 20% of the estimated burden of MDR/RR-TB patients currently being detected.[1]

The WHO's End TB Strategy[2] calls for the implementation of a package of interventions organized around the 3 pillars of integrated patient-centered care and prevention, bold policies and supportive systems, and intensified research and innovation that should be adapted at country level. Early diagnosis and the initiation of appropriate treatment and care for all persons of all ages who have any form of TB are among the core interventions described under pillar 1 of the strategy. This requires ensuring access to WHO-recommended rapid diagnostics and universal access to drug-susceptibility testing (DST) for all patients with

Global TB Programme, World Health Organization, 20 Avenue Appia, 1211 Geneva 27, Switzerland
* Corresponding author.
E-mail address: mirzayevf@who.int

Clin Chest Med 40 (2019) 755–762
https://doi.org/10.1016/j.ccm.2019.07.005
0272-5231/19/© 2019 The Authors. Published by Elsevier Inc. This is an open access article under the CC BY-NC-ND license (http://creativecommons.org/licenses/by-nc-nd/4.0/).

signs and symptoms of TB. The WHO defines universal access to DST as rapid DST for at least rifampicin among patients with bacteriologically confirmed TB, and further DST for at least fluoroquinolones among patients with rifampicin resistance.[3] The effective management of TB and MDR/RR-TB relies on the rapid diagnosis and effective treatment of resistant infections. Culture-based phenotypic DST methods are currently the gold standard for drug resistance detection, but these methods are time consuming and require sophisticated laboratory infrastructure, qualified staff, and strict quality control.[4]

THE ORIGINS OF THE SUPRANATIONAL REFERENCE LABORATORIES NETWORK

In 1994, the WHO TB Supranational Reference Laboratory Network (SRLN) was created to support the WHO Global Project on anti-TB drug resistance surveillance.[5] This network has extensively collaborated in the standardization of DST through technical support to countries in conducting national drug resistance surveys and ensuring the quality of laboratory testing.[6] Over the last 24 years, the project has systematically collected and analyzed data on drug resistance from 160 countries to enable reliable estimates of the magnitude of drug resistance globally and provide data to inform WHO policy decisions.[1] The reliability of data on drug resistance is, however, dependent on the quality of the DST being performed.

Proficiency testing is a fundamental tool that helps to ensure the accuracy of testing in different laboratories through interlaboratory comparisons of DST results on the same standardized panel of strains that can allow for an assessment of the general performance level of the laboratory's service, and detecting laboratory facilities with unacceptable levels of proficiency. The annual rounds of proficiency testing have provided an objective tool to monitor and improve performance of laboratories performing DST.[6,7] In 1994, there were only a few laboratories worldwide with the technical ability to perform DST for *Mycobacterium tuberculosis* (MTB) reliably or with the appropriate laboratory infrastructure and these were mostly in high-income, low TB burden settings in Europe and the United States. The first 5 rounds of proficiency testing were conducted between 1994 and 1998 and were coordinated through the Laboratory Center for Disease Control, Ottawa, Canada.[8,9] For each of these rounds of proficiency testing, different panels of 10 clinical isolates of MTB in blinded duplicates were sent to each participating laboratory.[9]

During these early rounds, technical difficulties in performing DST were identified and allowed for deficiencies to be corrected. Subsequent rounds have been coordinated through the Institute of Tropical Medicine (ITM) in Antwerp, Belgium. Initially strains were selected from the ITM collection, but in later rounds included strains representing a wider geographic representation and included a total of 30 strains, 10 strains in duplicate and 10 single strains.[6] From round 11 onward, mass culture from a single colony on subculture was used to minimize the risk of including a mixture of different strains or including strains with heteroresistance.[6]

EXPANSION OF THE SUPRANATIONAL REFERENCE LABORATORIES

Between 1994 and 2018, the SRLN was expanded from initial 14 to 32 Supranational Reference Laboratories (SRLs) and 4 National Centers of Excellence (NCE-SRLN), largely driven by regional initiatives and institutional interest in joining the WHO SRLN network (**Fig. 1**). The eligibility and inclusion criteria agreed during a consultation of the SRLN in 2010 required that each of the SRLs had a permanent functional TB laboratory officially recognized by the national health authority of the country and providing a range of laboratory tests for the detection of TB and drug resistance using both culture-based and molecular methods recommended for use by the WHO. It also required a commitment to support at least 2 countries with DST proficiency testing, to provide external quality assessment during drug resistance surveys, provide technical assistance and training on TB laboratory methods and DST as needed (**Box 1**).

In 2015, a new category of laboratory—the National Center of Excellence for the TB Supranational TB Reference Laboratory Network (NCE-SRLN)—was established specifically designed to recognize well performing laboratories in large middle-income countries (Brazil, Russia, India, China and South Africa). A designated NCE-SRLN has an equivalent status as an SRL within the network, but primarily works to build in-country laboratory capacity. Countries with laboratories currently eligible to apply for designation as an NCE-SRLN include Brazil, the Russian Federation, India, China, and South Africa. Four NCE-SRLN have been designated to date: 3 in the Russian Federation (Central Tuberculosis Research Institute in Moscow, the Novosibirsk Tuberculosis Research Institute in Novosibirsk, the Ural Research Institute for Phtysiopulmonology in Yekaterinburg), and the National Institute

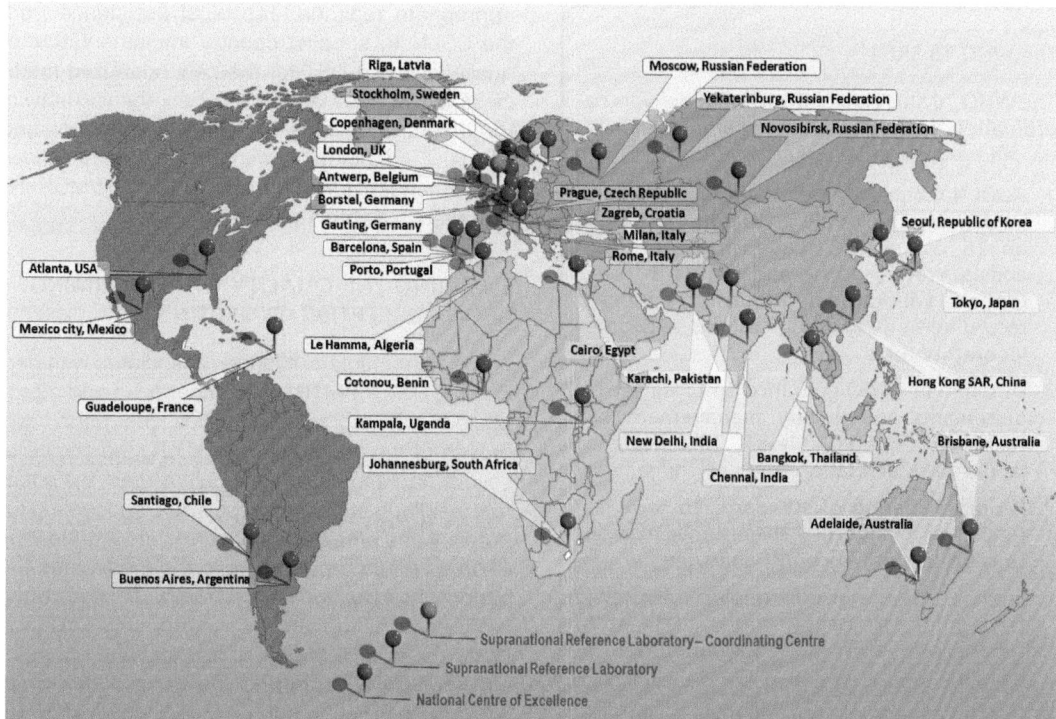

Fig. 1. The WHO TB SRLN as of December 2018.

of TB and Respiratory Diseases in New Delhi, India.

Well-performing TB reference laboratory can be designated an SRL through a mechanism where they are nominated as a candidate SRL to WHO and undergo a period of mentorship before being designated as a full member of the network. The 3 newest members of the SRLN, all on the African continent, were evaluated and designated using this mechanism. SRLs have now been established in Kampala, Uganda, Cotonou, Benin, and Johannesburg, South Africa. All these SRLs have formalized linkages for technical support with national TB reference laboratories in many countries across Africa, including Eastern, Southern, Western, and Central Africa.

VALUE OF THE SUPRANATIONAL REFERENCE LABORATORIES NETWORK

TB laboratory services have changed dramatically over the last 10 years and there is increasing recognition of the importance of reliable diagnosis of TB and drug-resistant TB are driving this change, with the SRLN serving as the backbone for both TB surveillance and diagnosis. Individual SRLs and the network are a great technical resource for laboratory scale-up and capacity development in countries, and provide unique

support to the reliable detection of drug resistance. Each SRL is linked to 1 or more countries with a formal collaboration agreement with the Ministry of Health and these links often reflect a long-standing and respected relationship with a history of multiple technical support events over many years. The SRL therefore represents the preferred technical partner identified by the Ministry of Health to develop national laboratory capacity for TB and strengthen drug-resistant TB surveillance and diagnosis.

The SRLN continues to support the WHO global TB drug resistance surveillance project, often leads the introduction of new TB diagnostics at country level and provides technical leadership to countries in building their laboratory capacity. Sustained and prolonged technical assistance is considered integral to the success of scaled-up laboratory services to support TB and drug-resistant TB treatment programs. SRLs are supporting primarily current drug resistance surveillance and quality assurance of DST activities and have not been sufficiently resourced to assist countries with the expansion of their routine diagnostic services, technology transfer, and implementation of novel, rapid TB diagnostics, external laboratory quality assurance, proficiency testing for DST or training. However, many SRLs have the capacity to provide extended and highly

Box 1
The WHO TB SRLN

The WHO TB SRLN is a platform that delivers co-ordination, identifies synergies among individual SRLs and serves as a platform to:

1. Assist National Reference Laboratories in the implementation of the WHO policy guidance on TB diagnostics, diagnostic algorithms, and laboratory norms and standards using Global Laboratory Initiative endorsed recording and reporting systems and other laboratory tools;

2. Disseminate WHO guidance on biosafety requirements and quality management systems for national level TB reference laboratories and laboratory networks;

3. Facilitate sharing of standardized technical reports from all technical assistance missions to counties with in-country partners;

4. Provide standardized quality assurance testing for microscopy, culture, DST of *M tuberculosis* and molecular methods as needed;

5. Coordinate among individual SRLs comparative evaluations of diagnostic tests and define priorities for evaluation of different as needed;

6. Oversee the pathway for the development of standardized protocols to test drug susceptibility against new and existing anti-TB drugs; and

7. Advocate with national TB programs to help ensure diagnosis and treatment of TB and drug resistant cases are aligned.

specialized technical assistance that no other technical partners or partner organizations can make available. The long-term history of interaction and assistance to the linked countries is an additional facilitating factor.

In 2018, the WHO issued new recommendations[10] that depart from previous approaches to treating MDR/RR-TB. Injectable agents are no longer among the priority medicines when designing longer MDR-TB regimens, with kanamycin and capreomycin not recommended any more. Fully oral regimens should thus become the preferred option for most patients. Three medicines—fluoroquinolones (levofloxacin or moxifloxacin), bedaquiline, and linezolid—are strongly recommended as part of a longer regimen, which is completed with other medicines ranked by a relative balance of benefits and harms. The new update reinforces the need for expanded access to quality DST to better triage the patients to an appropriate regimen. Technical assistance from the SRLN to support country implementation of quality assured DST for the new prioritized medicines will be a key laboratory strengthening activity for 2019 and beyond. Critical concentrations and clinical breakpoint concentrations for medicines recommended for the treatment of RR/MDR-TB are given in **Table 1**.[4]

ENSURING THE QUALITY OF PERFORMING DRUG-SUSCEPTIBILITY TESTING

There are multiple challenges associated with performing DST for MTB in a standardized and reproducible manner, which include the purity and growth of the culture used for DST, the choice of solid or liquid media, the inoculum used, the accurate weighing of pure drug powders accounting for potency, the preparation of correct concentrations of drugs for incorporation into the media, and the period of incubation of the media. To ensure the proficiency of the SRLN in performing DST, the WHO and several technical partners and donor institutions have supported the participation of all SRLs in conducting annual proficiency testing for DST using a well-characterized panel of strains of MTB. This has been a core activity of the SRLN and has contributed to an improved understanding of the strengths and limitations for performing different phenotypic and genotypic DST methods against different anti-TB medicines. The preparation and distribution of these methods have been facilitated each year by WHO over the last 2 decades. Since 1999, the coordinating SRL at ITM in Antwerp, Belgium, has been assigned the responsibility to select strains that are representative of susceptible and resistant TB strains, perform DNA sequencing of gene regions associated with drug resistance, ensure their purity, and prepare standardized panels that are distributed to SRLs and National Reference Laboratories and other reference laboratories in many countries (reaching a maximum distribution to 85 national and other reference laboratories for several years), besides analysis and reporting of the results.[6] Since 2007 (14th round) proficiency testing for second-line anti-TB medicines was incorporated, demonstrating the success of the network in producing a substantial improvement in performance.[7] Good performance in at least 1 recent proficiency testing round in a national reference laboratory is considered a positive indication of the laboratory's capacity for conducting a drug resistance survey, because it provides a minimum guarantee of the local quality of DST. Demonstrated proficiency in performing either genotypic or phenotypic DST methods is

Table 1
Critical concentrations (CC) and clinical breakpoints (CB) for medicines recommended for the treatment of RR-TB and MDR-TB

			CC (µg/mL) for DST by Medium			
Group	Medicine	Abbreviation	Löwenstein–Jensen[a]	Middlebrook 7H10[a]	Middlebrook 7H11[a]	BACTEC MGIT Liquid Culture[a]
Group A	Levofloxacin (CC)	LFX[b,c]	**2.0**	1.0	—	1.0
	Moxifloxacin (CC)	MFX2,3	**1.0**	0.5	0.5	0.25
	Moxifloxacin (CB)[d]		—	2.0	—	1.0
	Bedaquiline[e]	BDQ	—	—	**0.25**	**1.0**
	Linezolid[f]	LZD	—	1.0	1.0	1.0
Group B	Clofazimine	CFZ	—	—	—	**1.0**
	Cycloserine	CS	—	—	—	—
	Terizidone	TZD	—	—	—	—
Group C	Ethambutol[g]	E	2.0	5.0	7.5	5.0
	Delamanid[h]	DLM	—	—	**0.016**	**0.06**
	Pyrazinamide[i]	PZA	—	—	—	100.0
	Imipenem-cilastatin	IMP/CLN	—	—	—	—
	Meropenem	MPM	—	—	—	—
	Amikacin[j]	AMK	30.0	2.0	—	1.0
	(Or streptomycin)	(S)	4.0	2.0	2.0	1.0
	Ethionamide	ETO	40.0	5.0	10.0	5.0
	Prothionamide	PTO	40.0	—	—	2.5
	Para-aminosalicylic acid	PAS	—	—	—	—

Interim CC are highlighted in bold.

[a] The use of the indirect proportion method is recommended. Other methods using solid media (such as the resistance ratio or absolute concentration) have not been adequately validated for anti-TB agents.

[b] Testing of ofloxacin is not recommended because it is no longer used to treat drug-resistant TB and laboratories should transition to testing the specific fluoroquinolones (levofloxacin and moxifloxacin) used in treatment regimens.

[c] Levofloxacin and moxifloxacin interim CCs for Lowenstein-Jensen established despite very limited data.

[d] CB concentration for 7H10 and MGIT apply to high-dose moxifloxacin (ie, 800 mg/d).

[e] No evidence is available on the safety and effectiveness of BDQ beyond 6 months; individual patients who require prolonged use of BDQ will need to be managed according to off-label best practices.

[f] The optimal duration of use of LZD is not established. Use for at least 6 mo was shown to be highly effective, although toxicity may limit use for extended periods of time.

[g] DST not reliable and reproducible. DST is not recommended.

[h] The position of delamanid will be reassessed once individual patient data by Otsuka are available for review. No evidence is available on effectiveness and safety of DLM beyond 6 months; individual patients who require prolonged use of DLM will need to be managed according to off-label best practices.

[i] Pyrazinamide is only counted as an effective agent when DST results confirm susceptibility in a quality-assured laboratory. Its use with BDQ may be synergistic.

[j] Amikacin and streptomycin are only to be considered if DST results confirm susceptibility and high-quality audiology monitoring for hearing loss can be ensured. Streptomycin is to be considered only if amikacin cannot be used and if DST results confirm susceptibility. Streptomycin resistance is not detectable with second-line molecular line probe assays).

essential to assure the reliability of TB programs in the programmatic management of drug-resistant TB.

Performing genotypic methods in addition to phenotypic DST has allowed for improved knowledge regarding the molecular basis of resistance and the correlation with culture-based DST results. The findings from the rounds of proficiency testing have demonstrated a lack of consistency in performing phenotypic DST for ethambutol and streptomycin.[9] The proficiency testing panels have allowed for the recognition of discordant testing between genotypic and phenotypic DST, which is of particular importance for the disputed mutations in *rpo*B gene that have reportedly been associated with poor treatment outcomes.[11]

However, newer or repurposed drugs for the treatment of RR/MDR-TB, such as bedaquiline, linezolid, clofazimine, and delamanid, are recommended for use by the WHO under specific and relevant DST methods need to be incorporated into routine proficiency testing.

TUBERCULOSIS LABORATORY STRENGTHENING TECHNICAL ASSISTANCE

Sustained and prolonged technical assistance is considered integral to the success of scaled-up laboratory services to support TB and drug-resistant TB treatment programs. SRLs are supporting primarily current drug resistance surveillance and quality assurance of DST activities and have not been sufficiently resourced to fully assist countries with the expansion of routine diagnostic services, technology transfer, and the implementation of novel, rapid TB diagnostics, external laboratory quality assurance, or training. However, many SRLs have the capacity to provide extended and highly specialized technical assistance that no other technical partners or partner organizations can make available. The long-term history of interaction, technical partnership, and assistance to the linked countries is an additional facilitating factor. Specific areas of technical assistance required to build laboratory capacity in priority countries are described in **Box 2**.

Box 2
Specific technical assistance provided by the SRLN

- Developing and/or strengthening national TB laboratory strategic plans;

- Strengthening laboratory capacity at central, regional and peripheral levels for TB detection, drug resistance detection and treatment monitoring, including culture, DST and rapid molecular methods;

- In-country hands-on training with the monitoring of performance with implementation of these new tools through quality assurance mechanisms including proficiency testing and follow-up technical assistance visits;

- Strengthening the implementation of laboratory diagnostics by guiding improvements in specimen transport mechanisms, logistics and commodity management and recording and reporting systems;

- Mentoring junior/support consultants to provide technical assistance missions; and

- Assisting reference laboratories implement a quality management system toward accreditation.

DEVELOPMENT OF DRUG-SUSCEPTIBILITY TESTING METHODS FOR NEW DRUGS

In 2018, critical concentrations were revised or established for performing DST for the group of medicines that are strongly recommended to be used in the treatment of RR/MDR-TB. These include the later generation fluoroquinolones (levofloxacin and moxifloxacin), bedaquiline, and linezolid. A critical concentration for the oral core agent clofazimine was established for BACTEC MGIT medium only. Critical concentrations for the group of add-on agents (according to 2018 WHO guidelines) were established or validated for delamanid, amikacin, and pyrazinamide.[12]

The SRLN has the infrastructure, technical resources, and relevant expertise to provide support to validate these new DST methods. Implementing DST for the newer second-line anti-TB medicines should be introduced when proficiency has been demonstrated in performing DST for other anti-TB agents. Therefore, it is necessary to establish and validate high-quality DST procedures. For laboratories in resource-limited countries, this testing is usually done in collaboration with a member of the WHO SRLN. When introducing DST for second-line agents, it is necessary to follow the protocols for test validation and to establish a reproducible procedure (ie, ensure that intertest agreement is ≥95%) before beginning to test clinical isolates and report those results.

A technical manual for the DST of medicines use in the treatment of TB has now been developed that describes the standardized laboratory protocols for performing these tests for both first- and second-line anti-TB medicines.[4] It will now be essential that the proficiency testing panels incorporate strains that can certify the performance of DST against the newer medicines.

CHALLENGES AHEAD FOR THE SUPRANATIONAL REFERENCE LABORATORIES NETWORK

In most countries with a high burden of TB, there is not sufficient capacity for routine susceptibility testing for all patient strains to medicines used for treatment. In these settings, the extent of anti-TB drug resistance is estimated through periodic epidemiologic surveys, which have largely relied on conventional culture and DST by use of phenotypic methods. Drug resistance in MTB is mainly conferred through point mutations in specific gene targets. Next-generation sequencing offers great promise for rapid diagnosis of drug resistance although sequencing data interpretation is complex, and clear rules and criteria are needed to determine the clinical relevance of mutations detected. Sequencing has been shown to be a valuable surveillance tool and can be used to accurately predict drug resistance in low- and middle-income countries.[13] Next-generation sequencing has the potential to overcome the challenges of performing culture based DST methods by providing rapid and detailed sequence information for multiple gene regions associated with drug resistance or whole genomes of interest.[14] In many instances, SRLs are already performing next-generation sequencing for research and surveillance purposes and are well positioned to support country adoption of sequencing platforms in settings with a high burden of TB and drug-resistant TB.

The SRLs can play an important role in elucidating new or novel mechanisms of resistance for the new and repurposed drugs by supporting National Reference Laboratories to store and subsequent sequence strains isolated from persons on treatment with the newer medicines and especially in instances when patients are failing treatment. Both phenotypic and genotypic DST will need to be performed for the foreseeable future until the molecular basis of resistance and the association of specific mutations with increases in minimum inhibitory concentration for different anti-TB medicines are more completely understood and highly specialized technical support for both approaches is needed. Greater investment will be needed in bioinformatics to ensure a standardized interpretation of complex sequence data and allow for improved understanding of presence and frequency of certain mutations and the confidence of their association with drug resistance.

SUMMARY

The WHO TB SRLN has continuously supported the Global Project on Anti-Tuberculosis Drug Resistance Surveillance, which remains the oldest and largest initiative on the surveillance of antimicrobial resistance in the world.[5] It has been integral in building global knowledge around drug-resistant TB and its epidemiology. Funding for the SRLN has become increasingly challenging in recent years. Technical assistance from individual SRLs has been supported by a variety of mechanisms, such as the inclusion of specific laboratory strengthening activities in national and regional Global Fund grants or through direct funding from USAID and Challenge TB. It is essential that support from the SRLN be incorporated as an integral component into country laboratory strengthening plans especially in those with a high burden of RR/MDR-TB.

The timing is also right to expand the activities of the WHO TB SRLN to other diseases and, with adequate financial support, the SRLN could potentially become a resource for antimicrobial resistance surveillance or for surveillance of human immunodeficiency virus drug resistance, thereby contributing to the SDG goals for universal health coverage.

REFERENCES

1. Global tuberculosis report 2018. Geneva (Switzerland): World Health Organization; 2018. WHO/CDSTB/2018.20; Available at: https://www.who.int/tb/publications/global_report/en/. Accessed January 7, 2019.
2. The End TB Strategy: global strategy and targets for tuberculosis prevention, care and control after 2015. Geneva (Switzerland): World Health Organization; 2014. Available at: http://www.who.int/tb/strategy/End_TB_Strategy.pdf. Accessed January 7, 2019.
3. Compendium of WHO guidelines and associated standards: ensuring optimum delivery of the cascade of care for patients with tuberculosis. 2nd edition. Geneva (Switzerland): World Health Organization; 2018. Available at: http://apps.who.int/iris/bitstream/handle/10665/272644/9789241514101-eng.pdf. Accessed January 7, 2019.
4. Technical manual for drug susceptibility testing of medicines used in the treatment of tuberculosis Geneva: World Health Organization. Available at: https://www.who.int/tb/publications/2018/WHO_technical_drug_susceptibility_testing/en/. Accessed January 7, 2019.
5. Zignol M, Dean AS, Falzon D, et al. Twenty years of global surveillance of antituberculosis-drug resistance. N Engl J Med 2016;375(11):1081–9.
6. Van Deun A, Wright A, Zignol M, et al. Drug susceptibility testing proficiency in the network of supranational tuberculosis reference laboratories. Int J Tuberc Lung Dis 2011;5:116–24.
7. Hillemann D, Hoffner S, Cirillo D, et al. First evaluation after implementation of a quality control system for the second line drug susceptibility testing of Mycobacterium tuberculosis joint efforts in low and high incidence countries. PLoS One 2013;8(10): e76765.
8. Laszlo A, Rahman M, Raviglione M, et al. Quality assurance programme for drug susceptibility testing of Mycobacterium tuberculosis in the WHO/IUATLD Network of Supranational Reference Laboratory Network: first round of proficiency testing. Int J Tuberc Lung Dis 1997;1:231–8.
9. Laszlo A, Rahman M, Espinal M, et al. WHO/IUATLD Network of Supranational Reference

Laboratories. Quality assurance programme for drug susceptibility testing of Mycobacterium tuberculosis in the WHO/IUATLD Supranational Reference Laboratory Network: five rounds of proficiency testing, 1994–1998. Int J Tuberc Lung Dis 2002;6:748–56.

10. WHO treatment guidelines for multidrug- and rifampicin-resistant tuberculosis, 2018 update. Geneva (Switzerland): World Health Organization; 2018. Available at: https://www.who.int/tb/publications/2018/WHO.2018.MDR-TB.Rx.Guidelines.prefinal.text.pdf. Accessed January 7, 2019.

11. Van Deun A, Aung K, Bola V, et al. Rifampin drug resistance tests for tuberculosis: challenging the gold standard. J Clin Microbiol 2013;51(8):2633–40.

12. Technical report on critical concentrations for drug susceptibility testing of medicines used in the treatment of drug-resistant tuberculosis. Geneva (Switzerland): World Health Organization; 2018. Available at: http://apps.who.int/iris/bitstream/10665/260470/1/WHO-CDS-TB-2018.5-eng.pdf. Accessed January 7, 2019.

13. Zignol M, Cabibbe AM, Dean AS, et al. Genetic sequencing for surveillance of drug resistance in tuberculosis in highly endemic countries: a multi-country population-based surveillance study. Lancet Infect Dis 2018;18(6):675–83. https://doi.org/10.1016/S1473-3099(18)30073-2.

14. The use of next-generation sequencing technologies for the detection of mutations associated with drug resistance in Mycobacterium tuberculosis complex: technical guide. Geneva (Switzerland): World Health Organization; 2018. Available at: http://apps.who.int/iris/bitstream/handle/10665/274443/WHO-CDS-TB-2018.19-eng.pdf. Accessed January 7, 2019.

Treatment of Drug-Susceptible Tuberculosis

Beth Shoshana Zha, MD, PhD[a], Payam Nahid, MD, MPH[b],*

KEYWORDS

- Drug-susceptible *Mycobacterium tuberculosis* • *Mycobacterium tuberculosis* treatment regimen
- HIV and *Mycobacterium tuberculosis* co-infection
- *M tuberculosis* treatment supervision and patient-centered care

KEY POINTS

- *Mycobacterium tuberculosis* (tuberculosis) infection is a major public health concern and requires prompt treatment of identified patients to avoid ongoing transmission.
- Empiric treatment with a preferred regimen of isoniazid, rifampin, ethambutol, and pyrazinamide should be initiated for all patients with probable disease.
- Extrapulmonary tuberculosis disease is often treated similarly to pulmonary disease.
- All patients with treatment failure, relapse, or recurrence should have retreatment initiated under direct observation.
- Patients with human immunodeficiency virus infection and tuberculosis not currently on treatment should be started on antiretroviral therapy within 8 weeks of starting the tuberculosis regimen, unless the patient is diagnosed with tuberculosis meningitis.

INTRODUCTION

Mycobacterium tuberculosis (TB) remains the world's deadliest infectious disease and a tremendous public health concern. The goals of treatment include both curing the individual patient and protecting the community from ongoing TB transmission. To achieve durable cure, regimens must include multiple agents given concurrently and in a manner to ensure completion of therapy. This article focuses on summarizing the current guidelines by the American Thoracic Society, Centers for Disease Control and Prevention, and Infectious Diseases Society of America (ATS/CDC/IDSA) and World Health Organization (WHO) for the treatment of drug-susceptible TB.

DECISION TO TREAT

Patients with confirmed TB disease must be initiated on effective therapy as promptly as possible. However, clinical decision making is complicated when disease is suspected but unconfirmed. More frequently than not, empiric therapy should be started in patients suspected of having TB disease because delays in initiation of treatment have been associated with poor outcomes.[1,2] Strong factors favoring initiation include patients with a high risk of progression of disease (ie, immunosuppression), life-threatening illness, and those residing in high transmission risk settings (**Fig. 1**).[3] Once treatment is initiated, the results of additional diagnostics can help to inform whether to discontinue empiric therapy. Rapid

Disclosure Statement: None.
[a] Department of Pulmonary, Critical Care, Allergy and Sleep Medicine, University of California, San Francisco, Box 0111, 513 Parnassus Avenue, San Francisco, CA 94117, USA; [b] Department of Pulmonary, Critical Care, Allergy and Sleep Medicine, University of California, San Francisco, Box 0841 MD, 1001 Potrero Avenue, 5J6, San Francisco, CA 94110, USA
* Corresponding author.
E-mail address: pnahid@ucsf.edu

Clin Chest Med 40 (2019) 763–774
https://doi.org/10.1016/j.ccm.2019.07.006
0272-5231/19/© 2019 Elsevier Inc. All rights reserved.

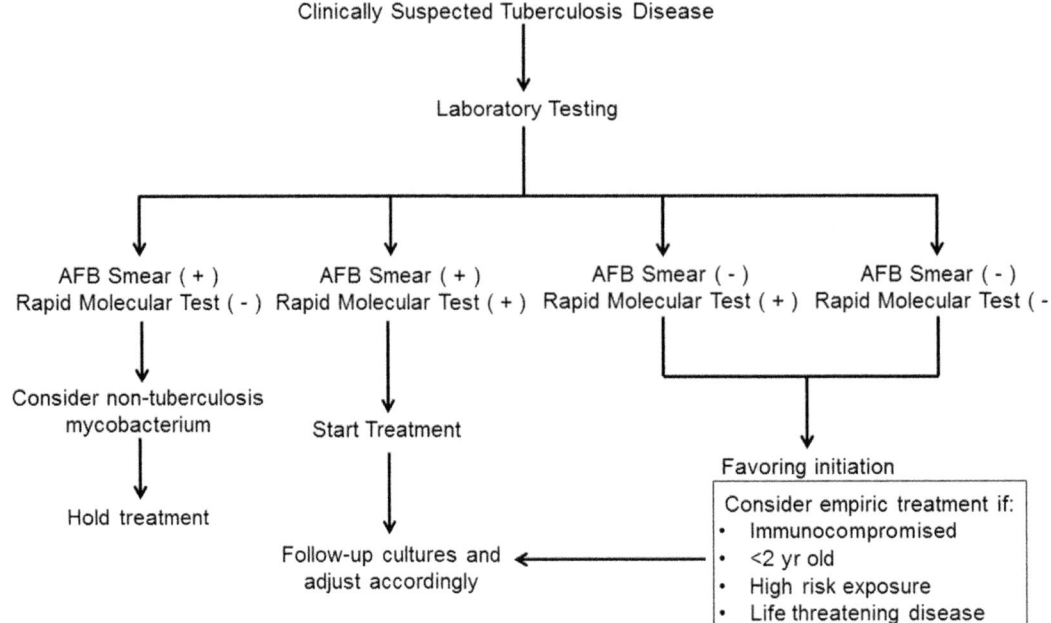

Clinically Suspected Tuberculosis Disease

↓

Laboratory Testing

| AFB Smear (+) | AFB Smear (+) | AFB Smear (-) | AFB Smear (-) |
| Rapid Molecular Test (-) | Rapid Molecular Test (+) | Rapid Molecular Test (+) | Rapid Molecular Test (-) |

Consider non-tuberculosis mycobacterium

↓

Hold treatment

Start Treatment

↓

Follow-up cultures and adjust accordingly

Favoring initiation

Consider empiric treatment if:
- Immunocompromised
- <2 yr old
- High risk exposure
- Life threatening disease

Fig. 1. Decision tree to initiate TB treatment. Flow diagram when to initiate therapy based on laboratory data. Strong indicators for initiation of empiric therapy are listed in bottom right panel. AFB, acid-fast bacilli.

molecular testing should be used whenever feasible[4,5] as molecular testing can identify TB in 50% to 80% of AFB smear-negative samples before culture positivity, significantly shortening time to diagnosis[4,6] (See Akos Somoskovi and Max Salfinger's article, "How Can the Tuberculosis Laboratory Aid in the Patient-Centered Diagnosis and Management of Tuberculosis?," in this issue).

Continuing empiric therapy depends on many factors, including clinical course, radiographic improvement, and whether TB is isolated through culture or molecular techniques. If the diagnosis is confirmed, a full treatment course is completed. However, if cultures or molecular assays are negative, or the patient does not improve on empiric therapies, alternative diagnosis must be considered. Culture-negative disease is not an uncommon phenomenon, representing disease phenotypes that have low bacillary burden, antibiotic use before obtaining samples, and issues in the processing of the sample that adversely affect yield of culture systems. Therefore, if there is clinical or radiographic evidence of improvement with empiric therapy, treatment may be completed even in the absence of isolating a pathogen. When there remains a strong suspicion of TB despite a lack of improvement or uncertainty of the diagnosis, practitioners should seek consultation with a TB expert through public health department TB control programs, referral to 1 of

the 4 CDC-supported TB Centers of Excellence (https://www.cdc.gov/tb/education/tb_coe) in the United States, or the electronic Consilium by the WHO/European Respiratory Society (www.tbconsilium.org).

If a patient is not felt to have active TB disease but has a positive tuberculosis test via interferon gamma release assay or purified protein derivative-tuberculosis skin test (PPD-TST), they should be treated for latent-TB infection. Multiple options for treatment of latent-TB exist, as discussed in Elisa H. Ignatius and Kelly E. Dooley's article, "New Drugs for the Treatment of Tuberculosis," in this issue, but of note, completion of the intensive phase of a drug-sensitive TB regimen usually suffices.

TREATMENT REGIMENS
Preferred Regimen

In drug-susceptible TB disease, the preferred regimen has remained unchanged since the 1970s. There are 2 phases of the regimen: intensive and continuation. The intensive phase is once daily 4-drug therapy for 2 months and allows for the rapid reduction of bacillary burden,[7] while the continuation phase is 2-drug therapy for 4 months required for complete sterilization and cure.[8,9] Although effective, this regimen is hampered by pill burden, prolonged duration, and numerous side effects that complicate patient and provider efforts to complete regimens or take medications consistently, increasing risks for failure, relapse, and the emergence of drug-resistant organisms.

In most cases, drug susceptibility is unknown at the time of therapy initiation. Unless there is identifiable risk of drug resistant organisms (eg, case contact with proven drug-resistant disease), patients can be empirically started on a drug-susceptible regimen with isoniazid (INH), rifampin (RIF), ethambutol (EMB), and pyrazinamide (PZA) while laboratory data are pending (**Tables 1** and **2**). This approach is particularly warranted in epidemiologic settings where there is a low proportion of drug resistant disease. Moreover, the decreased efficacy and increased toxicities of regimens aimed at resistant organisms limit their broad empiric use unless there is a risk for drug resistance (**Table 3**).[3,10] When drug resistance is suspected, an expanded empiric regimen should be prescribed to include INH, RIF, EMB, PZA, as well as a fluoroquinolone, injectable agent, or second-line multidrug resistant therapeutic while awaiting definitive drug susceptibility results (See Moises A. Huaman and Timothy R. Sterling's article, "Treatment of Latent Tuberculosis Infection – An Update," in this issue).

Each drug in the intensive phase regimen has a unique contribution to overall efficacy. By inhibiting cell wall production, INH has a remarkable bactericidal action on actively replicating bacilli[11] but leaves behind persistors. Conversely, PZA targets persistors, partially understood by altering intracellular pH.[12] RIF inhibits transcription and demonstrates exposure-dependent killing, which enhances sterilization.[13] The principle role of EMB is to protect against additional acquisition of resistance in the setting in which there is unrecognized monoresistance to INH by also acting at the cell wall.[14,15] However, EMB carries significant dose-dependent risks of visual changes and loss of color differentiation, and current practice in the United States is to discontinue EMB as soon as susceptibility to INH, RIF, and PZA is confirmed.

A continuation phase of 4 months is needed for multiple putative reasons, including the slow life cycle of TB,[16] the ability for bacilli to remain metabolically inactive,[9] and the accumulation of drug needed at the location of infection.[17,18] The recommended 4 months of continuation phase is therefore not exact. Therapy often needs to be extended in cavitary disease and those with a delay in culture conversion after the intensive phase.[3] Contemporary treatment duration shortening trials have identified characteristics in which shorter regimens are sufficient for cure, including low bacillary burden and lack of cavitation.[19] Further research is needed to select duration of treatment with greater precision than the current approach of one-size-fits-all regimens.

Alternative Composition

When intolerance or monoresistance is found, alternative regimens that can be considered include[3]:

- PZA cannot be used – use a 3-drug regimen with INH, RIF, and EMB during the intensive phase and extend the continuation phase to 7 months.

Table 1
Preferred treatment regimens for drug-susceptible TB

Regimen	1	2	3	4
Intensive phase	INH, RIF, EMB, PZA			
8 weeks	Daily (56 doses) or 5 d a week (40 doses)	Daily (56 doses) or 5 d a week (40 doses)	Thrice weekly (24 doses)	Daily for 14 doses then twice weekly for 12 doses
Continuation phase	INH, RIF			
18 Weeks	Daily (126 doses) or 5 d a week (90 doses)	Thrice weekly (54 doses)	Thrice weekly (54 doses)	Twice weekly (36 doses)
Notes	Preferred regimen	Consider if more frequent DOT is problematic	Use with caution in HIV co-infected patients or cavitary disease	Do not use in HIV co-infected patients or cavitary disease

Preferred regimen is daily dosing throughout, however, to accommodate systematic and patient barriers, other dosing regimens can be considered.
Abbreviation: DOT, directly observed therapy.

Table 2
Dosing of preferred treatment agents and rifamycin substitutes

Agent	Frequency	Adult Dose	Creatinine Clearance <30 mL/min	Pediatric Dose
INH	Daily	300 mg	No adjustment	10–15 mg/kg
	Intermittent	900 mg		20–30 mg/kg
RIF	Daily	600 mg	No adjustment	10–20 mg/kg
	Intermittent	600 mg		10–20 mg/kg
EMB[a]	Daily	800, 1200, 1600 mg	20–25 mg/kg three times weekly	20 mg/kg
	Intermittent	1200, 2000, 2400 mg[b] 2000, 2800, 4000 mg[c]		50 mg/kg
PZA[a]	Daily	1000, 1500, 2000 mg	25–35 mg/kg three times weekly	35 mg/kg
	Intermittent	1500, 2500, 3000 mg[b] 2000, 3000, 4000 mg[c]		50 mg/kg
Rifabutin	Daily	300 mg	No adjustment	Unknown, ~5 mg/kg
	Intermittent	Not recommended		Not recommended
Rifapentine	Weekly	10–20 mg/kg	No adjustment	10–20 mg/kg Not for <12 yo

Doses given are clarified according to daily or intermittent dosing frequency.
Abbreviation: YO, years old.
[a] EMB and PZA are weight stratified in 40 to 55, 56 to 75, and 76 to 90 kg groups.
[b] Thrice weekly dosing.
[c] Twice weekly dosing.

- EMB cannot be used – substitute with a fluoroquinolone and retain duration of therapy (4-month fluoroquinolone regimens are inferior to the standard 6-month regimen).[20–22]
- INH cannot be used – regimen remains controversial, with most experts using 6 months of EMB, RIF, and PZA with or without a fluoroquinolone.[3,10] Variations in the duration of components of the regimen[23] and novel regimens are also being considered.[22]

Patient-Centered Care and Supervision

Ensuring adherence to therapy is equally essential to prescribing the correct regimen. Lapses in treatment can lead to a lack of rapid decrease in bacillary burden and acquisition of drug resistance, placing both patient and the wider community at risk. To improve treatment investment, patient-centered approaches are key to the management of TB disease[24] and emphasized in the ATS/CDC/IDSA and WHO guidelines.

Patient-centered care empowers the patient by facilitating the incorporation of needs, including access barriers and quality of life.[25] In the United States, this issue is best addressed by formulating an individualized care plan with input from the patient, care providers, and an assigned case manager.[26] One major focus is the route of administration being either directly observed therapy (DOT) or self-administered therapy (SAT). The current ATS/CDC/IDSA guidelines support the use of DOT, whereas the

Table 3
Risk factors for drug-resistant TB disease: when to consider an expanded regimen

Factor	Medium Risk	High Risk
Environment	Reside or emigrated from drug-resistant prevalent area	Household contact with proven drug-resistant disease
Patient characteristics	Limited respiratory reserve Central nervous system involvement	Impaired immunity and worsening clinical disease
Previous treatment	Interruption or relapse	Treatment failure Use of second-line drugs

Data from Refs.[3,87,88]

WHO guidelines remain equivocal as there is currently low supportive evidence, largely owing to inability to study and confirm efficacy in any meaningful randomized trial.[27] Populations with the most benefit of DOT include those with human immunodeficiency virus infection (HIV) co-infection and those with previous treatment interruptions.[28–30] The decision to use DOT should be made in concert with the patient, with the use of mobile messaging and video observation considered when appropriate.[31–33]

Drug Dosing

The frequency of dosing is largely determined by the method of administration. For any patient undergoing SAT, it is recommended all medications are prescribed for daily dosing throughout treatment to prevent confusion and mixed administration. Historically when undergoing DOT, dosing 5 days per week was viewed as noninferior to 7 days per week. In fact, current ATS/IDSA/CDC guidelines include this grade of intermittent dosing as an option.[3] Although there are no randomized trials comparing 5 versus 7 day a week dosing, analysis of individual participant datasets from 3 recent trials demonstrated an increase in unfavorable outcomes (including death, treatment failure, and recurrence) in any regimen with less than 7 day a week dosing.[19] In fact, missing just 1 in 10 doses significantly increased risk. When daily dosing is simply not feasible in the setting of DOT, some programs even use thrice weekly dosing during the continuation phase in non–HIV-infected patients with noncavitary disease,[34] but with these new data such a regimen should be used with caution and never used in HIV-infected patients or those with cavitary disease.[35,36]

Monitoring Outcomes

Monitoring response to treatment is essential to ensure rapid bacillary clearance, verify diagnosis, and ensure there is no development of drug resistance. In pulmonary disease, sputum samples are generally collected at least monthly until 2 consecutive cultures are negative. To determine the time of conversion even more accurately, some experts obtain samples every 2 weeks. Such detail is desired to understand if the continuation phase should be extended, as conversion by the end of the intensive phase correlates with risk of relapse.[26,37] Reasons to extend the continuation phase include[26,38–40]:

- Positive culture at 2 months and cavitation on initial chest radiograph

- Positive culture at 2 months or cavitation on initial chest radiograph plus one of the following:
  - Greater than 10% below ideal body weight
  - Active smoker
  - Diabetes mellitus
  - HIV co-infection or another immunosuppressive condition
  - Extensive disease on initial imaging

Repeat imaging can also be helpful in following treatment response, but it is not viewed as essential. The most useful times to obtain imaging is paucibacillary tuberculosis to ensure improvement before ending therapy[41] and spinal disease.[42] If symptoms are persistent, imaging should also be obtained to ensure a concurrent disease process is not occurring. That being said, many programs obtain an end of treatment chest radiograph to establish a baseline for the patient should they re-present.

Interruptions in Therapy

Interruption in TB treatment is a common occurrence, with etiologies including drug side effects, feeling improved on therapy with subsequent nonadherence, the complexities of substance abuse, and the patient-experienced costs of prolonged treatment, among other reasons.[43,44] The decision on how to restart therapy depends on when and how long the interruption occurred. If treatment is stopped for less than 2 weeks, most experts resume the regimen from when it was interrupted. However, if the lapse is more than 2 weeks in the first month of therapy or more than 1 month thereafter, most experts restart a full course of therapy. Lapses of 2 to 4 weeks in duration after the first month of therapy require a sputum smear, cultures, and more thorough workup to determine the next best step (**Table 4**). In all circumstances, most experts implement DOT to enhance likelihood of successfully completing treatment.

Failure and Recurrence

In patients in whom slow treatment response or failure is suspected, the etiology must be investigated promptly to direct subsequent medical management (**Table 5**). Specific definitions need to first be understood in narrowing the cause:

- Slow response: cultures remain positive after complete dosing for the intensive phase
- Treatment failure: cultures are positive at 4 months (United States) or 5 months (Europe/WHO) after initiation of therapy

Table 4
Managing treatment interruptions in new patients

Treatment Length Before Interruption	Length of Interruption	Next Step	Notes
<4 wk	<14 d >14 d	Resume Restart	If >8 wk of lapse, obtain sensitivity testing
4–8 wk	<14 d 14–28 d >28 d	Resume Smear negative = resume Smear positive = restart Restart	Perform sensitivity testing if smear positive or >28 d of interruption
>8 wk	<14 d 14–28 d >28 d	Resume Smear negative = resume Smear positive = restart Restart	Perform sensitivity testing if smear positive or >28 d of interruption

- Recurrence: cultures were stably negative at the end of continuation phase but return positive after discontinuation of therapy
- Relapse: recurrence by the same strain confirmed by genotyping,[23] as opposed to new infection

Treatment adherence and insufficient drug exposure can underlie these issues. Beyond discussing with patients the importance of adherence, providers should enquire about other drugs that may result in drug–drug interactions (DDIs), as well as evaluating for signs of malabsorption issues such as short gut syndrome, chronic diarrhea, or gastroparesis. Therapeutic drug monitoring can help to determine if a low drug concentration underlies the poor response. To determine the maximum serum concentration, drug levels are taken at time of dosing and at 2 and 6 hours after the medication is ingested in a fasting state. Dosing is subsequently adjusted by an expert, although this is currently imprecise.[45–47] In addition to slow responders and recurrence, therapeutic drug monitoring can also be considered earlier in the treatment course in patients taking antiretroviral therapy (ART) owing to DDIs, on second-line therapeutics given unclear pharmacokinetics, and possibly in diabetes mellitus[48] and other comorbidities.[49] However, therapeutic drug monitoring is not recommended for the general

Table 5
Key factors associated with poor TB treatment outcomes

Category	Attribute	Potential Adverse Events
Bacteria characteristics	Drug tolerance	Drug resistance
Genetic factors	Metabolism and pharmacokinetics	Decreased drug concentration Increased side effects
Microbiologic data	Baseline colony forming units Culture positivity after intensive phase	Slow response Relapse
Patient characteristics	Age Alcohol use Comorbid conditions Immunologic factors Nutritional status	Relapse Therapy interruption
Programmatic issues	Dosing frequency Patient support Regimen adherence	Drug resistance Relapse
Radiographic findings	Cavitary disease Extensive Disease	Slow response Relapse
Regimen Factors	Bactericidal and Sterilizing Potency Duration of therapy Synergy and antagonism	Treatment failure

population given unclear precise goal drug levels in those with adequate clinical response[45] and a global lack of testing on programmatic scales.[50]

When a regimen is demonstrating evidence of failure and the patient is on SAT, DOT should be initiated because studies show that there is a higher rate of resistance in the setting of SAT.[51,52] Of critical importance, providers should not add a single agent to a failing regimen,[53] but rather adjust the therapy with multiple agent modifications while repeat drug susceptibility tests are pending.

TREATMENT IN SPECIAL POPULATIONS
HIV Infection

HIV–TB co-infection complicates treatment regimens owing to DDIs, cost, and programmatic challenges. Fortunately, successful cure in HIV patients on ART is similar to the rate of non–HIV-infected individuals.[54] For those not on ART at time of the TB diagnosis, several randomized clinical trials have conclusively addressed to start ART early, demonstrating a higher rate of mortality when initiation of ART therapy is postponed.[55–58]

The mortality benefit of earlier initiation of ART significantly outweighs any risk of starting therapy concurrently, the major of which is immune reconstitution inflammatory syndrome (IRIS).[58–61] Current guidelines recommend starting ART within 8 weeks of TB treatment initiation,[3,10] and if the CD4 count is less than 50 cells/μL, initiating within 2 weeks because the greatest mortality benefit is noted in this subpopulation.[62] The exception is in TB–meningitis co-infection, for which ART should be delayed by 8 weeks owing to higher consequences of IRIS in central nervous system disease. That being said, although an overall mortality benefit is noted with earlier initiation of ART, the risk of IRIS is doubled regardless of CD4 count.[63] One recent randomized controlled trial has demonstrated a significant decrease in the risk of TB-associated IRIS when given low-dose prednisone for the first month of ART initiation.[64] Hopefully, the potential benefit of concurrent use of steroids with early initiation of ART will be addressed in coming guidelines.

Other recommendations to consider in the HIV–TB co-infected patient are:

- RIF has DDIs with many ART drugs owing to its induction of the cytochrome P450 family of enzymes.[64] Rifabutin is a less potent inducer of cytochrome P450 enzymes and should be considered as a substitute of RIF. Appropriate dose adjustments when

concurrently prescribing ART and TB therapy can be found through the CDC and the US Food and Drug Administration.
- The continuation phase should be extended for an additional 3 months in those not on ART owing to risk of recurrence and reinfection.[65,66]
- Intermittent dosing should not be prescribed to HIV–TB co-infected patients because there is an unacceptably high rate of failure at any phase of therapy.[52,67]
- Co-trimoxazole prophylaxis should be prescribed for all patients especially with CD4 counts of less than 200 cells/μL.[68,69]

Pregnant, Breastfeeding, and Pediatric Patients

Prompt diagnosis and treatment of TB in pregnant patients is essential to reduce the risk of complications to the child. Fortunately, all 4 first-line TB drugs are considered safe in pregnancy.[70–72] Of note, in the United States some providers exclude PZA in the regimen owing to a lack of studies on fetal malformations. However, its use is recommended by the WHO, and it is recommended by experts to be included in the regimen.[10] Breastfeeding should also not be discouraged or interrupted while on TB therapy, because drug concentrations in breast milk are small and no evidence has emerged of toxic effects to infants for the first-line drugs.[73]

In children, the diagnosis of TB is challenging. Children commonly develop primary disease characterized by intrathoracic lymphadenopathy with or without lung opacities,[74] rather than the characteristic upper lobe opacities and cavitation seen in adults. Such paucibacillary phenotypes of TB disease decreases the ability to obtain adequate samples and the yield of existing diagnostic assays.[75] In part because of the poor performance of currently available diagnostic tools in children, when TB is suspected empiric treatment should be started as the disease can rapidly disseminate. Because children are usually secondary cases in a household or other contact investigation, the composition of the treatment regimen can be determined based on the drug susceptibilities of the presumed source case. However, if resistance is suspected or no case identified, obtaining direct culture data from the patient is extremely important. This task can be approached by gastric lavage, sputum induction, bronchoalveolar lavage, or even tissue biopsy.

There is no difference of the preferred regimen for children in either pulmonary or extrapulmonary drug-susceptible disease.[75,76] However, it is difficult for young children to receive eye examinations to monitor for EMB toxicity, and therefore some clinicians use a 3-drug intensive phase regimen for 3 months (INH, RIF, PZA) to avoid EMB in low-risk patients. Drug tolerance must be monitored closely no matter which regimen is chosen.

Monitoring the success of therapy in children is also challenging. Weight gain and monitoring of developmental benchmarks can be informative, but these parameters should not be used in isolation for modifications to the prescribed regimen. Rather, most providers use a combination of clinical and radiographic findings, as well as obtaining additional cultures whenever feasible.

EXTRAPULMONARY DISEASE

Regimens for extrapulmonary disease do not differ significantly from standard pulmonary treatment. In drug-susceptible disease, there is no difference in the intensive phase. The continuation phase can be extended up to 9 months if deemed necessary, but 6 months is often determined adequate. The one exception is meningitis, for which therapy is extended given the less than ideal blood–brain barrier penetrance and drug accumulation confounded with a high risk of relapse.[77,78]

There are no randomized controlled trials investigating the use of intermittent dosing in extrapulmonary TB, and therefore daily therapy is the only recommended regimen at this time. Unless concurrent pulmonary disease exists, response to treatment should be followed on clinical and radiologic findings rather than repeat specimen sampling.

Key notes about specific extrapulmonary diseases include:

- Meningitis: TB meningitis has a high morbidity and mortality, making this entity the most worrisome extrapulmonary infection. Although the exact duration of the continuation phase is not yet determined, current recommendations are at least 7 months. In addition, corticosteroids should be given upfront for 6 to 8 weeks.[77–80]
- Lymphadenitis: excision is not indicated, but consider aspiration if the node is fluctuant or otherwise worrisome.
- Bone, joint, and spine: owing to difficulties of repeat sampling to rule out cure, most practitioners extend the total regimen to 9 months, and 12 months if hardware is involved. Surgery should be considered only if there is a

poor response to therapy, or vertebral compression or spinal instability is present.[81,82]
- Pericardial tuberculosis: the need for corticosteroid use remains unclear and the routine use of steroids in all patients is not recommended in the current guidelines.[83]
- Pleura: if an empyema forms, it should be drained.
- Disseminated infection: despite more complex disease, 6-month therapy is still recommended.
- Genitourinary: surgery is indicated if an obstruction is leading to renal injury. Of note, dose adjustments will be needed if renal dysfunction is present.
- Abdominal: clinicians should keep a high index of suspicion for infection in the abdomen because there are often nonspecific presentations and no clear findings on imaging/examinations.[84]

ADVERSE EFFECTS

The most common, and often limiting, side effects of antituberculosis agents are gastrointestinal. However, there are many more potential and significant adverse effects, and therefore patients must be monitored frequently. The most common adverse events are listed in **Table 6**.

One of the most worrisome of these is hepatotoxicity, defined as an alanine aminotransferase of 3 or more times the upper limit of normal with hepatitis symptoms, or 5 or more times the upper limit of normal without symptoms.[85] When present, all hepatotoxic agents should be stopped immediately, and other causes of abnormal liver function tests, such as viral hepatitis, alcohol use, herbal/dietary supplements, and biliary tract disease, should be ruled out. Once the alanine aminotransferase is less than 2 times upper limit of normal or near baseline, medications can be restarted individually (preferably RIF, INH, then PZA in increment intervals of 1 week).

Rash is a significant side effect of TB drugs.[86] More serious reactions include a petechial rash with thrombocytopenia from RIF, Stevens-Johnson syndrome, toxic epidermal necrosis, eosinophilia with systemic symptoms, and drug hypersensitivity syndrome. In thrombocytopenia by a rifamycin, the agent cannot be reintroduced. For most other reactions, a repeat challenge with close monitoring can be considered, but permanently stop the agent if the reaction occurs again.

Table 6
Adverse events of preferred regimen agents

Adverse Effect	Potential Agent	Recommended Testing	Interventions
Cutaneous reactions	All	Complete blood count	See text
Drug fever	All	Rule out other infection	Hold drugs until fever resolves Restart individually every 2–3 d
Gastrointestinal upset	All	Liver function testing	Take pills with snack Split dosing Proton pump inhibitor
Gouty arthritis flare	PZA		Consider drug substitution in patient with history of severe gout
Hepatotoxicity	INH PZA RIF	Liver function testing Viral hepatitis panel	Hold drugs until resolving Resume individually in 1 wk increments (see text)
Lupus-like syndrome	INH	Antinuclear antibodies Double strand DNA	Discontinue INH
Orange body fluids	RIF		Warn patient Consider avoiding contact lenses
Optic neuritis	EMB INH (rare)	Visual acuity Color discrimination	Stop EMB If no improvement, hold INH
Peripheral neuropathy	INH		Pyridoxine 25–50 mg/d prophylaxis 100 mg/d treatment
Polyarthralgia	PZA		Nonsteroidal anti-inflammatory

Listed are major known side effects of first-line agents and potential interventions if they occur.

SUMMARY AND FUTURE DIRECTIONS

When there is a suspicion for TB disease, an empiric preferred 4-drug regimen should be initiated without awaiting definitive results of diagnostic studies. Patient-centered approaches should be used to enhance the likelihood of completion and achieving durable cure. A significant research focus in TB therapeutics remains the shortening of regimens through the use of new chemical entities and optimizing drug dosing. Although novel drugs with new mechanisms of action are being evaluated, for now the 6-month 4-drug regimen of INH, RIF, PZA, and EMB administered daily achieves high rates of cure despite its numerous shortcomings and remains the current standard of care for drug-susceptible TB in the United States and worldwide.

REFERENCES

1. Asres A, Jerene D, Deressa W. Delays to treatment initiation is associated with tuberculosis treatment outcomes among patients on directly observed treatment short course in Southwest Ethiopia: a follow-up study. BMC Pulm Med 2018;18(1). https://doi.org/10.1186/s12890-018-0628-2.

2. Virenfeldt J, Rudolf F, Camara C, et al. Treatment delay affects clinical severity of tuberculosis: a longitudinal cohort study. BMJ Open 2014;4(6): e004818.

3. Nahid P, Dorman SE, Alipanah N, et al. Executive summary: official American Thoracic Society/Centers for Disease Control and Prevention/Infectious Diseases Society of America clinical practice guidelines: treatment of drug-susceptible tuberculosis. Clin Infect Dis 2016;63(7):853–67.

4. Guerra RL, Hooper NM, Baker JF, et al. Use of the amplified Mycobacterium tuberculosis direct test in a public health laboratory: test performance and impact on clinical care. Chest 2007; 132(3):946–51.

5. Centers for Disease Control and Prevention (CDC). Updated guidelines for the use of nucleic acid amplification tests in the diagnosis of tuberculosis. MMWR Morb Mortal Wkly Rep 2009;58:7–10.

6. Moore DF, Guzman JA, Mikhail LT. Reduction in turn-around time for laboratory diagnosis of pulmonary tuberculosis by routine use of a nucleic acid amplification test. Diagn Microbiol Infect Dis 2005;52(3): 247–54.

7. Diacon AH, Donald PR. The early bactericidal activity of antituberculosis drugs. Expert Rev Anti Infect Ther 2014;12(2):223–37.

8. Connolly LE, Edelstein PH, Ramakrishnan L. Why is long-term therapy required to cure tuberculosis? PLoS Med 2007;4(3):e120.

9. Mitchison DA. The diagnosis and therapy of tuberculosis during the past 100 years. Am J Respir Crit Care Med 2005;171(7):699–706.

10. World Health Organization. Guidelines for treatment of drug-susceptible tuberculosis and patient care. Switzerland: World Health Organization; 2017.

11. Global Alliance for TB Drug Development. Isoniazid. Tuberculosis 2008;88(2):112–6.

12. Global Alliance for TB Drug Development. Pyrazinamide. Tuberculosis 2008;88(2):141–4.

13. Global Alliance for TB Drug Development. Rifampin. Tuberculosis 2008;88(2):151–4. Available at: http://www.cdc.gov/mmwR/preview/.

14. Global Alliance for TB Drug Development. Ethambutol. Tuberculosis 2008;88(2):102–5.

15. Sarkar S, Suresh MR. An overview of tuberculosis chemotherapy-a literature review. J Pharm Pharm Sci 2011;14:148–61. Available at: www.cspsCanada.org.

16. Koul A, Arnoult E, Lounis N, et al. The challenge of new drug discovery for tuberculosis. Nature 2011; 469(7331):483–90.

17. Cazzola M, Blasi F, Terzano C, et al. Delivering antibacterials to the lungs. Am J Respir Med 2002;1(4):261–72.

18. Chiu LM, Amsden GW. Intrapulmonary pharmacokinetics of antibacterial agents. Am J Respir Med 2002;1(3):201–9.

19. Imperial MZ, Nahid P, Phillips PPJ, et al. A patient-level pooled analysis of treatment-shortening regimens for drug-susceptible pulmonary tuberculosis. Nat Med 2018;24(11):1708–15.

20. Merle CS, Fielding K, Sow OB, et al. A four-month gatifloxacin-containing regimen for treating tuberculosis. N Engl J Med 2014;371(17):1588–98.

21. Gillespie SH, Crook AM, McHugh TD, et al. Four-month moxifloxacin-based regimens for drug-sensitive tuberculosis. N Engl J Med 2014;371(17):1577–87.

22. Jindani A, Harrison TS, Nunn AJ, et al. High-dose rifapentine with moxifloxacin for pulmonary tuberculosis. N Engl J Med 2014;371(17):1599–608.

23. Center for Disease Control Advisory Group on Tuberculosis Genotyping NTCA. Guide to the application of genotyping to tuberculosis prevention and control handbook for TB controllers, epidemiologists, laboratorians, and other program staff 2004. Atlanta (GA). Available at: https://www.cdc.gov:443/tb/programs/genotyping/manual/htm.

24. Hopewell PC, Fair EL, Uplekar M. Updating the international standards for tuberculosis care: entering the era of molecular diagnostics. Ann Am Thorac Soc 2014;11(3):286–95.

25. The TB Control Assistance Program. Patient centered approach strategy 2010. Available at: https://www.challengetb.org/?s=Patient+Centered+Approach+Strategy&category_name=tool.

26. McLaren ZM, Milliken AA, Meyer AJ, et al. Does directly observed therapy improve tuberculosis treatment? More evidence is needed to guide tuberculosis policy. BMC Infect Dis 2016;16(1). https://doi.org/10.1186/s12879-016-1862-y.

27. Reis-Santos B, Pellacani-Posses I, Macedo LR, et al. Directly observed therapy of tuberculosis in Brazil: associated determinants and impact on treatment outcome. Int J Tuberc Lung Dis 2015;19(10):1188–93.

28. Ershova JV, Podewils LJ, Bronner LE, et al. Evaluation of adherence to national treatment guidelines among tuberculosis patients in three provinces of South Africa. S Afr Med J 2014;104(5):362–8.

29. Kibuule D, Verbeeck RK, Nunurai R, et al. Predictors of tuberculosis treatment success under the DOTS program in Namibia. Expert Rev Respir Med 2018; 12(11):979–87.

30. Mirsaeidi M, Farshidpour M, Banks-Tripp D, et al. Video directly observed therapy for treatment of tuberculosis is patient-oriented and cost-effective. Eur Respir J 2015;46(3):871–4.

31. Hoffman JA, Cunningham JR, Suleh AJ, et al. Mobile direct observation treatment for tuberculosis patients. a technical feasibility pilot using mobile phones in Nairobi, Kenya. Am J Prev Med 2010; 39(1):78–80.

32. Holzman SB, Zenilman A, Shah M. Advancing patient-centered care in tuberculosis management: a mixed-methods appraisal of video directly observed therapy. Open Forum Infect Dis 2018;5(4). https://doi.org/10.1093/ofid/ofy046.

33. Johnston JC, Campbell JR, Menzies D. Effect of intermittency on treatment outcomes in pulmonary tuberculosis: an updated systematic review and metaanalysis. Clin Infect Dis 2017;64(9):1211–20.

34. Menzies D, Benedetti A, Paydar A, et al. Effect of duration and intermittency of rifampin on tuberculosis treatment outcomes: a systematic review and meta-analysis. PLoS Med 2009;6(9). https://doi.org/10.1371/journal.pmed.1000146.

35. Vashishtha R, Mohan K, Singh B, et al. Efficacy and safety of thrice weekly DOTS in tuberculosis patients with and without HIV co-infection: an observational study. BMC Infect Dis 2013;13(1). https://doi.org/10.1186/1471-2334-13-468.

36. Horne DJ, Royce SE, Gooze L, et al. Sputum monitoring during tuberculosis treatment for predicting outcome: systematic review and meta-analysis. Lancet Infect Dis 2010;10(6):387–94.

37. Mitchison DA. Assessment of new sterilizing drugs for treating pulmonary tuberculosis by culture at 2 months. Am Rev Respir Dis 2013;147(4):1062–3.

38. Leung CC, Yew WW, Chan CK, et al. Smoking adversely affects treatment response, outcome and relapse in tuberculosis. Eur Respir J 2015; 45(3):738–45.

39. Baker MA, Harries AD, Jeon CY, et al. The impact of diabetes on tuberculosis treatment outcomes: a systematic review. BMC Med 2011;9. https://doi.org/10.1186/1741-7015-9-81.

40. Khan A, Sterling TR, Reves R, et al. Lack of weight gain and relapse risk in a large tuberculosis treatment trial. Am J Respir Crit Care Med 2006;174(3): 344–8.

41. Gordin FM, Slutkin G, Schecter G, et al. Presumptive diagnosis and treatment of pulmonary tuberculosis based on radiographic findings. Am Rev Respir Dis 1989;139(5):1090–3.

42. Skoura E, Zumla A, Bomanji J. Imaging in tuberculosis. Int J Infect Dis 2015;32:87–93.

43. Martha S, Gorityala S, Mateti U, et al. Assessment of treatment interruption among pulmonary tuberculosis patients: a cross-sectional study. J Pharm Bioallied Sci 2015;7(3):226. https://doi.org/10.4103/0975-7406.160034.

44. Dooley KE, Lahlou O, Ghali I, et al. Risk factors for tuberculosis treatment failure, default, or relapse and outcomes of retreatment in Morocco. BMC Public Health 2011;11. https://doi.org/10.1186/1471-2458-11-140.

45. Verbeeck RK, Günther G, Kibuule D, et al. Optimizing treatment outcome of first-line anti-tuberculosis drugs: the role of therapeutic drug monitoring. Eur J Clin Pharmacol 2016;72(8): 905–16.

46. Sekaggya-Wiltshire C, Lamorde M, Kiragga AN, et al. The utility of pharmacokinetic studies for the evaluation of exposure-response relationships for standard dose anti-tuberculosis drugs. Tuberculosis 2018;108:77–82.

47. Peloquin C. The role of therapeutic drug monitoring in mycobacterial infections. Microbiol Spectr 2017; 5(1). https://doi.org/10.1128/microbiolspec.tnmi7-0029-2016.

48. Dekkers BGJ, Akkerman OW, Alffenaar JWC. Role of therapeutic drug monitoring in treatment optimization in tuberculosis and diabetes mellitus comorbidity. Antimicrob Agents Chemother 2019;63(2). https://doi.org/10.1128/AAC.

49. Alsultan A, Peloquin CA. Therapeutic drug monitoring in the treatment of tuberculosis: an update. Drugs 2014;74(8):839–54.

50. Heysell SK, Moore JL, Keller SJ, et al. Therapeutic drug monitoring for slow response to tuberculosis treatment in a state control program, Virginia, USA. Emerg Infect Dis 2010;16(10):1546–53.

51. Mishra P, Hansen EH, Sabroe S, et al. Adherence is associated with the quality of professional-patient interaction in Directly Observed Treatment Short-course, DOTS. Patient Educ Couns 2006;63(1–2): 29–37.

52. Burman W, Benator D, Vernon A, et al. Acquired rifamycin resistance with twice-weekly treatment of HIV-related tuberculosis. Am J Respir Crit Care Med 2006;173(3):350–6.

53. Seung KJ, Gelmanova IE, Peremitin GG, et al. The effect of initial drug resistance on treatment response and acquired drug resistance during standardized short-course chemotherapy for tuberculosis. Clin Infect Dis 2004;39(9):1321–8.

54. Mfinanga SG, Kirenga BJ, Chanda DM, et al. Early versus delayed initiation of highly active antiretroviral therapy for HIV-positive adults with newly diagnosed pulmonary tuberculosis (TB-HAART): a prospective, international, randomised, placebo-controlled trial. Lancet Infect Dis 2014;14(7):563–71.

55. Karim SS, Naidoo K, Grobler A, et al. Timing of initiation of antiretroviral drugs during tuberculosis therapy. N Engl J Med 2010;362(8):697–706.

56. Blanc F-X, Sok T, Laureillard D, et al. Earlier versus later start of antiretroviral therapy in HIV-infected adults with tuberculosis. N Engl J Med 2011; 365(16):1471–81.

57. Amogne W, Aderaye G, Habtewold A, et al. Efficacy and safety of antiretroviral therapy initiated one week after tuberculosis therapy in patients with CD4 counts < 200 cells/µL: TB-HAART study, a randomized clinical trial. PLoS One 2015;10(5). https://doi.org/10.1371/journal.pone.0122587.

58. Havlir DV, Kendall MA, Ive P, et al. Timing of antiretroviral therapy for HIV-1 infection and tuberculosis. N Engl J Med 2011;365(16):1482–91.

59. Manosuthi W, Mankatitham W, Lueangniyomkul A, et al. Time to initiate antiretroviral therapy between 4 weeks and 12 weeks of tuberculosis treatment in HIV-infected patients: results from the TIME Study. J Acquir Immune Defic Syndr 2012;60(4):377–83. Available at: www.jaids.com.

60. Naidoo K, Yende-Zuma N, Padayatchi N, et al. The immune reconstitution inflammatory syndrome after antiretroviral therapy initiation in patients with tuberculosis: findings from the SAPiT Trial. Ann Intern Med 2012;157(5):313–24.

61. Luetkemeyer AF, Kendall MA, Nyirenda M, et al. Tuberculosis immune reconstitution inflammatory syndrome in A5221 STRIDE. JAIDS J Acquir Immune Defic Syndr 2014;65(4):423–8.

62. World Health Organization. Consolidated guidelines on the use of antiretroviral drugs for treating and preventing HIV infection. 2nd edition. Geneva (Switzerland): World Health Organization; 2016.

63. Uthman OA, Okwundu C, Gbenga K, et al. Optimal timing of antiretroviral therapy initiation for HIV-infected adults with newly diagnosed pulmonary tuberculosis: a systematic review and meta-analysis. Ann Intern Med 2015;163(1):32–9.

64. Division of TB Elimination Office of Infectious Diseases C for DC and P. Managing drug interactions in the treatment of HIV-related tuberculosis 2013. Available at: http://www.cdc.gov/tb/TB_HIV_Drugs.

65. Fitzgerald DW, Desvarieux M, Severe P, et al. Effect of post-treatment isoniazid on prevention of recurrent tuberculosis in HIV-1-infected individuals: a randomised trial. Lancet 2000;356(9240):1470–4.

66. Ahmad Khan F, Minion J, Al-Motairi A, et al. An updated systematic review and meta-analysis on the treatment of active tuberculosis in patients with hiv infection. Clin Infect Dis 2012;55(8):1154–63.

67. Vernon A, Burman W, Benator D, et al. Acquired rifamycin monoresistance in patients with HIV-related tuberculosis treated with once-weekly rifapentine and isoniazid. Lance 1999;353:1843–7.

68. Nunn AJ, Mwaba P, Chintu C, et al. Role of co-trimoxazole prophylaxis in reducing mortality in HIV infected adults being treated for tuberculosis: randomised clinical trial. BMJ 2008;337(7663):220–3.

69. Suthar AB, Granich R, Mermin J, et al. Effect of co-trimoxazole on mortality in HIV-infected adults on antiretroviral therapy: a systematic review and meta-analysis. Bull World Health Organ 2012;90(2):128–38.

70. Bothamley G. Drug treatment for tuberculosis during pregnancy. Drug Saf 2001;24(7):553–65.

71. Nguyen HT, Pandolfini C, Chiodini P, et al. Tuberculosis care for pregnant women: a systematic review. BMC Infect Dis 2014;14(1). https://doi.org/10.1186/s12879-014-0617-x.

72. Czeizel AE, Rockenbauer M, Olsen J, et al. A population-based case-control study of the safety of oral anti-tuberculosis drug treatment during pregnancy to study the human teratogenic potential of isoniazid and other anti-tuberculosis drug treatment during pregnancy. cases from a large population-based dataset at the Hungarian case-control surveil-lance of congenital abnormalities, and controls from the national. Int J Tuberc Lung Dis 2001;5(6):564–8.

73. Aquilina S, Winkelman T. Tuberculosis a breast-feeding challenge. J Perinat Neonatal Nurs 2008;22(3):205–13.

74. Perez-Velez CM, Marais BJ. Tuberculosis in children. N Engl J Med 2012;367(4):348–61.

75. McAnaw SE, Hesseling AC, Seddon JA, et al. Pediatric multidrug-resistant tuberculosis clinical trials: challenges and opportunities. Int J Infect Dis 2017;56:194–9.

76. WHO Global TB Programme, Stop TB partnership (World Health Organization), Childhood TB Subgroup, World Health Organization. Guidance for national tuberculosis programmes on the management of tuberculosis in children. Int J Tuberc Lung Dis 2006.

77. Critchley JA, Young F, Orton L, et al. Corticosteroids for prevention of mortality in people with tuberculosis: a systematic review and meta-analysis. Lancet Infect Dis 2013;13(3):223–37.

78. Thwaites GE, Duc Bang N, Huy Dung N, et al. Dexamethasone for the treatment of tuberculous meningitis in adolescents and adults. N Engl J Med 2004;17. Available at: www.nejm.org.

79. Dooley DP, Carpenter JL, Rademacher S. Adjunctive corticosteroid therapy for tuberculosis: a critical reappraisal of the literature. Pediatr Infect Dis J 1998;17(3):270.

80. Kumarvelu S, Prasad K, Khosla A, et al. Randomized controlled trial of dexamethasone in tuberculous meningitis. Tuber Lung Dis 1994;75(3):203–7.

81. Kotil K, Rvet A, Bilge T. Medical management of Pott disease in the thoracic and lumbar spine_ a prospective clinical study. J Neurosurg Spine 2007;6(3):222–8.

82. Nene A, Bhojraj S, Ortho D. Results of nonsurgical treatment of thoracic spinal tuberculosis in adults. Spine J 2005;5(1):79–84.

83. Wiysonge CS, Ntsekhe M, Thabane L, et al. Interventions for treating tuberculous pericarditis. Cochrane Database Syst Rev 2017;2017(9). https://doi.org/10.1002/14651858.CD000526.pub2.

84. Rasheed S, Zinicola R, Watson D, et al. Intra-abdominal and gastrointestinal tuberculosis. Color Dis 2007;9(9):773–83.

85. Saukkonen JJ, Cohn DL, Jasmer RM, et al. An official ATS statement: hepatotoxicity of antituberculosis therapy. Am J Respir Crit Care Med 2006;174(8):935–52.

86. Lehloenya RJ, Dheda K. Cutaneous adverse drug reactions to anti-tuberculosis drugs: state of the art and into the future. Expert Rev Anti Infect Ther 2012;10(4):475–86.

87. Brown EG, Dooley DS, Smith K. Drug-resistant tuberculosis: a survival guide for clinicians. San Francisco (CA): Curry International Tuberculosis Center and State of California; 2016.

88. World Health Organization. Management of MDR-TB: a field guide a companion document to guidelines for the programmatic management of drug-resistant tuberculosis. Geneva (Switzerland): World Health Organization; 2009.

Treatment of Drug-Resistant Tuberculosis

Sundari R. Mase, MD, MPH[a], Terence Chorba, MD, DSc[b],*

KEYWORDS

- Tuberculosis • Drug resistance • Treatment • Management • Regimen • Adverse drug reactions

KEY POINTS

- A patient-centered approach with case management strategies should be used in the care of drug-resistant (DR) tuberculosis (TB) with attention to patient preferences; social, cultural, and environmental aspects of care; comorbid conditions, adherence strategies, patient monitoring for clinical response and safety, and the need for palliative care.
- There are 2 World Health Organization–recommended treatment options for multidrug-resistant (MDR) or extensively DR (XDR) TB that can be decided on based on extent of resistance, availability of drug susceptibility testing (DST) results, and patient preference:
  a. If the clinician and patient opt for an individualized, longer treatment regimen, MDR-TB/XDR-TB should be treated with at least 4 drugs for the first 6 months, followed by 3 drugs for a total duration of 18 to 20 months depending on extent and severity of disease; drug history; and clinical, bacteriologic, and radiographic response.
  b. If none of the exclusion criteria for the standardized shorter regimen are met and the clinician and patient opt for this regimen, MDR-TB/XDR-TB should be treated for 9 to 12 months with the standardized medications and duration of treatment specified in the shorter regimen.
- The choice of drugs for the treatment of DR-TB should be guided by known effectiveness of given drugs, propensity for adverse drug reactions/drug-drug interactions, and DST, excluding all drugs to which the isolate shows resistance. If DST is only partially available or not available, or if an empiric DR-TB regimen must be started before DST results are available, the regimen should consist of drugs that are highly likely to be susceptible, based on previous treatment history, pattern of resistance of the presumed source case, and patterns of resistance found from national or regional drug-resistance surveys.
- An all-oral treatment regimen including new and repurposed drugs is the preferable strategy for most patients; injectable agents should be avoided whenever possible, especially in children.
- Expert consultation from a recognized DR-TB expert should be sought whenever possible in the treatment of patients with MDR-TB/XDR-TB or patients in whom issues of drug resistance or drug intolerance may complicate care.

Disclaimer: References in this article to any specific commercial products, process, service, manufacturer, or company do not constitute any endorsement or recommendation by the US government or the US Centers for Disease Control and Prevention (CDC). The findings and conclusions are those of the authors and do not necessarily represent the views of the CDC or other funding agencies.

[a] World Health Organization, Southeast Asian Regional Office, World Health House, Indraprastha Estate, Mahatma Gandhi Marg, New Delhi 110 002, India; [b] Field Services Branch, Division of Tuberculosis Elimination, National Center for HIV/AIDS, Viral Hepatitis, STD, and TB Prevention, Centers for Disease Control and Prevention, 1600 Clifton Road NE (MS: US 12-4), Atlanta, GA 30329, USA
* Corresponding author.
E-mail address: TLC2@CDC.GOV

chestmed.theclinics.com

INTRODUCTION
Background

The development of drug-resistant (DR) tuberculosis (TB) has become an increasing concern over the past few decades as the result of numerous factors, including widespread inappropriate or ineffectual use of antimicrobials to treat TB in the absence of drug-susceptibility testing (DST), lack of adequate uptake of systematic approaches to the treatment of drug-susceptible (DS) TB and DR-TB, introduction of human immunodeficiency virus (HIV) into areas with preexisting DR-TB, provider error, poor adherence to treatment, lack of availability of effective drugs, and transmission of DR strains.[1] The World Health Organization (WHO) has estimated that annually there are over half a million new cases of rifampicin-resistant (RR) and multidrug-resistant (MDR) TB; that is, disease caused by *Mycobacterium tuberculosis* with resistance to isoniazid and rifampin. Globally, 156,000 persons with MDR-TB or RR-TB began treatment in 2018, but the latest data show that only 56% completed treatment successfully.[2] Such poor treatment completion rates are the result of treatment for a longer duration with second-line anti-TB drugs (SLDs), which are less effective and have greater toxicity than the 4 drugs most commonly used to treat DS-TB. However, treatment performance has been shown to be much better when regimens are designed carefully and ensure good retention, under both trial and programmatic conditions.[3,4]

Definitions

There are many forms of DR-TB (**Box 1**). Definitions for extensively DR (XDR) TB and pre–XDR-TB need to be modified as all-oral regimens become standard of care.

Guidelines Development

The treatment and management of DR-TB has evolved significantly in the past decade with the advent of rapid molecular diagnostic tests, new and repurposed drugs, results based on individual patient data meta-analysis (IPD-MA),[5–12] and a strategy to decentralize patient care in line with a patient-centered approach, including in high burden settings.[13] The WHO has recently published an evidence-based update to its MDR-TB treatment guidelines,[14] introducing new regimens, enhanced monitoring strategies, and a feasible implementation plan, based on an IPD-MA of data from recently completed phase III trials of delamanid and a shorter MDR-TB regimen; an IPD-MA with more than 13,100 records from

---

Box 1
Drug-resistant tuberculosis definitions

- Monodrug-resistant TB: TB caused by organisms that show resistance to a single anti-TB drug (eg, isoniazid, rifampin, ethambutol, or pyrazinamide).
- Isoniazid-resistant TB: TB caused by organisms that show resistance to isoniazid (rifampin susceptible).
- Rifampin-resistant TB (RR-TB): TB caused by organisms that show resistance to rifampin, but may be susceptible to isoniazid, or resistant to isoniazid (ie, MDR-TB), or resistant to other first-line TB medicines (polydrug resistant) or second-line TB medicines (eg, extensively drug-resistant TB [XDR-TB]).
- Polydrug-resistant TB (PDR-TB): TB caused by organisms that show resistance to more than 1 anti-TB drug, but not including both isoniazid and rifampin.
- MDR-TB: TB caused by organisms that show resistance to at least isoniazid and rifampin.
- Preextensively drug-resistant TB (pre–XDR-TB): TB caused by organisms that show multidrug resistance, and resistance to any fluoroquinolone or a second-line injectable (SLI) agent (ie, amikacin, kanamycin, or capreomycin).
- Extensively DR TB (XDR-TB): TB caused by organisms that show multidrug resistance, and resistance to any fluoroquinolone and at least 1 of the SLI agents.
- Primary or newly diagnosed DR-TB: DR-TB in a person who has previously received no or less than 1 month of anti-TB treatment (ATT).
- Acquired or previously treated DR-TB: TB in a person who has previously received at least 1 month of ATT.

---

patients treated with longer MDR-TB regimens in 40 countries; another IPD-MA with more than 2600 records from patients treated with the 9-month to 12-month shorter MDR-TB regimens from 15 countries; and pharmacokinetic and safety data from trials of bedaquiline and delamanid in patients less than or equal to 18 years old.[14] These guidelines are intended to be applicable to low-resource countries. The American Thoracic Society (ATS), the Centers for Disease Control and Prevention (CDC), the European Respiratory Society (ERS), and the Infectious Disease Society of America (IDSA) are also collaborating to develop guidelines for low-incidence, high-resource countries, which they will publish in 2019, using published IPD-MA data from more than 12,000 patients treated with MDR-TB regimens from 25 countries in 50 studies.[8] At the time of the writing of this article, those guidelines have not been finalized, but will be based principally on a published IPD-MA[8] and will be intended for settings in which mycobacterial cultures, phenotypic and molecular DST, and radiographic resources are readily available.

New Recommendations from the World Health Organization (2019)

The new WHO recommendations are a departure from previous approaches to treat MDR-TB/RR-TB in several regards:

- Injectables are no longer considered priority medicines when designing longer MDR-TB regimens. Kanamycin and capreomycin are no longer recommended.
- Oral regimens are preferred for most patients.
- Fluoroquinolones (levofloxacin or moxifloxacin), bedaquiline, and linezolid are strongly recommended for all longer regimens (unless contraindicated), with other medicines ranked by a relative balance of benefits to harms.
- Most regimens should include at least 4 drugs that are likely to be effective in the first 6 months, and 3 drugs thereafter.
- The total duration of longer MDR-TB regimens should be 18 to 20 months, modified depending on patient response.
- A standardized, shorter MDR-TB regimen may be offered to eligible patients who agree to a briefer treatment (9–12 months) if they are cognizant that this may be less effective than an individualized longer regimen and of the inconvenience/risks associated with the daily injectable agent needed for 4 to 6 months.
- It is strongly recommended that MDR-TB regimens should be monitored with cultures rather than merely with sputum microscopy, and it is preferred that cultures are performed monthly to diagnose treatment failure, relapse, or unidentified/acquired drug resistance in a timely fashion.
- Bedaquiline may be given to children greater than or equal to 6 years old and delamanid to those greater than or equal to 3 years old.
- Regimens that vary substantially from the recommended composition and duration can be explored under operational research conditions.
- Patient-centered support for medication adherence (including the use of digital technologies where feasible) and active TB drug-safety monitoring and management (aDSM)

are essential for anyone starting an MDR-TB regimen.

Key Principles/Best Practices

Several best-practices statements can readily be derived for diagnosing, treating, monitoring, and providing case management for DR-TB, based on expert opinion and on the IPD-MAs that have served as the basis for development of the 2019 WHO guidelines[14]:

- Treatment should follow evidence-based up-to-date guidelines of WHO or of other organizations with similar levels of expertise.
- Diagnosis, treatment, and management strategies differ depending on the epidemiology of TB, programmatic resources, and characteristics of different patient populations.
- Treatment and management of DR-TB or cases in which drug intolerance may complicate care should be done in consultation with an expert in the management of these complex cases.
- Quality-assured laboratory testing, including culture and DST, should be available for optimal patient care.
- Choice of drugs should be informed by quality-assured laboratory testing, including culture and DST, with avoidance of drugs to which there is documented resistance (individualized treatment).
- If possible, testing for rapid detection for molecular evidence of drug resistance in conjunction with growth-based DST should be performed when DR-TB is suspected, whether such suspicion has an epidemiologic or clinical basis.
- In using a longer treatment regimen, 5 drugs may be used rather than 4 drugs for the first 6 months of treatment (when using bedaquiline or in the initiation phase if an injectable agent is used) and 4 drugs rather than 3 drugs after 6 months (or during the continuation phase if an injectable agent is used) if it is deemed medically necessary and if resources allow.
- Treatment choice and duration should be determined in conjunction with the strength of the drugs used for treatment, extent and severity of disease, and the treatment response as shown bacteriologically, clinically, and radiographically. Where possible, monthly cultures should be obtained during treatment. Weight should be monitored monthly.
- Never add a single drug to a failing regimen (as manifested by persistent culture positivity, or clinical or radiographic deterioration).

- If a shorter MDR-TB regimen (9–12 months) is to be implemented, it should be in countries where a longer regimen (18–20 months) is not feasible.
- An uninterrupted supply of quality-assured drugs should be ensured.
- Active pharmacovigilance for serious adverse events (SAEs) and passive pharmacovigilance for adverse drug reactions (ADRs) are crucial. At each patient contact while on treatment, patients should be asked about possible ADRs, with attention to identification of toxicities or other evidence of issues in tolerability of the anti-TB drugs and any ADRs or SAEs should be reported immediately. All ADRs merit investigation and early action to limit harms. Collection of detailed data on SAEs may help patients and programs to improve performance.
- Treatment adherence should be ensured through directly observed therapy (DOT) or supported using information communication technology (ICT)–based adherence strategies.[15]
- A patient-centered approach with case management strategies (incentives and enablers) should be used, with attention to the social, cultural, and environmental aspects of care, treatment of comorbid conditions such as HIV, malnutrition, diabetes, smoking and alcoholism, and palliative care if needed.
- Posttreatment monitoring should be performed at regular intervals (eg, every 6 months) for 1 to 2 years to evaluate for relapse or recurrence.
- DR-TB contacts should be evaluated to exclude TB disease and offered treatment of latent TB infection (LTBI) tailored to the susceptibility pattern of the source-case isolates whenever possible.

For use of rapid molecular diagnostic tests, see Michelle K. Haas and Robert W. Belknap's article, "Diagnostic Tests for Latent Tuberculosis Infection," in this issue. For treatment of HIV, see the article in this issue on treatment of HIV.

CLASSIFICATION OF DRUGS

In 2018, WHO revised the classification of anti-TB drugs based on a recent IPD-MA analyzing the relative risk of treatment failure or relapse versus treatment success, death versus treatment success, and the SAEs for each individual drug.[5,8,10] This classification (**Table 1**) is used to devise the longer-treatment WHO regimen (lasting for a total treatment duration of 20 months), because the standardized shorter treatment regimen (lasting 12 months or less) is composed of a fixed regimen of drugs that cannot be substituted unless done in a research mode.[14]

The key recommendations in the new WHO reclassification scheme for anti-TB drugs are as follows:

- Fluoroquinolones (levofloxacin and moxifloxacin), bedaquiline, and linezolid (group A) were

Table 1
Grouping of medicines recommended for use in longer multidrug-resistant tuberculosis regimens

Groups and Steps	Medicine	Acronym
Group A: include all 3 medicines	Levofloxacin, or	Lfx
	Moxifloxacin	Mfx
	Bedaquiline	Bdq
	Linezolid	Lzd
Group B: add 1 or both medicines	Clofazimine	Cfz
	Cycloserine, or	Cs
	Terizidone	Trd
Group C: add to complete the regimen and when medicines from groups A and B cannot be used	Ethambutol	E
	Delamanid	Dlm
	Pyrazinamide	Z
	Imipenem-cilastatin, or	Ipm-Cln
	Meropenem	Mpm
	Amikacin, or	Am
	Streptomycin	S
	Ethionamide, or	Eto
	Prothionamide	Pto
	para-Aminosalicylic acid	PAS

From the WHO treatment guidelines for DR-TB: 2019 update. https://www.who.int/tb/publications/2019/consolidated-guidelines-drug-resistant-TB-treatment/en/.

considered highly effective and are strongly recommended to be included in an MDR-TB regimen unless contraindicated.

- Clofazimine and either cycloserine or terizidone (group B) are conditionally recommended as second-choice drugs.
- Drugs are in group C ranked by the balance of benefit to harm and can be considered when group A or B drugs are not available to build an adequate multidrug regimen.
- Injectable agents, amikacin and streptomycin, have been downgraded to group C and are not included if an adequate regimen can be built without them. Kanamycin and capreomycin are no longer recommended for use.
- Gatifloxacin and thioacetazone are either not available or not being used, and therefore are not included in the recommendations.
- High-dose isoniazid may have a role when there is confirmed isoniazid susceptibility or when only an inhA mutation is detected in longer MDR regimens and is a standard drug in the shorter MDR regimen.
- Clavulanic acid (only available in the combination amoxicillin-clavulanic acid form [Augmentin]) should only be given with a carbapenem (eg, meropenem) and should not be individually counted as an anti-TB drug.
- There is no recommendation for the use of 4-thioureidoiminomethyl pyridinium perchlorat interferon-gamma, or sutezolid and no evidence that they increase likelihood of cure.
- Bedaquiline can be given to children greater than or equal to 6 years of age.
- Delamanid can be given to children greater than or equal to 3 years of age.
- There is no recommendation for giving bedaquiline and delamanid together.
- Bedaquiline and delamanid should be given for 6 months and, if extended, would be considered off-label use.
- Pyrazinamide should only be counted in the regimen if susceptibility is shown.
- Amikacin and streptomycin should only be used if susceptibility is confirmed (phenotypic conformation for streptomycin) and if high-quality audiology monitoring is available.

These results reflect analyses from 3 IPD-MA cohorts.[14] ATS/CDC/ERS/IDSA guidelines are being developed using data from a single IPD-MA[8] with a patient cohort (overlapping, but not identical) similar to that of one of the cohorts used in developing the WHO guidelines.[14]

The results of the IPD-MA used in developing the ATS/CDC/ERS/IDSA guidelines differed from that used in developing the WHO treatment guidelines in the following ways:

1. Amikacin and streptomycin showed better effectiveness if susceptibility was confirmed.
2. Treatment outcomes were significantly worse for patients treated with drugs for which there was documented resistance.
3. Fewer data were available on bedaquiline, resulting in a less pronounced effect of bedaquiline on treatment outcome.

In turn, these findings and other differences, such as the availability of rapid molecular testing for the detection of drug resistance, phenotypic DST for additional SLD, and therapeutic drug monitoring, may lead to some differences in recommendations in treatment approaches for low-incidence settings.

BUILDING A TREATMENT REGIMEN

MDR-TB/XDR-TB should always be treated with a multidrug regimen consisting of drugs to which the patient's isolate is susceptible, excluding all drugs to which the isolate shows resistance. If DST is not available or an empiric DR-TB regimen must be started before DST results are available, the regimen should consist of drugs that are highly likely to be susceptible or effective, based on previous treatment history, pattern of resistance of the presumed source case, potential for cross-resistance with drugs for which DST is available (see **Table 9**), and patterns of resistance found from national or regional drug-resistance surveys (DRSs) that tend to indicate the local effectiveness of different drugs. In addition, when only rapid molecular testing for rifampin resistance is available (eg, Xpert MTB/RIF assay, Cepheid, Sunnyvale, CA),[16] RR-TB should be treated as if it were MDR-TB.[14] However, in the United States and other low-prevalence countries, false resistance is common with Xpert MTB/RIF assay (low PPV); in such settings, sequencing is recommended to confirm rpoB mutation and assess for potential mutations conferring isoniazid resistance to diagnose MDR-TB.

When treated with an inadequate treatment regimen, DR mutant strains of M tuberculosis in the bacterial population are favored, leading to treatment failure, relapse, further acquired drug resistance, and potentially death. According to the new 2019 updated WHO DR-TB guidelines, a longer MDR-TB regimen can be used for MDR/RR-TB, lasts for at least 18 months, and can be either standardized or individualized. A shorter MDR-TB regimen can be used for MDR/RR-TB, is largely standardized, and is given for 9 to 12 months (**Fig. 1** shows the choice of longer vs shorter regimens).

Longer Treatment Regimen

According to the new WHO guidelines, a longer treatment regimen (preferably all oral) should be designed using the following principles.

Recommendations

- Recommendation 1: if an injectable agent is used, the duration of the intensive phase should be 6 to 7 months (**Box 2**).
- Recommendation 2: a total duration of 18 to 20 months is recommended.
- Recommendation 3: treatment duration of 15 to 17 months after culture conversion is recommended.
- Other recommendations:
  - All 3 group A drugs and at least 1 group B drug should be included for a total of at least 4 drugs given for 6 months until bedaquiline is stopped and a total of at least 3 drugs for the remainder of the treatment duration (**Table 2**).
  - If 1 or 2 group A drugs cannot be included, the remaining group A drugs, both group B drugs and group C drugs (if needed) should be added (in order of ranking) to achieve at least 4 drugs at start of treatment.
  - If 1 or 2 group A drugs cannot be included and 1 or both group B drugs cannot be included, group C drugs should be added (in order of ranking) to achieve at least 4 drugs at start of treatment.
  - If 2 agents are likely to be stopped before the end of treatment (eg, bedaquiline at 6 months and linezolid because of toxicity), 5 agents may be given at start of treatment to ensure that 3 agents can be given for the duration of treatment.
  - Duration of treatment depends on the drugs used in the regimen and may be decreased or extended depending on the patient's response to treatment.

Implementation considerations

- When there is additional resistance to simple MDR-TB, a longer regimen may be preferable to a shorter regimen.
- An all-oral regimen should be the preferred choice for most patients.
- Ideally, all drugs used in a regimen should have confirmed susceptibility.
- Ideally, all patients with RR-TB should have DST to isoniazid to exclude non-MDR RR-TB or polydrug-resistant (PDR) TB.
- Ideally, all patients with MDR-TB should have DST to a fluoroquinolone, and, if an injectable is to be used, DST to second-line injectable (SLI) agents.

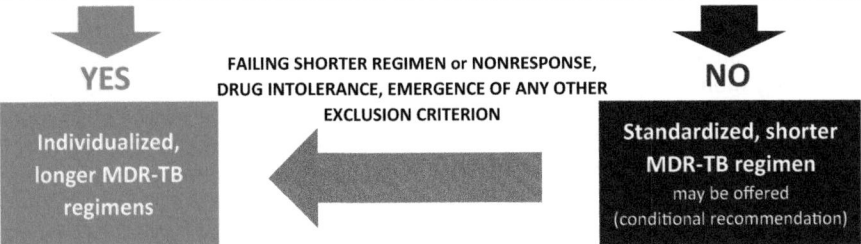

Is any of the following present?

- Preference by the clinician and patient for a longer MDR-TB regimen
- Confirmed resistance or suspected ineffectiveness to a medicine in the shorter MDR-TB regimen (except isoniazid resistance)[a]
- Exposure to one or more second-line medicines in the shorter MDR-TB regimen for >1 mo (unless susceptibility to these second-line medicines is confirmed)
- Intolerance to medicines in the shorter MDR-TB regimen or risk of toxicity (eg, drug-drug interactions)
- Pregnancy
- Disseminated, meningeal, or central nervous system TB
- Any extrapulmonary disease in a person living with HIV
- One or more medicines in the shorter MDR-TB regimen not available

YES

FAILING SHORTER REGIMEN or NONRESPONSE, DRUG INTOLERANCE, EMERGENCE OF ANY OTHER EXCLUSION CRITERION

NO

Individualized, longer MDR-TB regimens

Standardized, shorter MDR-TB regimen
may be offered
(conditional recommendation)

Fig. 1. Criteria to decide when the shorter MDR-TB regimen may be offered.[14] [a] Strains from patients with MDR-TB/RR-TB should ideally be tested for resistance to fluoroquinolones and other regimen components regardless of the type of MDR-TB treatment regimen offered. (*From* the WHO treatment guidelines for DR-TB: 2019 update. https://www.who.int/tb/publications/2019/consolidated-guidelines-drug-resistant-TB-treatment/en/.)

Box 2
Duration of treatment of longer multidrug-resistant tuberculosis regimen (refer to recommendations 1–3, given earlier, in building a treatment regimen)

- When an injectable agent[a] is used, all 3 recommendations apply for duration of treatment.
- When an all-oral regimen is used, recommendations 2 and 3 apply for duration of treatment.
- With extrapulmonary disease, only recommendation 3 applies for the duration of treatment.
- Changes to the recommended duration of treatment should be tailored to the patient's bacteriologic, clinical, and radiographic response.

[a] Injectable agent here does not refer to meropenem and imipenem-cilastatin; this term is used to refer to amikacin or streptomycin (kanamycin and capreomycin are no longer recommended).

- Ideally, DST for bedaquiline, delamanid, linezolid, and pyrazinamide should be performed.
- Ideally, patients should have molecular testing for inhA and katG mutations to look for ethionamide/low-dose isoniazid resistance and high-dose isoniazid resistance respectively.
- DST to other SLDs should be obtained where available and quality assured.
- When DST is not available, selection of drugs should be based on DST pattern of presumed source case, treatment history, cross-resistance between drugs, and surveillance data from national or regional DRS.
- Although the GenoType MTBDRsl (Hain Lifescience GmbH, Nehren, Germany) assay, the only rapid commercial test for detection of resistance to the principal SLDs, may correlate well with phenotypic resistance to ofloxacin and levofloxacin, moxifloxacin resistance is best confirmed through phenotypic testing.
- When there is uncertainty about the efficacy of a particular drug, it can be included as part of the regimen, but not included numerically as one of the effective drugs.
- Five drugs rather than 4 may be started with initial treatment if:
  - Two of the 4 drugs are likely to be stopped before completion of treatment.
  - There is a question as to the efficacy of 1 or more drugs because of lack of quality DST and high level of resistance to that drug, or 1 of the drugs in the regimen shows

Table 2
Stepwise algorithm for building a multidrug-resistant/extensively drug-resistant tuberculosis treatment regimen

Step 1: choose all 3 group A drugs (if possible)	Levofloxacin/moxifloxacin, bedaquiline, linezolid
Step 2: choose both of these prioritized drugs	Clofazimine Cycloserine/terizidone
Step 3: if a regimen cannot be assembled with 4 effective oral drugs, and the isolate is likely susceptible, add group C drugs in the order of ranking until a regimen with ≥4 drugs can be constructed	Ethambutol Delamanid Pyrazinamide Imipenem/cilastatin or meropenem/clavulanate Amikacin (or streptomycin) Ethionamide or prothionamide para-aminosalicylic acid
Step 4: if needed, and the isolate is susceptible, may use the following drug	High-dose isoniazid
The following drugs are no longer recommended for inclusion in DR-TB regimens	Capreomycin and kanamycin Amoxicillin/clavulanate (when used without a carbapenem) Azithromycin and clarithromycin Azithromycin and clarithromycin
The following drugs have no data for or against use	Perchlozone, interferon-gamma, or sutezolid

Adapted and updated from the Curry International Tuberculosis Center DR-TB Survival Guide.[17] http://www.currytbcenter.ucsf.edu/products/view/drug-resistant-tuberculosis-survival-guide-clinicians-3rd-edition.

cross-resistance with another drug for which there is known or suspected resistance.
- ○ The regimen is unlikely to be successful based on a factor such as the extent of resistance.
- ○ All 3 group A drugs are not used.

Clinical strategy to build an individualized treatment regimen
Principles
- Build a regimen using greater than or equal to 4 drugs to which the isolate is susceptible (or has low likelihood of resistance), preferably with drugs that have not been used to treat the patient previously.
- Choice of drugs depends on DST, previous treatment history, the pattern of resistance of the presumed source case, patterns of resistance found from national or regional DRS capacity to appropriately monitor for significant adverse effects, patient comorbidities and preferences/values (choices therefore subject to program and patient safety limitations).
- In children with TB disease who are contacts of infectious MDR-TB source cases, the source case's isolate DST result should be used if no isolate is obtained from the child.
- TB expert medical consultation is recommended.

Shorter Regimen

Per WHO guidelines, if a shorter treatment regimen is implemented, it should be designed using the following principles.

Recommendations
- The shorter regimen consists of 4 to 6 months of moxifloxacin, amikacin, ethionamide, clofazimine, high-dose isoniazid, pyrazinamide, and ethambutol (depending on smear conversion at 4 months), followed by 5 months of moxifloxacin, clofazimine, pyrazinamide, and ethambutol.
- The shorter regimen may be considered for patients who desire a shorter duration of treatment despite the use of an injectable agent and who do not have the exclusion criteria noted in **Box 3**.
- Patients should only be started on the shorter regimen if they have confirmed susceptibility to fluoroquinolones and SLI agents by molecular or phenotypic DST.
- Ideally, patients should have molecular testing for inhA and katG mutations to look

---

Box 3
Exclusion criteria for the shorter regimen

- Resistance to or suspected ineffectiveness to a medicine in the shorter MDR-TB regimen (except isoniazid resistance)
- Exposure to 1 or more second-line medicines in the regimen for greater than 1 month (unless susceptibility to these second-line medicines is confirmed)
- Intolerance to any medicine in the shorter MDR-TB regimen or risk of toxicity from a medicine in the shorter regimen (eg, drug-drug interactions)
- Pregnancy
- Disseminated, meningeal, or central nervous system TB
- Any extrapulmonary disease in patients with HIV

---

for ethionamide/low-dose isoniazid resistance and high-dose isoniazid resistance respectively; if both mutations are present, a longer MDR-TB regimen should be considered.
- Ideally, patients should also have phenotypic DST to pyrazinamide before starting the shorter regimen, but this should not preclude the use of the regimen if needed.

Implementation considerations
- Patients eligible for shorter regimens may still opt for a longer regimen if they want to avoid SLI agents on the understanding that they need a much more protracted course of medication.
- Kanamycin should be replaced by amikacin.
- If any drug in the regimen or essential monitoring (especially audiometry) are unavailable, a longer regimen should be used.
- If an all-oral shorter regimen (eg, replacing kanamycin with bedaquiline) is implemented, this should be done in an operational research mode because there are no data on an all-oral shorter regimen.
- If DRS results show high levels of resistance to any drug in the shorter regimen, especially ethionamide, fluoroquinolone, or pyrazinamide, a longer regimen should be considered.
- The shorter regimen should be given by DOT or an information and ICT-based adherence method.[18]

Rifampin-Resistant Tuberculosis (Isoniazid Susceptible)

In cases with rifampin resistance in which susceptibility to isoniazid is confirmed:

Recommendations

- Expert opinion customarily holds that a longer or shorter MDR-TB regimen may be used with the addition of high-dose isoniazid if there is no DST for ethambutol and/or pyrazinamide and if there is a high level of baseline resistance to either drug based on surveillance data.
- If DST to all first-line drugs and fluoroquinolones is available, please refer to **Table 3** for a DST-driven treatment regimen.

Implementation considerations

- The regimen used for RR-TB depends on the availability to perform molecular or phenotypic DST to the other first-line drugs and fluoroquinolones, and the availability of quality-assured drugs in country.
- Wherever possible, molecular or phenotypic DST should be performed for isoniazid to confirm lack of MDR-TB.

Isoniazid-Resistant Tuberculosis (Rifampin Susceptible)

In cases with isoniazid-resistant TB in which susceptibility to rifampin is confirmed:

Recommendations

- Treatment with rifampin, ethambutol, pyrazinamide, and levofloxacin recommended for a duration of 6 months.[14]
- The 4-drug HREZ fixed-dose combination (FDC) with isoniazid, rifampin, ethambutol, and pyrazinamide may be used (because there is no approved rifampin-ethambutol-pyrazinamide FDC available) to limit the need for using single drugs.
- Drug susceptibility to fluoroquinolones should preferably be confirmed ahead of start of treatment.
- It is generally not recommended to add streptomycin or other injectable agents to the treatment regimen.

Implementation considerations

- If isoniazid resistance is confirmed before start of treatment, follow the recommendations outlined earlier.
- If isoniazid resistance is suspected (based on source-case isolate), start isoniazid, rifampin, ethambutol, and pyrazinamide empirically, and add a fluoroquinolone only after RR-TB has been reliably excluded; if isoniazid susceptibility is confirmed, change to standard 4-drug regimen for DS-TB.
- If isoniazid resistance is confirmed after treatment start (either because of unidentified resistance at treatment start or acquired resistance), exclude rifampin resistance immediately through molecular testing and, if rifampin susceptible, change regimen to rifampin, ethambutol, pyrazinamide, and a fluoroquinolone for 6 months; if rifampin resistance is found, start treatment of MDR-TB.
- If isoniazid resistance is diagnosed 4 to 5 months after treatment start, treatment should be based on patient's clinical, bacteriologic, and radiographic response and further DST results.
- Ideally, fluoroquinolone resistance should be excluded before starting this regimen using a line probe assay to detect resistance to SLDs, especially in countries with high levels of fluoroquinolone resistance based on DRS.
- Levofloxacin is the recommended fluoroquinolone based on its safety profile and fewer drug-drug interactions, particularly with antiretrovirals.
- Moxifloxacin should be considered if only levofloxacin or low-level moxifloxacin resistance is confirmed (moxifloxacin less than or equal to 1.0 μg/mL Lowenstein-Jensen; less than or equal to 0.5 μg/mL Middlebrook 7H10/7H11; ≤0.25 μg/mL BACTEC MGIT).[19]
- A fluoroquinolone should be used unless any of the following are present:
  ○ Resistance to rifampin cannot be excluded (ie, unknown susceptibility to rifampin; indeterminate/error results on GeneXpert MTB/RIF).
  ○ Known or suspected resistance to levofloxacin; moxifloxacin may be considered (discussed earlier).
  ○ Known intolerance to fluoroquinolones.
  ○ Known or suspected risk for prolonged QT interval, or high risk for or known aortic aneurysm.[20]
  ○ In pregnancy or during breastfeeding (not an absolute contraindication).
- If a fluoroquinolone cannot be used, isoniazid, rifampin, ethambutol, and pyrazinamide can be given for 6 months.
- The duration of treatment can be extended based on delayed clinical, bacteriologic, and radiographic response.
- The addition of isoniazid is based on FDC use and there are no data on added efficacy; if

Table 3
Treatment regimens for the management of monoresistant and polyresistant tuberculosis pattern of drug resistance

Pattern of Drug Resistance	Suggested Regimen	Minimum Duration of Treatment (mo)	Comments
Isoniazid (±streptomycin)	Rifampin, pyrazinamide, ethambutol, and fluoroquinolone	6–9	Levofloxacin or moxifloxacin may be used. Consider high- dose isoniazid if inhA mutation
Isoniazid and ethambutol	Rifampin, pyrazinamide, and fluoroquinolone	6–9	A longer duration of treatment should be used for patients with extensive disease. Consider high-dose isoniazid if inhA mutation
Isoniazid and pyrazinamide	Rifampin, ethambutol, and fluoroquinolone	9–12	A longer duration of treatment should be used for patients with extensive disease. Consider high-dose isoniazid if inhA mutation
Isoniazid, ethambutol, pyrazinamide (±streptomycin)	Rifampin, fluoroquinolone, plus 1–2 oral second-line agents (linezolid, cycloserine)	9–12	A longer duration of treatment should be used for patients with extensive disease. An injectable may strengthen the regimen for patients with extensive disease
Rifampin	Isoniazid, ethambutol, fluoroquinolone, plus at least 2 mo of pyrazinamide. Or a fully oral MDR-TB regimen per WHO guidelines (see text)	12–18	A longer duration of treatment should be used for patients with extensive disease. An injectable drug may strengthen the regimen for patients with extensive disease. For additional options, see text
Rifampin and ethambutol (±streptomycin)	Isoniazid, pyrazinamide, fluoroquinolone, plus an injectable agent for at least the first 2–3 mo. Or a fully oral MDR-TB regimen per WHO guidelines	18	A longer course (6 mo) of the injectable may strengthen the regimen for patients with extensive disease
Rifampin and pyrazinamide (±streptomycin)	Isoniazid, ethambutol, fluoroquinolone, plus an injectable agent for at least the first 2–3 mo. Or a fully oral MDR-TB regimen per WHO guidelines	18	A longer course (6 mo) of the injectable may strengthen the regimen for patients with extensive disease
Pyrazinamide	Isoniazid, rifampin	9	Most commonly seen in *Mycobacterium bovis* infections

Adapted and updated from the Curry International Tuberculosis Center DR-TB Survival Guide.[17] http://www.currytbcenter.ucsf.edu/products/view/drug-resistant-tuberculosis-survival-guide-clinicians-3rd-edition.

there are side effects attributed to isoniazid, single drugs (rifampin, ethambutol, pyrazinamide, fluoroquinolone) should be used.

- Streptomycin or other injectable agents can be added to the regimen in certain exceptional circumstances (see **Table 3**).
- If DST to all first-line drugs and fluoroquinolones is available, please refer to **Table 3**.

Polydrug Resistance (Isoniazid Susceptible)

Recommendations

For patients with PDR-TB for whom DST to all first-line drugs and fluoroquinolones is available, treatment decisions must be guided largely by expert opinion, rather than through recommendations developed through the GRADE (Grading of Recommendations Assessment, Development and Evaluation) methodology[21,22] because of the paucity of available data to inform such a process. **Table 3** shows adapted and updated recommendations for individualized treatment (primarily based on expert opinion) from the Curry International Tuberculosis Center DR-TB Survival Guide.[17]

Implementation considerations

- These recommendations are primarily applicable when DST is available for all first-line drugs and fluoroquinolones.
- As with MDR-TB, for RR-TB (isoniazid susceptible) with or without additional resistance,

clinicians and patients may prefer an all-oral MDR-TB regimen, incorporating bedaquiline, rather than an injectable-containing regimen.

- In countries or settings where DST to ethambutol and pyrazinamide are not available:
  - Treat RR-TB as if it were MDR-TB, and
  - Treat any isoniazid-resistant TB per WHO guidelines as set out in relation to treatment of isoniazid-resistant TB.

TREATMENT IN SPECIAL SITUATIONS
Extrapulmonary Tuberculosis

- The longer MDR-TB regimen may be given in extrapulmonary TB; TB meningitis should be treated with a regimen of drugs that achieve effective drug levels in the central nervous system (CNS) (**Table 4**) and should be directed by DST.
- In culture-negative extrapulmonary TB or when culture conversion cannot be shown because of inability to obtain a specimen, a total duration of treatment of 18 to 20 months is recommended; if an injectable agent is used, it should be given for 6 to 7 months based on clinical response.
- The shorter regimen should be avoided in patients with disseminated or CNS disease and in persons living with HIV.
- There is no difference in other regimens for other forms of DR-TB specific to extrapulmonary TB.

Table 4
Central nervous system (blood-brain barrier) penetration of antituberculosis drugs[23–25]

Drug	CNS Penetration	Notes
Fluoroquinolones (moxifloxacin, levofloxacin)	Good	—
Ethionamide/prothionamide	Good	—
Cycloserine/terizidone	Good	—
Clofazimine	No data	—
Imipenem/cilastatin Meropenem	Poor	Imipenem/cilastatin more likely to cause seizures in children than meropenem
Linezolid	Good	—
High-dose isoniazid	Moderate	Need high dose to be 15–18 mg/kg
Pyrazinamide	Moderate	—
para-Aminosalicylic acid	Negligible	Use is not advised
Ethambutol	Negligible	Use is not advised
Amikacin/streptomycin	Negligible	Only in the presence of meningeal inflammation; in general, use is not advised
Bedaquiline	No data	—
Delamanid	No data	—

- Monthly cultures may not be possible in extrapulmonary TB; therefore, monitoring for response to therapy may be based on clinical and/or radiographic response.

Pregnancy

There is a paucity of data on the treatment of DR-TB in pregnancy. Untreated MDR-TB during pregnancy can be associated with adverse maternal and fetal outcomes.

- The benefits of treatment of DR-TB to mother, child, and the community outweigh the harms.
- An all-oral individualized longer regimen is preferable in order to avoid drugs that may be teratogenic (Table 5).
- The shorter regimen should be avoided in pregnancy.
- Patients on treatment of DR-TB should be counseled to avoid pregnancy and a birth control method should be recommended; oral contraceptives should be avoided as the method for birth control if rifampin is to be used in the regimen, because of drug-drug interactions rendering oral contraceptive pills less effective.

Children

There is a paucity of data on the treatment of DR-TB in children, so many of the recommendations made for adults have been extrapolated to children.[10]

- The longer oral MDR-TB regimen is recommended in children. Injectable agents are used only when other drugs cannot be used because of resistance or toxicity.
- Injectable agents are avoided whenever possible because of the adverse side effect of hearing loss, painful injections, and because children often have paucibacillary disease.
- Given that children are often culture negative, a total treatment duration of 18 to 20 months should be given with a low threshold to decrease the duration in the case of children with less extensive or severe disease.

Table 5
Teratogenicity of antituberculosis drugs[26]

Drug	FDA Category/Teratogenicity	Notes
Isoniazid	C/Safe	—
Rifampin	Safe	—
Fluoroquinolones (levofloxacin, moxifloxacin)	Possible	Arthropathy in puppy models, but wide use in humans shows no negative effect
Ethionamide/ prothionamide	Possible	Associated with congenital defects
Clofazimine	No data	—
Cycloserine/ terizidone	Unlikely	Animal models show no toxicity
Imipenem-cilastatin Meropenem	No data	—
Linezolid	Possible	High dose has shown toxicity in animal models
High-dose isoniazid	No data	—
Pyrazinamide	No data	—
para-Aminosalicylic acid	Unlikely	Animal models show no toxicity
Ethambutol	Safe	—
Amikacin/streptomycin	Documented	Eighth nerve toxicity
Bedaquiline	No data	—
Delamanid	No data	—

Abbreviation: FDA, US Food and Drug Administration.
Adapted from Table 1 in Gupta A, et al. Toward earlier inclusion of pregnant and postpartum women in tuberculosis drug trials: Consensus statements from an international expert panel. Clinical Infectious Diseases 2016;62:762-769.

- A shorter MDR-TB regimen may be given in children, although avoiding the injectable agent may be factored into the decision between the longer and the shorter regimens.
- Gastric aspirates should be obtained for diagnosis and follow-up in young children who cannot produce sputa.
- Child-friendly formulations should be given whenever possible, and breaking of adult-sized pills should be minimized because the efficacy of drugs may be affected by altering the physical properties of the drug.

Comorbid Conditions

The treatment of DR-TB in the setting of comorbid conditions such as diabetes mellitus, tobacco use, alcoholism, and drug use is similar to the treatment of DS-TB in these settings except for the need for dose adjustment of SLDs in the case of renal or hepatic insufficiency. An expert in the management of DR-TB should be consulted in these circumstances.

TREATMENT OF DRUG-RESISTANT TUBERCULOSIS CONTACTS

The treatment of DR-TB contacts seems to have some efficacy in preventing progression to TB disease.[27–29] DR-TB contacts should be evaluated to exclude TB disease and offered treatment of LTBI tailored to the susceptibility pattern of the source-case isolates whenever possible. **Table 6** shows the treatment patterns for appropriate drug choices in this setting.[17]

There are currently 3 ongoing randomized controlled trials evaluating the efficacy of treating contacts of persons with MDR-TB/XDR-TB.[30,31] Close contacts to patients with DR-TB may be considered for prophylactic treatment using the principles set out in **Box 4**:

MONITORING AND EVALUATION
Response to Treatment

- Patients being treated for DR-TB should be closely monitored for treatment failure, acquired drug resistance, loss to follow-up, and potential ADRs.
- Patients should be followed at regular intervals clinically, radiographically (if pulmonary disease), and bacteriologically.
- Monthly cultures should be obtained throughout the treatment duration, and, if still positive at 3 to 4 months,[14,32] or reverts to positive after conversion, DST should be obtained right away to exclude acquired resistance.
- When feasible, an end-of-treatment culture should be obtained to show and document treatment cure.
- Patients should be monitored posttreatment completion at regular intervals for 1 to 2 years for relapse.

Table 6
Treatment of latent tuberculosis infection in contacts of patients with drug-resistant tuberculosis, according to susceptibility pattern of the source-case isolates

Resistance Pattern	LTBI Treatment Options
Isoniazid (rifampin susceptible)	Rifampin 4 mo (adults and children)
Isoniazid, rifampin, ethambutol	Fluoroquinolone, fluoroquinolone + ethambutol
Isoniazid and rifampin, pyrazinamide	Fluoroquinolone, fluoroquinolone + ethionamide
Isoniazid and rifampin, ethambutol, pyrazinamide	Fluoroquinolone, fluoroquinolone + ethambutol
Isoniazid and rifampin, ethambutol, pyrazinamide, ± injectable	Fluoroquinolone, fluoroquinolone + ethionamide
Isoniazid and rifampin, ethambutol, pyrazinamide, injectable, ethionamide	Fluoroquinolone, fluoroquinolone + cycloserine
Isoniazid and rifampin, ethambutol, pyrazinamide, fluoroquinolone	No treatment, clinical monitoring (in select cases, cycloserine + *para*-aminosalicylic acid, *para*-aminosalicylic acid + ethionamide, or ethionamide + cycloserine may be considered)

From Curry International Tuberculosis Center DR-TB Survival Guide.[17] http://www.currytbcenter.ucsf.edu/products/view/drug-resistant-tuberculosis-survival-guide-clinicians-3rd-edition.

Box 4
Principles for the treatment of drug-resistant tuberculosis contacts

- Contacts to DR-TB should have a positive test for LTBI and have TB disease excluded before receiving treatment of presumed MDR LTBI.
- Treatment with 1 to 2 drugs to which the presumed source-case isolate shows susceptibility may be given for a period of 6 to 12 months (see **Table 6**).
- For isoniazid-resistant or PDR-TB (rifampin susceptible), rifampin may be given for a period of 4 months.
- For RR-TB or PDR-TB (isoniazid susceptible), isoniazid may be given for 6 to 9 months.
- For MDR-TB, 6 to 12 months of treatment can be given with a fluoroquinolone alone or with a second drug, based on source-case isolate DST.
- When 2 drugs are used, based on evidence of increased toxicity, ADR, and discontinuations, expert opinion is that pyrazinamide should not be routinely used as the second drug.
- In lieu of fluoroquinolone-based treatment, there are few data for the use of other second-line medications and, because of toxicity, they are not recommended by experts.
- For contacts to fluoroquinolone-resistant, pre–XDR-TB, pyrazinamide and ethambutol may be an effective option, if source-case isolate DST shows susceptibility to these drugs.
- For contacts to fluoroquinolone-resistant, pre–XDR-TB with resistance to all first-line drugs, consider ethionamide/p-aminosalicylic acid or the newer drugs bedaquiline or delamanid. Studies are underway with delamanid.
- In children, TB drugs are generally better tolerated, and levofloxacin is preferred because of the availability of an oral suspension formulation.

Adverse Drug Reaction Monitoring

One of the biggest obstacles to successful completion of treatment and cure is unrecognized/unmanaged or mismanaged ADRs. Early detection and appropriate management of ADRs minimize treatment interruptions, loss to follow-up, and poor treatment outcomes such as treatment failure, relapse, and acquired drug resistance.

- Per WHO, TB programs need to have comprehensive pharmacovigilance programs in place with aDSM to ensure early detection, timely reporting, and appropriate management of ADRs and SAEs, as the standard of care for all patients on any MDR regimen.[33]
- Training and education of field staff is necessary for proper management of ADRs.
- A list of common ADRs and associated TB drugs is provided in **Table 7**.
- Routine monitoring for ADRs and SAEs should be performed while patient is on treatment (see **Table 7**; **Table 8**).
- Note that intolerance to 1 drug in a drug class does not automatically imply intolerance to all drugs in the drug class (eg, rifabutin may be tolerated when rifampin is not).

ADDITIONAL CONSIDERATIONS
Selection of Drugs

The following principles apply when building a DR-TB treatment regimen:

- Cross-resistance: avoid using drugs that have known cross-resistance to other drugs to which the isolate shows resistance (eg, isoniazid and ethionamide) (**Table 9**).
- Avoid previously used drugs (based on history): avoid using drugs that the patient has taken for greater than or equal to 1 month previously unless DST shows the drug organism to be fully susceptible to the drug.
- Consider side effects: chose drugs that will not potentiate or worsen underlying illnesses or symptoms (eg, cycloserine if the patient has underlying mental illness).
- Drug-drug interactions: avoid drugs that have known interactions with other drugs that the patient is taking (eg, bedaquiline and efavirenz).

Administration of Medications

Adherence to the complete DR-TB treatment regimen for the full duration is crucial for relapse free cure. Minimizing treatment interruptions caused by ADRs/SAEs and loss to follow-up requires patient education, good case management, active pharmacovigilance, adherence strategies, and a patient-centered approach to care.

- Dose escalation: one of the measures that may minimize side effects such as nausea and vomiting is the dose escalation method when beginning DR-TB drugs such as ethionamide, para-aminosalicylic acid, and cycloserine (**Fig. 2**). Escalating the dose of drugs over a week allows the patient to get used to the drug and mitigate side effects.

Table 7
Common adverse drug reactions (ADRs) and associated antituberculosis drugs

ADR	Drug	Management[b]
Nausea/vomiting/gastritis	Ethionamide/prothionamide, linezolid, *para*-aminosalicylic acid, pyrazinamide, fluoroquinolones, bedaquiline, clofazimine, delamanid, imipenem-cilastatin, meropenem	Antiemetics; drug ramping; twice-daily dosing
Hepatotoxicity	Isoniazid, rifampin, ethionamide/prothionamide, bedaquiline, moxifloxacin, *para*-aminosalicylic acid	See DR-TB survival guide[17] Stop drugs when liver function tests $\geq5\times$ upper limit of normal or >3× upper limit of normal if symptoms present
Diarrhea	*para*-Aminosalicylic acid, linezolid	Antidiarrheals; drug ramping
CNS side effects	Cycloserine, terizidone, ethionamide/prothionamide, high-dose moxifloxacin	Pyridoxine; psychiatric evaluation
Peripheral neuropathy	Linezolid, isoniazid	Pyridoxine
Bone marrow suppression	Rifampin, linezolid, high-dose isoniazid	Granulocyte-macrophage colony-stimulating factor; erythropoietin
Electrolyte imbalance	Amikacin, streptomycin	Electrolyte replenishment
Renal toxicity	Amikacin, streptomycin	Drug holiday[a]
Eighth nerve toxicity	Amikacin, streptomycin	Drug holiday[a]
Visual toxicity	Ethambutol, linezolid, ethionamide (rare), rifabutin (uveitis)	Stop drug
Rash	Any drug	Topical steroid; oral antihistamine; hospitalization if severe with involvement of mucous membranes (Stevens-Johnson syndrome)
Skin discoloration	Clofazimine	Reversible
Hypothyroidism	*para*-Aminosalicylic acid, ethionamide/prothionamide	Reversible
Cardiac (QT-interval prolongation)	Bedaquiline, delamanid, fluoroquinolones, clofazimine	Depends on extent of prolongation
Arthralgias/myalgias	Pyrazinamide, bedaquiline fluoroquinolones	Exclude gout, symptomatic management
Tendon rupture/aortic aneurysm rupture	Fluoroquinolones	Stop drug

[a] Stopping the offending drug for a short while (<1 week) to evaluate for resolution or improvement of ADR, with low threshold to withdraw offending drug if ADR recurs.
[b] For detailed management of ADRs, see Curry International Tuberculosis Center DR-TB Survival Guide.[17] (http://www.currytbcenter.ucsf.edu/products/view/drug-resistant-tuberculosis-survival-guide-clinicians-3rd-edition).

- Adherence measures/patient-centered approach: a patient-centered approach considers the values and preferences of the patient during treatment. It is the approach that is likely to result in the most humane and effective treatment strategy to ensure cure and other good outcomes.[13]
  o Ideally medication should be given once daily via DOT.
  o Twice-daily dosing is generally discouraged because of the challenge posed for full adherence.
- Intermittent dosing is not advised except in the case of an injectable agent that can be decreased in frequency of dosing to twice or thrice weekly after sputum culture conversion has occurred, generally after 2 to 3 months of therapy, to minimize the potential for toxicity.

Table 8
Monitoring schedule for common adverse drug reactions

Test	Frequency	Drug
Complete blood count	Baseline and monthly	Rifampin, linezolid
Electrolytes, blood urea nitrogen, creatinine	Baseline and monthly	Amikacin, streptomycin
Liver function tests	Baseline and monthly	Isoniazid, rifampin, pyrazinamide, ethionamide/prothionamide, para-aminosalicylic acid, moxifloxacin, bedaquiline
Audiogram	Baseline and monthly	Amikacin, streptomycin
Electrocardiogram	Daily for 2 wk, then monthly	Bedaquiline, delamanid, linezolid, combinations of QT interval–prolonging drugs
Mini mental status examination	Weekly	Cycloserine, terizidone
Neuroexamination	Weekly	Isoniazid, linezolid
Eye examination	Monthly	Ethambutol, linezolid
Skin examination	Monthly	Clofazimine
Thyroid-stimulating hormone	Monthly	para-Aminosalicylic acid, ethionamide

Table 9
Cross-resistance between recommended antituberculosis drugs

Drug	Cross-Resistance	Comments
Isoniazid	Ethionamide	Cross-resistance to ethionamide is common (up to 70%) when there is low-level resistance to isoniazid caused by a mutation in inhA promoter region
Rifampin	Rifamycins	Cross-resistance among the rifamycin class of drugs is typical
Ethambutol	None	—
Pyrazinamide	None	—
Cycloserine	Terizidone	—
para-Aminosalicylic acid	None	—
Ethionamide	Isoniazid	Low-level cross-resistance to isoniazid may occur because of mutation in inhA promoter region
Clofazimine	Bedaquiline	Cross-resistance has been shown in both directions through efflux-based resistance
Linezolid	None	—
Bedaquiline	Clofazimine	Cross-resistance has been shown in both directions through efflux-based resistance
Delamanid	None	—
Fluoroquinolones	Other fluoroquinolones	Data suggest that moxifloxacin may continue to show some activity despite resistance to ofloxacin or levofloxacin[34]

From the Curry International TB Center DR TB survival guide.[17] http://www.currytbcenter.ucsf.edu/products/view/drug-resistant-tuberculosis-survival-guide-clinicians-3rd-edition.

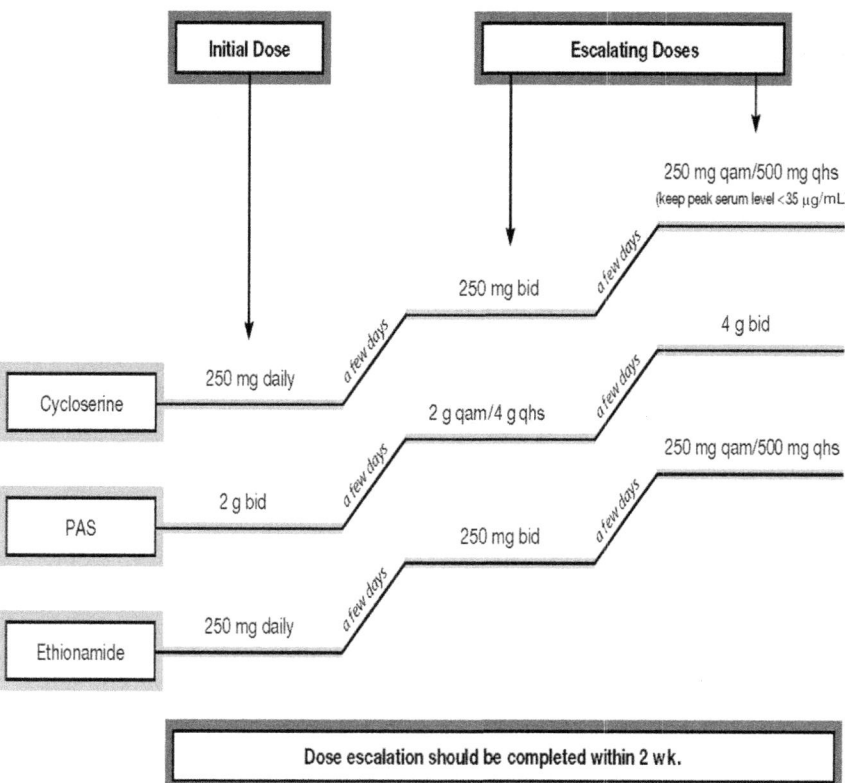

Fig. 2. Dose escalation. The patient is begun on a low starting dose and the dose is increased every few days until the targeted dose is reached. The dose escalation should be completed within 2 weeks. Some patients will tolerate consolidation of cycloserine to once-daily dosing, which can enhance adherence. bid, twice daily; PAS, *para*-aminosalicylic acid; qam, every morning; qhs, at hour of sleep. (*From* the Curry International TB Center DR TB survival guide.[17] http://www.currytbcenter.ucsf.edu/products/view/drug-resistant-tuberculosis-survival-guide-clinicians-3rd-edition.)

- Intermittent dosing may be required with clofazimine in children (see online Table).[35]
- Palliative care: when there is no treatment option available because of extensive resistance and disease, the patient must receive palliative measures such as pain management and management of dyspnea to provide the most humane care possible. It is also necessary to follow infection control practices to minimize transmission of DR-TB to family members and the community.

THERAPEUTIC DRUG MONITORING

Therapeutic drug monitoring (TDM), or the measurement of serum levels of drugs, can be an important test to check for treatment adherence (confirming ingestion of TB drugs), for adequate dosing of TB drugs, and to maximize efficacy and minimize toxicity of TB drugs.[36]

- A quality-assured laboratory is required for TDM.

- A pharmacology specialist is required for performing TDM and interpreting the results.
- TDM may be helpful in the following situations:
  - For dosage of toxic drugs like amikacin, linezolid, cycloserine.
  - In renal insufficiency, diabetes mellitus, HIV infection, and other comorbid conditions that may affect the absorption or excretion of drugs.
  - For patients with evidence of treatment failure or relapse while on an appropriate treatment regimen.
  - When patients have few effective drugs in the treatment regimen based on DST results.
  - When drug-drug interactions are likely.

SURGERY

Patients with extensive resistance, extensive disease, or localized disease may benefit from surgical resection in addition to treatment[37] with a DR-TB treatment regimen, especially when there

Table 10
Outcomes for patients with rifampin-resistant/multidrug-resistant/extensively drug-resistant tuberculosis treated using second-line treatment

Treatment Outcome	Current WHO Definition
Cured	Treatment completed as recommended by the national policy without evidence of failure, and 3 or more consecutive cultures taken at least 30 d apart are negative after the intensive phase[a]
Completed	Treatment completed as recommended by the national policy without evidence of failure, but no record that 3 or more consecutive cultures taken at least 30 d apart are negative after the intensive phase[a]
Treatment failure (RR-TB/MDR-TB/XDR-TB)	Treatment terminated or need for permanent regimen change of at least 2 anti-TB drugs because of: • Lack of conversion[b] by the end of the intensive phase[a], or • Bacteriologic reversion[b] in the continuation phase after conversion[b] to negative, or • Evidence of additional acquired resistance to fluoroquinolones or SLI drugs, or • ADRs
Died	A patient who dies for any reason during the course of treatment
Lost to follow-up	A patient whose treatment was interrupted for 2 consecutive months or more
Not evaluated	A patient for whom no treatment outcome is assigned (this includes cases transferred out to another treatment unit and whose treatment outcome is unknown)
Treatment success	The sum of cured and treatment completed

[a] For treatment failed, lack of conversion by the end of the intensive phase implies that the patient does not convert within the maximum duration of intensive phase applied by the program. If no maximum duration is defined, an 8-month cutoff is proposed. For regimens without a clear distinction between intensive and continuation phases, a cutoff 8 months after the start of treatment is suggested to determine when the criteria for cured, treatment completed, and treatment failed start to apply.

[b] The terms conversion and reversion of culture as used here are defined as follows. Conversion (to negative) means that culture is considered to have converted to negative when 2 consecutive cultures, taken at least 30 days apart, are found to be negative. In such a case, the specimen collection date of the first negative culture is used as the date of conversion. Reversion (to positive) means that culture is considered to have reverted to positive when, after an initial conversion, 2 consecutive cultures, taken at least 30 days apart, are found to be positive. For the purpose of defining treatment failed, reversion is considered only when it occurs in the continuation phase.

From the WHO Definitions and Reporting Framework for Tuberculosis, 2013 revision. https://www.who.int/tb/publications/definitions/en/.

is a high risk of relapse or treatment failure with chemotherapy alone.

- Patients should have preoperative evaluation to determine that they are good surgical candidates, to ensure that they will have adequate lung capacity after surgery, and to ensure that they are not at risk for pulmonary hypertension after surgery.
- Lobectomy or wedge resection is the procedure of choice.
- Surgery should be performed by a surgeon with expertise in TB surgery.
- Proper infection control mechanisms should be in place during surgery (ultraviolet light, personal protective equipment).
- An appropriate treatment regimen should be given in conjunction with surgery, because surgery alone is not curative.

DRUG DOSAGES

In the recent updated WHO DR-TB guidelines, adult and pediatric drug dosages have been revised. The revised dosages may be found in on-line Table.[35]

WORLD HEALTH ORGANIZATION TREATMENT OUTCOMES

A recent publication from the Global TB Network[38] suggests several proposed revisions to the current WHO definitions of TB treatment outcomes to address some of the recent changes in treatment regimens (eg, all-oral regimens) and evolution in programmatic definitions for treatment outcomes. **Table 10** highlights current WHO treatment outcome definitions.[14]

RESEARCH PRIORITIES

Like numerous other pathogens, *M tuberculosis* complex has a remarkable ability to evolve and adapt to the presence of antimicrobials, developing virulence or resistance to commonly used drugs and rendering them ineffective. From programmatic and clinical perspectives, there are several areas in which research will continue to be needed for addressing drug resistance of TB. From a programmatic perspective, it is important that strategies are developed to improve appropriate antimicrobial use and ways of achieving adherence. From a clinical perspective, it is important that clinical trials are conducted to validate use of existing and new drugs and regimens and improve on the methods for conducting surveillance and monitoring of drug resistance. Over the past decade, the products of several comprehensive efforts to identify research priorities for TB have been published.[39–41] These areas of research include:

- Randomized controlled trials, including new drugs and shorter all-oral regimens.
- Studies to include children, pregnant women, extrapulmonary disease, persons living with HIV, patients with other comorbid conditions.
- Pharmacokinetic studies to determine optimal dosing and safety of drugs.
- Documentation of ADRs and SAEs through programmatic pharmacovigilance.
- Shorter MDR-TB regimens and their use in subgroups such as children, pregnant women, and patients with extrapulmonary disease.
- Optimal duration of the longer MDR-TB regimen.
- Predictors and biomarkers of treatment failure and relapse.
- Studies on optimal methods to achieve patient adherence.
- Optimal duration of posttreatment monitoring for relapse.
- Optimal regimen and duration of treatment of MDR-TB contacts.

APPENDIX 1: RESOURCES FOR THE MANAGEMENT OF DRUG-RESISTANT TUBERCULOSIS

1. Four regionally assigned CDC-supported TB Centers of Excellence (COEs), formerly known as Regional Training and Medical Consultation Centers. The TB COEs support domestic TB prevention and control efforts by increasing knowledge, skills, and abilities through communication, education, and training activities, and by improving evidence-based TB clinical practices and patient care through the provision of expert medical consultation (https://npin.cdc.gov/featured-partner/tb-regional-training-and-medical-consultation-centers-rtmccshttps://sntc.medicine.ufl.edu/rtmccproducts.aspx).
   a. Curry International Tuberculosis Center, part of the University of California at San Francisco (https://www.currytbcenter.ucsf.edu/)
   b. Global Tuberculosis Institute at Rutgers, the State University of New Jersey (http://globaltb.njms.rutgers.edu/)
   c. Heartland National Tuberculosis Center in San Antonio, part of the University of Texas Health Science Center at Tyler (https://www.heartlandntbc.org/)
   d. Southeastern National Tuberculosis Center at the University of Florida in Gainesville, Florida (https://sntc.medicine.ufl.edu/home/index#/)
2. Curry International Tuberculosis Center Drug-Resistant TB Survival Guide https://www.currytbcenter.ucsf.edu/products/view/drug-resistant-tuberculosis-survival-guide-clinicians-3rd-edition
3. European Respiratory Society Consultation service (http://www.waidid.org/site/clinicalIntro)
4. CA State MDR-TB Consultation Service (https://www.cdph.ca.gov/Programs/CID/DCDC/CDPH%20Document%20Library/TBCB-MDR-Fact-Sheet.pdf)

SUPPLEMENTARY DATA

Supplementary data to this article can be found online at https://doi.org/10.1016/j.ccm.2019.08.002.

REFERENCES

1. Salomon N, Perlman DC. Editorial response: multidrug-resistant tuberculosis – globally with us for the long haul. Clin Infect Dis 1999;29:93–5.
2. World Health Organization. Global tuberculosis report 2019. Geneva (Switzerland): World Health Organization; 2019. Available at: http://www10.who.int/tb/publications/global_report/en/.
3. von Groote-Bidlingmaier F, Patientia R, Sanchez E, et al. Efficacy and safety of delamanid in combination with an optimised background regimen for treatment of multidrug-resistant tuberculosis: a multicentre, randomised, double-blind, placebo-controlled, parallel group phase 3 trial. Lancet Respir Med 2019;7:249.
4. Nunn AJ, Philipps P, Meredith S, et al. A trial of a shorter regimen for rifampin-resistant tuberculosis.

N Engl J Med 2019. https://doi.org/10.1056/NEJMoa1811867.

5. Ahuja SD, Ashkin D, Avendano M, et al. Multidrug resistant pulmonary tuberculosis treatment regimens and patient outcomes: an individual patient data meta-analysis of 9,153 patients. PLoS Med 2012; 9(8):e1001300.

6. Falzon D, Gandhi N, Migliori GB, et al. Resistance to fluoroquinolones and second-line injectable drugs: impact on multidrug-resistant TB outcomes. Eur Respir J 2013 Jul;42(1):156–68.

7. Bastos ML, Lan Z, Menzies D. An updated systematic review and meta-analysis for treatment of multidrug-resistant tuberculosis. Eur Respir J 2017; 49(3) [pii:1600803].

8. Collaborative Group for the Meta-Analysis of Individual Patient Data in MDR TB Treatment-2017, Ahmad N, Ahuja SD, Akkerman OW, et al. Treatment successful correlates of outcomes in pulmonary multidrug-resistant tuberculosis: an individual patient data meta-analysis. Lancet 2018;392(10150):821–34.

9. Fregonese F, Ahuja SD, Akkerman OW, et al. Comparison of different treatments for isoniazid-resistant tuberculosis: an individual patient data meta-analysis. Lancet Respir Med 2018;6(4):265–75.

10. Harausz EP, Garcia-Prats AJ, Law S, et al. Treatment and outcomes in children with multidrug-resistant tuberculosis: a systematic review and individual patient data meta-analysis. PLoS Med 2018;15(7): e1002591.

11. Fox GJ, Mitnick CD, Benedetti A, et al. Surgery as an adjunctive treatment for multidrug-resistant tuberculosis: an individual patient data metaanalysis. Clin Infect Dis 2016;62(7):887–95.

12. Ahmad Khan F, Salim MAH, du Cros P, et al. Effectiveness and safety of standardised shorter regimens for multidrug-resistant tuberculosis: individual patient data and aggregate data meta-analyses. Eur Respir J 2017;50(1) [pii:1700061].

13. Reid MJA, Goosby E. Patient-centered tuberculosis programs are necessary to end the epidemic. J Infect Dis 2017;216(suppl_7):S673–4.

14. World Health Organization. WHO consolidated guidelines on guidelines on drug-resistant tuberculosis treatment. Geneva (Switzerland): World Health Organization; 2019. Available at: https://www.who.int/tb/publications/2019/consolidated-guidelines-drug-resistant-TB-treatment/en/.

15. World Health Organization. Guidelines for the treatment of drug-susceptible tuberculosis and patient care, 2017 update. Geneva (Switzerland): World Health Organization; 2017 (WHO/HTM/TB/2017.05). Available at: http://apps.who.int/iris/bitstream/10665/255052/1/9789241550000-eng.pdf.

16. American Public Health Laboratories (APHL). Laboratory considerations for use of Cepheid Xpert® MTB/RIF assay. Silver Spring (MD): APHL; 2013. Available at: https://www.aphl.org/AboutAPHL/publications/Documents/ID_2013Nov_Cepheid-Xpert-Fact-Sheet.pdf.

17. Curry International Tuberculosis Center and California Department of Public Health. Drug-resistant tuberculosis: a survival guide for clinicians. 3rd edition. San Francisco (CA): Francis C Curry International Tuberculosis Center; 2016.

18. World Health Organization. Handbook for the use of digital technologies to support tuberculosis medication adherence. Geneva (Switzerland): World Health Organization; 2018. Available at: https://apps.who.int/iris/bitstream/handle/10665/259832/9789241513456-eng.pdf.

19. World Health Organization. Technical manual for drug susceptibility testing of medicines used in the treatment of tuberculosis. Geneva (Switzerland): World Health Organization; 2018. Available at: https://apps.who.int/iris/bitstream/handle/10665/275469/9789241514842-eng.pdf?ua=1.

20. Meng L, Huang J, Jia Y, et al. Assessing fluoroquinolone-associated aortic aneurysm and dissection: data mining of the public version of the FDA adverse event reporting system. Int J Clin Pract 2019;73(5):e13331.

21. Schunemann HJ, Jaeschke R, Cook DJ, et al. An official ATS statement: grading the quality of evidence and strength of recommendations in ATS guidelines and recommendations. Am J Respir Crit Care Med 2006;174:605–14.

22. Guyatt GH, Oxman AD, Vist GE, et al. GRADE: an emerging consensus on rating quality of evidence and strength of recommendations. BMJ 2008;336: 924–6.

23. Donald PR. Cerebrospinal fluid concentrations of antituberculosis agents in adults and children. Tuberculosis 2010;90(5):279–92. ISSN 1472-9792.

24. Tsona A, Metallidis S, Foroglou N, et al. Linezolid penetration into cerebrospinal fluid and brain tissue. J Chemother 2010;22(1):17–9.

25. Blassmann U, Roehr AC, Frey OR, et al. Cerebrospinal fluid penetration of meropenem in neurocritical care patients with proven or suspected ventriculitis: a prospective observational study. Crit Care 2016; 20(1):343.

26. Gupta A, Mathad JS, Abdel-Rahman SM, et al. Toward earlier inclusion of pregnant and postpartum women in tuberculosis drug trials: consensus statements from an international expert panel. Clin Infect Dis 2016;62(6):761–9.

27. Bamrah S, Brostrom R, Dorina F, et al. Treatment for LTBI in contacts of MDR-TB patients, Federated States of Micronesia, 2009-2012. Int J Tuberc Lung Dis 2014;18(8):912–8.

28. Marks SM, Mase SR, Morris SB. Systematic review, meta-analysis, and cost-effectiveness of treatment of latent tuberculosis to reduce progression to

multidrug-resistant tuberculosis. Clin Infect Dis 2017;64(12):1670–7.

29. Sterling TR. Fluoroquinolones for the treatment and prevention of multidrug-resistant tuberculosis. Int J Tuberc Lung Dis 2016;20(12):42–7.

30. Seddon JA, Garcia-Prats AJ, Purchase SE, et al. Levofloxacin versus placebo for the prevention of tuberculosis disease in child contacts of multidrug-resistant tuberculosis: study protocol for a phase III cluster randomised controlled trial (TB-CHAMP). Trials 2018;19(1):693.

31. Dheda K, Gumbo T, Maartens G, et al. The epidemiology, pathogenesis, transmission, diagnosis, and management of multidrug-resistant, extensively drug-resistant, and incurable tuberculosis. Lancet Respir Med 2017;5(4):291–360.

32. Nahid P, Dorman SE, Alipanah N, et al. Official American Thoracic Society/Centers for Disease Control and Prevention/Infections Diseases Society of America Clinical Practice Guidelines: treatment of drug-susceptible tuberculosis. Clin Infect Dis 2016;63: e147–95.

33. World Health Organization. Companion Handbook to the WHO guidelines for programmatic management of drug-resistant tuberculosis. Geneva (Switzerland): World Health Organization; 2014. Available at: https://www.ncbi.nlm.nih.gov/books/NBK247420/pdf/Bookshelf_NBK247420.pdf.

34. Sirgel FA, Warren RM, Streicher EM, et al. gyrA mutations and phenotypic susceptibility levels to ofloxacin and moxifloxacin in clinical isolates of mycobacterium tuberculosis. J Antimicrob Chemother 2012;67:1088–93.

35. World Health Organization. Dosage by weight band for medicines used in MDR-TB regimens, adults and children. Geneva (Switzerland): World Health Organization; 2019. Annex 2 in reference 14 above.

36. Peloquin CA. Therapeutic drug monitoring in the treatment of tuberculosis. Drugs 2002;62: 2169–83.

37. Marrone MT, Venkataramanan V, Goodman M, et al. Surgical interventions for drug-resistant tuberculosis: a systematic review and meta-analysis. Int J Tuberc Lung Dis 2013;17(1):6–16.

38. Migliori GB, The Global Tuberculosis Network (GTN). Evolution of programmatic definitions used in tuberculosis prevention and care. Clin Infect Dis 2019;68(10):1787–9.

39. World Health Organization. Priorities for tuberculosis research: a report of the disease reference group report on TB, leprosy and Buruli ulcer. Geneva (Switzerland): World Health Organization; 2013. Available at: https://www.who.int/tdr/publications/tuberculosis_research/en/.

40. Rylance J, Pai M, Lienhardt C, et al. Priorities for tuberculosis research: a systematic review. Lancet Infect Dis 2010;10:886–92.

41. Lienhardt C, Lonnroth K, Menzies D, et al. Translational research for tuberculosis elimination: priorities, challenges, and actions. PLoS Med 2016. https://doi.org/10.1371/journal.pmed.100196.

Management of Children with Tuberculosis

Ameneh Khatami, BHB, MBChB, MD*, Philip N. Britton, MBBS, PhD,
Ben J. Marais, BMedSc, MBChB, MMed, PhD

KEYWORDS

• Child • Tuberculosis • Multi-drug resistant • *Mycobacterium tuberculosis* • Prevention • Diagnosis
• Treatment • Management

KEY POINTS

• Tuberculosis in children is often undiagnosed and unreported, but contributes to significant childhood morbidity and mortality globally.
• In the absence of preventive therapy, young children have a high risk of rapid disease progression after primary infection and can develop severe forms of tuberculosis.
• Signs and symptoms of tuberculosis in children are often nonspecific and very young children can present acutely.
• Microbiological confirmation should be sought in all instances, but in the absence of microbiological confirmation children should be treated according to the drug susceptibility pattern of the most likely source case.
• The principles of tuberculosis (including drug-resistant tuberculosis) treatment in children are similar to adults, although drugs are usually better tolerated and outcomes are better, especially for drug-resistant disease.

INTRODUCTION

In recent years there has been renewed interest in pediatric tuberculosis (TB) with growing awareness that more children have TB than was previously thought. TB is a significant cause of childhood morbidity and mortality in endemic areas, making a major contribution to global under 5 mortality with most affected children remaining undiagnosed and untreated.[1] However, a precise estimate of the global burden of TB in children is difficult, owing to challenges in case ascertainment and weak surveillance systems in many high TB incidence countries.[2] Pediatric TB is thought to represent less than 5% of all TB cases in low incidence settings, but at least 10% to 20% of all TB cases in areas with poor epidemic control.[3,4] The World Health Organization (WHO) estimates that in 2015, of the 10.4 million new TB cases, 10% (approximately 1 million cases) occurred in children.[5]

Overall, 5% to 15% of the estimated 2 to 3 billion people infected with *Mycobacterium tuberculosis* will develop TB in their lifetime; however, this risk is higher in young children and people with immune compromise, such as people living with human immunodeficiency virus (HIV).[6] Disease onset in children generally occurs within 1 year of primary infection.[7] As such, the incidence of pediatric TB is an indirect indicator of epidemic control and the effectiveness of TB control programs.[3,8] For example, the occurrence of drug-resistant (DR) TB in children reflects recent transmission of drug resistant strains in the community. Pediatric

Conflicts of interest: None to declare.
The Children's Hospital at Westmead Clinical School, Level 3 Children's Hospital Westmead, Locked Bag 4001, Hawkesbury Road, Westmead, New South Wales 2145, Australia
* Corresponding author. Department of Infectious Diseases and Microbiology, Children's Hospital Westmead, Locked Bag 4001, Hawkesbury Road, Westmead, New South Wales 2145, Australia.
E-mail address: Ameneh.khatami@gmail.com

Clin Chest Med 40 (2019) 797–810
https://doi.org/10.1016/j.ccm.2019.08.003
0272-5231/19/Crown Copyright © 2019 Published by Elsevier Inc. All rights reserved.

multidrug-resistant (MDR) TB cases have now been identified in every country where adult MDR TB cases have been diagnosed, with estimates that around 30,000 children develop MDR TB every year.[9,10]

PREVENTION

At a population level, the most effective means to limit TB transmission is early diagnosis and prompt initiation of appropriate treatment in all infectious cases.[11] Improving epidemic control is critical to prevent TB infection and subsequent disease in children.[3,12] Traditional passive case finding efforts are not sufficient to limit TB transmission in high incidence settings[13] and active case finding efforts in high-risk populations (eg, among people living with HIV) and in geographic disease hot spots seems to be essential to improve epidemic control. In addition, population-based approaches to target the social determinants of disease, including poverty and inequality, cigarette smoke exposure and indoor air pollution, as well as major comorbidities are crucial.[14]

Infection Control

Infection control failures within health care facilities can also fuel TB spread. TB endemic areas are often poorly equipped to implement appropriate infection control precautions, which results in significant risk to vulnerable young children who come in contact with coughing adolescents or adults who may have infectious TB. Robust measures require attention to building design, air flow, and air disinfection, as well as patient flows and management, such as triage of coughing patients, use of face masks, and effective respiratory isolation of potentially infectious patients.[15]

Bacille Calmette-Guerin Vaccination

Where there is failure of epidemic control, primary prevention of TB in children relies on bacille Calmette-Guerin (BCG) vaccination. Although BCG vaccination offers little protection against adult forms of disease and has limited epidemic impact,[16] it provides strong (approximately 80%) protection against disseminated (miliary) TB and TB meningitis in infants and young children[17]; offering protection against both drug-susceptible (DS) and DR-TB. Reports on the duration of protection provided by BCG vary, range from less than 10 to more than 50 years.[18] In general, the protective effect and duration of protection seems to increase with increasing latitude.[19] Owing to the risk of disseminated BCG disease[20] and lack of protective efficacy in HIV-infected infants,[21] BCG

vaccination is not recommended in this group.[22] In practice, this risk is minimized by well-functioning prevention of mother to child (vertical) HIV transmission programs. It is important to ensure high BCG coverage rates in all settings with uncontrolled TB transmission.[23]

Countries with minimal TB transmission, like the United States, often do not provide BCG vaccination at birth. It is important to recognize that unvaccinated young children are highly vulnerable and may be exposed to TB when immigrant families visit their country of origin (so-called visiting friends and relatives travel). Risk factors identified in a case series from Sydney, Australia,[24,25] included children born in a high TB incidence country (especially recent migrants), or having at least 1 parent born in a high TB incidence country, as well as children from a refugee background. Recent travel to a high TB incidence country, recent close contact with TB, and a lack of BCG vaccination were additional risk factors identified. Previous concern that BCG vaccination may interfere with future TB infection testing, is no longer valid now that more specific interferon-γ release assays (IGRAs) are available.

Preventive Therapy

Secondary prevention of TB involves screening of close contacts of infectious TB cases with provision of preventive therapy to infected individuals. Standard guidelines advise preventive therapy for all immunocompromised individuals and children aged less than 5 years (irrespective of immune status) after TB infection or close contact with an infectious TB case.[26,27] The most recent WHO guidance expands this to all infected contacts.[28] However, this is rarely implemented in TB endemic settings and considerable policy–practice gaps remain.[29] The WHO estimates that only a small fraction of exposed children around the world are provided preventive therapy (2.3% in South East Asia, 5.6% in Africa, 12% in the Eastern Mediterranean region, 13% in the Western Pacific region, 42% in Europe, and 67% in the Americas).[5]

Even in TB endemic settings, where the protective effect might be transient (given the high likelihood of future reinfection), preventive therapy is important to cover periods of high vulnerability, such as infection in young children or HIV-infected adults.[30] Without preventive therapy, there is a high risk of disease progression after primary M tuberculosis infection in young children,[7] as recently demonstrated in an observational study from Victoria, Australia.[31]

Preventive therapy, most commonly with isoniazid (INH) for 6 months, has been shown to be effective in preventing TB disease and mortality in children,[6] including those with HIV coinfection.[32] Short-course preventive therapy options, including INH and rifampin (RIF) or rifapentine (for children >2 years) for 3 months,[28] or RIF alone for 4 months,[33] have demonstrated equivalent efficacy with improved treatment adherence and reduced adverse effects (**Table 1**).

Either the tuberculin skin test (TST) or IGRAs may be used to diagnose latent TB infection, depending on local availability and relevant patient factors.[34] Neither the TST nor IGRAs can reliably differentiate TB infection from active disease. For young children, exclusion of active disease on the basis of a symptom screen, if access to chest radiography is limited, has been shown to be sufficient before commencing preventive therapy.[35] Furthermore, because preventive therapy is well-tolerated in children, its use in vulnerable young children with significant recent TB exposure is appropriate, even in the absence of TST/IGRA results (particularly in resource-limited settings).[36]

There is also general consensus to provide preventive therapy to infected young children (<5 years of age) in close contact with an infectious MDR-TB case, using newer generation fluoroquinolones (moxifloxacin or levofloxacin) or based on the drug resistance profile of the presumptive source case. WHO guidance requires consideration on a case-by-case basis,[28] and similar to the US Centers for Disease Control and Prevention[37] and European guidelines[38] offer alternatives of periodic screening or preventive therapy. Even if preventive therapy is given, because clear

evidence of effectiveness is not yet available, infected contacts of MDR-TB patients should be followed for at least 2 years.

DIAGNOSIS

It is now recognized that TB represents a dynamic continuum from a robust immunologic response, wherein all infecting bacteria are cleared, sometimes even without stimulation of acquired immunity, to uncontrolled bacterial replication and fulminant (disseminated) disease (**Fig. 1**). Cohort studies from low transmission settings indicate that 5% to 15% of recently infected individuals will develop TB disease during their lifetime, with the highest risk among those with recent primary infection (during the past 2 years).[31] Individuals with significant immunologic impairment have a particularly high risk of both early disease progression and later disease reactivation.

Young children are at high risk of disease progression based on both immunologic immaturity and recency of infection. Without BCG vaccination, approximately 50% of infants who become infected with M tuberculosis will progress to disease; 10% to 20% will develop disseminated disease.[39] TB disease risk declines to a nadir around 5 to 10 years of age, after which the risk to develop adult-type TB starts to increase. The disease spectrum in children is broad and varies to some extent with age. The rates of lymph node involvement and disseminated disease are highest in young children, whereas adult-type cavitary lung disease predominates after puberty.[40] Around 15% to 25% of disease in children younger than 15 years is extrapulmonary,[1] with lymphadenopathy being the most common manifestation (67%), followed by central nervous system (CNS) involvement (13%), pleural (6%), miliary/disseminated (5%), and skeletal (4%) TB.[39]

Establishing a TB diagnosis requires consideration of the clinical features of disease (including symptoms), and an epidemiologic link to TB exposure or proof of infection (**Fig. 2**). Identifying risk factors for TB disease progression will influence the urgency of diagnostic evaluation. Although TB usually presents as a subacute or chronic illness, it can present acutely in very young or immunocompromised children. In the early stages of disease there may not be sufficient findings to make a presumptive TB diagnosis and careful clinical follow-up is warranted. In the majority of uncertain cases, there is no urgency to initiate TB treatment and the natural evolution of symptoms and signs, or response to alternative therapies, may provide important clues to guide TB treatment decisions.

Table 1
Options for LTBI treatment in children

HIV Uninfected	HIV Infected	After MDR-TB Exposure
6 or 9 H (daily)	9 H (daily)	Only if considered to be at high risk of TB disease progression
3 HR (daily)		
4 R (daily)		1–2 drugs (including moxi/levofloxacin) for 6 mo based on DST of the likely source case
3 HP[a] (weekly)		

Abbreviations: DST, drug susceptibility test; H, isoniazid; LTBI, latent tuberculosis infection; P, rifapentine; R, rifampin.
[a] In children older than 2 y of age.

Symptoms of tuberculosis
Infection cleared by innate immunity
Adaptive immune response
Early disease, minimal symptoms
Advanced disease

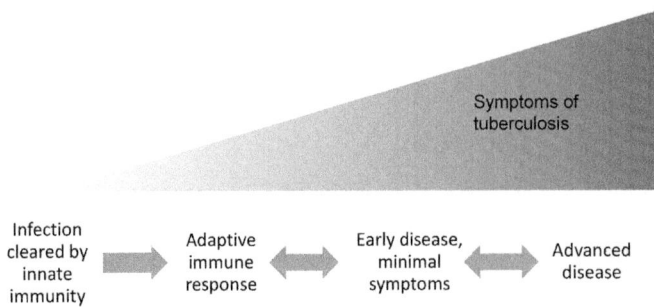

Fig. 1. The spectrum of TB from infection to disease. *Adapted from* Fox GJ, Dobler CC, Marais BJ, et al. Preventive therapy for latent tuberculosis infection-the promise and the challenges. *Int J Infect Dis.* 2017;56:68-76.

Clinical Assessment

Exposure history

Given their limited mobility and social contact, very young children (<3 years of age) usually acquire TB infection from people living in the same household.[41] As children's social interactions outside the household increases with age and independence, their risk of acquiring TB from the community increases, depending on levels of TB transmission within the community.[41] A detailed TB exposure history should explore recent (within the past 1–2 years) contact with confirmed TB cases, people with unexplained chronic cough, or anyone who died with an unexplained chronic

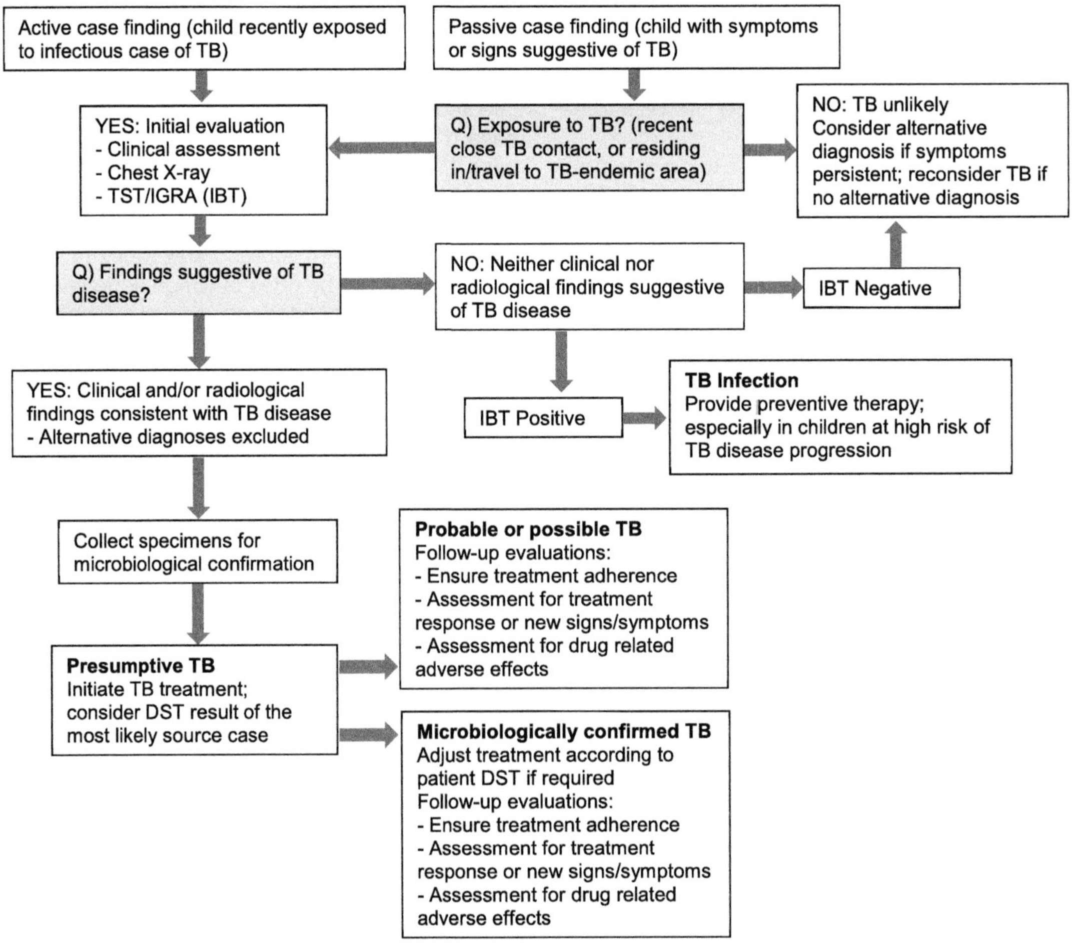

Active case finding (child recently exposed to infectious case of TB)
Passive case finding (child with symptoms or signs suggestive of TB)
YES: Initial evaluation
- Clinical assessment
- Chest X-ray
- TST/IGRA (IBT)
Q) Exposure to TB? (recent close TB contact, or residing in/travel to TB-endemic area)
NO: TB unlikely
Consider alternative diagnosis if symptoms persistent; reconsider TB if no alternative diagnosis
Q) Findings suggestive of TB disease?
NO: Neither clinical nor radiological findings suggestive of TB disease
IBT Negative
YES: Clinical and/or radiological findings consistent with TB disease
- Alternative diagnoses excluded
IBT Positive
TB Infection
Provide preventive therapy; especially in children at high risk of TB disease progression
Collect specimens for microbiological confirmation
Probable or possible TB
Follow-up evaluations:
- Ensure treatment adherence
- Assessment for treatment response or new signs/symptoms
- Assessment for drug related adverse effects
Presumptive TB
Initiate TB treatment; consider DST result of the most likely source case
Microbiologically confirmed TB
Adjust treatment according to patient DST if required
Follow-up evaluations:
- Ensure treatment adherence
- Assessment for treatment response or new signs/symptoms
- Assessment for drug related adverse effects

Fig. 2. Diagnosis of TB in children. DST, drug susceptibility testing; IBT, immune-based testing; NAAT, nucleic acid amplification test; Q, question; TB, tuberculosis. *Adapted from* Roya-Pabon CL, Perez-Velez CM. Tuberculosis exposure, infection and disease in children: a systematic diagnostic approach. Pneumonia (Nathan). 2016 Nov 24;8:23. https://doi.org/10.1186/s41479-016-0023-9. eCollection 2016.

illness.[41] It is important to consider the infectiousness of possible source cases, as well as the proximity, duration, and recency of contact, because most children who progress to active disease do so within 12 months after exposure or infection.

Symptoms and signs

Symptoms and signs of TB are often nonspecific and include fever (sometimes with night sweats), failure to thrive or weight loss, and fatigue or lethargy. Typical TB symptoms, such as a cough for longer than 2 weeks, are less sensitive in young or immunocompromised children.[42] For example, young children may present with bronchodilator-nonresponsive wheezing owing to airway compression from enlarged intrathoracic lymph nodes. In addition, a discrepancy between relatively mild clinical and severe radiologic signs is often suggestive of TB. TB lymphadenitis, which is the most common extrapulmonary manifestation of TB in children, often presents as a unilateral, nonpainful, matted lymph node mass in the cervical or supraclavicular region.[43]

Imaging

The spectrum of radiologic abnormalities in TB is broad and signs can be nonspecific.[44] Standard chest radiography, with a lateral projection, is useful in children for detecting enlarged hilar lymph nodes that may be obscured by the thymic shadow or other anatomic structures on the frontal view[45] (**Fig. 3**). A computed tomography scan of the chest allows a more detailed assessment, but routine use is discouraged owing to high radiation exposure. Similarly, bronchoscopy may assist in the diagnosis and management of complicated cases with tracheobronchial disease, but is not routinely indicated.[46] Ultrasound examination may be useful to evaluate pleural or pericardial fluid collections and lymph nodes.

Laboratory Tests

The most common nonspecific findings on full blood count in TB are mild anemia, neutrophilia, and monocytosis.[47] Body fluid (eg, pleural, pericardial, or cerebrospinal fluid [CSF]) cell counts and chemistry can be highly suggestive of TB; however, disease caused by other mycobacteria or fungal infections may present with similar findings. In general, nonturbid yellow fluid collected from a pleural or pericardial tap with moderately raised cell counts (predominantly lymphocytic, but may be neutrophilic early in the disease), elevated protein and reduced glucose is suggestive of TB.[48] A similar profile in the CSF is seen in TB meningitis.[49] In addition, biochemical markers such as lactate dehydrogenase and especially adenosine deaminase can strongly support a TB diagnosis. In adult studies, the sensitivity and specificity of adenosine deaminase values that are 40 U/L or greater is around 90% and 92%, respectively, with pleural effusions, and 88% and 83% with pericardial effusions.[50] Increased adenosine deaminase levels in CSF are also highly associated with TB meningitis.[51]

Immune-based Testing

TB infection is diagnosed by measuring immune sensitization to M tuberculosis proteins. The TST or Mantoux test is an in vivo measure of delayed type hypersensitivity to subcutaneously injected purified protein derivative, which has been used to diagnose TB infection for more than a century. However, the test is difficult to standardize and operator dependent, with false-negative test results possible owing to inadequate purified protein derivative storage, poor administration technique, overwhelming TB disease (eg, miliary disease), and other causes of immunosuppression such as severe malnutrition, HIV, or recent measles infection. In addition, the purified protein derivative contains antigens that cross-react with other mycobacteria and false-positive results may occur owing to BCG vaccination or after exposure (and especially disease) caused by nontuberculous mycobacteria (NTM).[52] The immune responses induced by the BCG vaccination at birth wane fairly rapidly[53] and it remains the most widely used test, owing to its low cost, relative ease of use,[54] and comparable diagnostic performance compared with IGRAs.[55]

IGRAs are in vitro tests that quantify interferon-gamma production by sensitized T cells after stimulation by TB-specific antigens.[56] These tests, including the commercially available enzyme-linked immunospot assay-based T-SPOT.TB (Oxford Immunotec USA, Inc, Marlborough, MA) and the enzyme-linked immunosorbent assay-based QuantiFERON Gold In-Tube and QuantiFERON Gold Plus (Qiagen, Hilden, Germany), offer increased specificity compared with the TST as they include antigens (CFP-10 and ESAT-6) rarely found in NTM, although Mycobacterium bovis, Mycobacterium kansasii, Mycobacterium szulgai, and Mycobacterium marinum do express CFP-10 and ESAT-6, which can lead to false-positive results.[57] However, IGRAs are more expensive and technically challenging to implement, with more variable reactions around specified cut-off values.

Both TST and IGRA tests reflect memory T-cell responses and are unable to differentiate current from previous TB disease or recent from remote

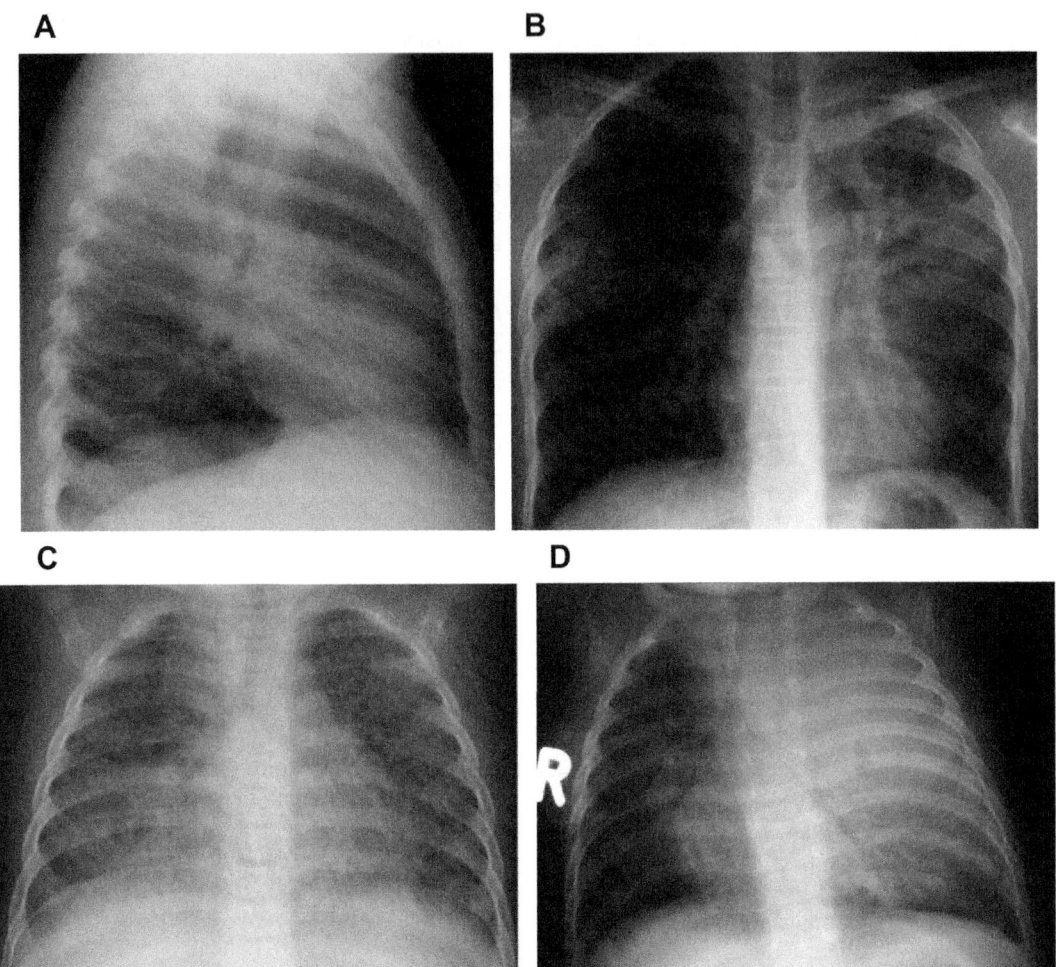

Fig. 3. Examples of findings on chest radiography in children with TB. (*A*) Intrathoracic lymph node disease: a density can be seen behind and below the carina. The dense circular ring around the hilum ("doughnut sign") is indicative of perihilar lymph node involvement. (*B*) Adult-type disease only emerges with the onset of puberty around 8 to 10 years of age and seems to be associated with an excessive and poorly regulated immune response. (*C*) Disseminated (miliary) disease: usually in very young children (<2–3 years of age) or severely immune compromised children, occurs within 6 months after primary infection. The spread of *M tuberculosis* via the bloodstream results in tubercles throughout the lungs and other organs and is frequently associated with TB meningitis. (*D*) Caseating (expansile) pneumonia: rupture of a TB-infected lymph node into the airway (with sinus formation) may result in aspiration of caseous material and development of dense (expansile) caseating pneumonia.

M tuberculosis infection.[58] More important, they fail to make the distinction between *M tuberculosis* infection, which is very common in TB endemic settings, and TB disease.[59] Furthermore, owing to suboptimal sensitivity, a negative immune-based test cannot be used to rule out TB disease.[60]

Microbiological Studies

Microbiological studies should always be carried out to the extent possible, because it allows bacteriologic confirmation and drug susceptibility testing. Although microbiological confirmation

of TB is possible in the majority of children with advanced disease, this occurs less frequently than in adults[61] owing to challenges that include the inability of young children to produce sputum[2] with limited health care worker training and available resources to obtain adequate samples.[62]

Specimen collection

M tuberculosis can be detected in a variety of respiratory specimens that should be collected before starting treatment. Yield can be maximized by collecting at least 2 high-quality and -quantity specimens. Early morning specimens generally give the best bacteriologic results, and pooled specimens may improve yield[63,64] and reduce cost. Older children (>8 years of age) can usually expectorate sputum on request, whereas younger children require sputum induction with suctioning of secretions from the laryngopharynx.[65] Alternatively, lower respiratory tract secretions that have reached the nasopharynx can be suctioned (nasopharyngeal aspirate).

Because young children reflexively swallow their respiratory secretions and M tuberculosis is an acid-resistant organism, an alternative respiratory specimen is a gastric aspirate or lavage. A string test can also be used to capture swallowed sputum using a highly absorbent nylon yarn that is swallowed within a gelatine capsule by cooperative children more than 4 years of age.[66] Given that swallowed sputum passes through the gastrointestinal tract, stool may contain swallowed M tuberculosis and bacteriologic confirmation of TB has been achieved with Xpert MTB/RIF (Cepheid, Sunnyvale, CA) using stool samples in more than 40% of children with probable TB.[67] Bronchoalveolar lavage should only be performed if bronchoscopy is required for another reason, because it is an invasive procedure and the bacteriologic yield is equivalent to a series of induced sputum or gastric aspirate specimens.[68]

Enlarged peripheral lymph nodes (usually cervical) in children can be sampled by fine-needle aspiration biopsy. Culture yields are excellent and Xpert MTB/RIF has a sensitivity of more than 80% compared with culture.[69] The biopsy material can also be sent for cytopathologic analysis to exclude alternative diagnoses, such as lymphoma. Mycobacterial testing and histopathology should be performed on any relevant tissue sample (eg, bone or synovial biopsy). The culture yield of serosal fluid increases with immediate bedside inoculation, although tissue generally has a higher yield.[70] Pleural or pericardial fluid should be sent for nucleic acid amplification tests, cytopathology, IGRA, and biochemistry testing. In suspected miliary TB, mycobacterial cultures can be performed on blood, bone marrow, and urine. If TB meningitis is suspected, the CSF should be sent culture and Xpert Ultra,[71] as well as cell counts and biochemistry testing.

Acid-fast staining

Smear microscopy for acid-fast bacilli is a rapid and inexpensive test, but sensitivity is highly dependent on the bacillary load, which explains its poor sensitivity in young children with paucibacillary TB. Given its inability to differentiate M tuberculosis from other mycobacteria

commonly found in tap water, its use is not advised in specimens such as gastric aspirates.

Nucleic acid amplification tests

The Xpert MTB/RIF assay is a fully automated platform that uses real-time polymerase chain reactions to simultaneously detect the presence of M tuberculosis and RIF resistance (mutations in the rpoB gene). It has a high sensitivity (pooled estimate, 95%–96%) in smear-positive sputum samples using culture as a reference standard, but only moderate sensitivity (pooled estimate, 55%–62%) in smear-negative sputum samples.[72]

Sensitivity in children with paucibacillary disease is suboptimal,[73] but far better than smear microscopy.[74] Studies in children have demonstrated results similar to those achieved in sputum smear-negative adults (approximately 70% sensitivity compared with culture). Since 2013, the WHO has recommended Xpert MTB/RIF to be used for diagnosis of TB in children[5] particularly in those with HIV infection or suspected DR-TB.[72] The new Xpert Ultra is expected to have increased sensitivity and may be of particular value in children with paucibacillary disease. The inability of Xpert MTB/RIF to detect INH resistance is a major concern, because this is an important risk factor for treatment failure[75] and a precursor for the development of MDR-TB.[76] Another risk is the selection of RIF-resistant strains with mutations outside the RIF resistance-determining region detected by Xpert MTB/RIF, resulting in delayed diagnosis and ongoing transmission of these strains.[77]

Several commercial line probe assays have also been approved for the detection of drug-resistant M tuberculosis, as well as common NTM. GenoType MTBDRplus or Genoscholar NTM + MDRTB simultaneously assess INH and RIF resistance in smear-positive sputum samples or cultured isolates.[78]

Mycobacterial culture

Culture remains the reference standard for microbiological confirmation. In hospital-based studies culture yields in children with probable TB ranged from 25% to 75%, depending on disease severity and method of specimen collection. After successful mycobacterial culture, definitive M tuberculosis complex identification can be undertaken by phenotypic analysis, antigen tests (such as MPT64) or molecular-based methods (using line probe assays, matrix-assisted laser desorption/ionization time-of-flight mass spectrometry, or whole genome sequencing).

Histopathology

Any tissue sampled should be sent for histopathology review to help confirm a mycobacterial etiology and to exclude differential diagnoses such as fungal infection or malignancy. Multiple granulomas in various stages of development, some with central caseous necrosis, is suggestive of TB; however, granulomatous inflammation can also be due to infection with NTM, fungi, bartonella (cat scratch disease), helminths (eg, schistosomiasis) or protozoa (eg, toxoplasmosis), as well as autoimmune or idiopathic diseases (eg, sarcoidosis) and foreign bodies.

TREATMENT

When the decision has been made to treat a child for TB, several considerations should be taken into account, including disease phenotype, likely organism load, and the possibility of drug resistance. Other issues to consider are potential adverse effects and treatment adherence. The goals of TB treatment are to cure the individual child, limit ongoing transmission, and prevent the emergence of drug resistance.[26,79] TB treatment regimens must include a combination of drugs to which the infecting strain is either known to be, or is highly likely to be, susceptible, while maintaining a high barrier to selecting for drug resistance.

TB treatment is divided into an intensive and continuation phase. The intensive phase aims to achieve rapid killing of actively metabolizing bacilli to decrease symptoms, prevent ongoing respiratory transmission, and decrease the population of organisms from which drug resistance may emerge. Given the capacity of M tuberculosis to maintain itself in a low/intermittent metabolic state, the continuation phase aims to achieve sterilization of tissues to prevent relapse. A high organism load should be anticipated where there is cavitation or extensive multilobar involvement on chest radiography. Additionally, a higher organism load should be suspected in children with HIV or other immunocompromise. Involvement of anatomic locations with variable or lower drug penetration, such as the brain and CSF or bones and joints, also affects treatment choice and duration.

Table 2 summarizes dosage and adverse effects of antituberculous antimicrobials used for both DS- and DR-TB.[80,81] Directly observed therapy is generally preferred, but patient-centered care also requires a strong focus on patient and family education, counseling, and provision of material and psychological support.[82,83] This process

Table 2
Overview of first-line drugs used for TB treatment in children

Drug	Recommended Dose[a]	Adverse Effects	Additional Notes
Rifampin (R)	10–20 mg/kg/d (maximum 900 mg)	Hepatitis, orange discoloration of secretions, rash	Multiple drug–drug interactions; see summary in Nahid et al,[83] 2016
Isoniazid (H)	7–15 mg/kg/d neonates 5–10 mg/kg/d; high dose 15–20 mg/kg/d (max 600 mg)	Hepatitis, peripheral neuropathy, rash	Pyridoxine (5–25 mg/d) in selected children reduces the risk of peripheral neuropathy
Pyrazinamide (Z)	30–40 mg/kg/d (max 2000 mg)	Arthritis/arthralgia, hepatitis, rash	Most common cause of hepatotoxicity
Ethambutol (E)	15–25 mg/kg/d (max 1200 mg)	Optic neuritis	Vision/color vision review if available
Rifapentine (Rpt)	Preventive therapy, once weekly dosing: 10–14 kg 300 mg; >14–25 kg 450 mg; >25–32 kg 600 mg; >32–50 kg 750 mg; >50 kg 900 mg	Hepatitis, discoloration of secretions, gastrointestinal disturbance	Only approved in children ≥2 y
Rifabutin (Rfb)	5 mg/kg daily or 3 ×/wk (max 300 mg)	Uveitis, myelosuppression	Dosing in children not established

[a] Unless stated otherwise, use adult doses for children greater than 30 kg.

Data from Outhred AC, Britton PN, Marais BJ. Drug-Resistant tuberculosis - primary transmission and management. *J Infect.* 2017;74 Suppl 1:S128-S135 and Schaaf HS, Marais BJ, Carvalho I, Seddon JA. Challenges in childhood tuberculosis. In: Migliori GB, Bothamley G, Duarte R, Rendon A, eds. *Tuberculosis.* United Kingdom: European Respiratory Society; 2018 includes a focus on flexible options for treatment administration, such as community- or home-based treatment.

Standard Treatment

A minimum of 3 drugs (INH, RIF, pyrazinamide [PZA]) is advised during the 2-month intensive phase, with ethambutol (EMB) included as a fourth drug in cases with extensive pulmonary disease, and a continuation phase usually composed of INH and RIF for a further 4 months.[26,83] This applies where disease is either microbiologically confirmed to be DS or, in the absence of microbiological confirmation, if there are no risk factors for drug resistance. Child-friendly, water dispersible fixed-dose combinations of first-line TB drugs are available through the Global Drug Facility.[84] All children should receive daily treatment during the intensive phase and preferably throughout treatment. A Cochrane review found a lack of evidence to support or refute the use of intermittent treatment over daily treatment regimens in children with DS-TB.[85] The WHO conditionally recommends a 3 times per week dosing during the continuation phase in children who are HIV negative, and where adherence can be ensured.[26]

Treatment of Tuberculous Meningitis and Osteoarticular Tuberculosis

The optimal drug regimen and treatment duration are not as well established for tuberculous meningitis (TBM). WHO recommends treatment with a 4-drug regimen (INH, RIF, PZA, EMB) for 2 months, followed by 2 drugs (INH, RIF) for 10 months using the same doses as for pulmonary TB.[26] INH and PZA penetrate the CSF very well, but RIF less so, although it is considered essential to lower mortality in TBM.[79,86] Alternatives to the WHO regimen include high-dose INH, RIF, and PZA with ethionamide or levofloxacin as a complementary fourth drug[79,86] for the entire treatment course. Such a 6-month short course (9-month for HIV-infected children) TBM regimen produced excellent outcomes in South Africa[87,88] and is now supported by a systematic review, albeit of observational data.[89]

Corticosteroids are an essential adjunct to TB treatment in children with meningitis. A systematic review and meta-analysis concluded that corticosteroids improved outcome in HIV-negative children and adults with TBM.[90] Several dosing schedules have been used in clinical trials. In summary, 2 to 4 mg/kg/d prednisolone (or equivalent dexamethasone) is generally recommended for a minimum of 4 weeks, weaned over 2 to 6 weeks.[26,86,90] Additional immunosuppressive medications may be used for tuberculomas, or where corticosteroid response is inadequate.[86] The WHO recommends the same treatment regimen for osteoarticular disease as for TBM.[26]

Treatment of Drug-Resistant Tuberculosis

DR-TB should be suspected where there has been a failure to respond to first-line treatment or known contact with a DR-TB case. Other concerning features in the contact history include a person who died on TB treatment, was known to be poorly adherent, or required more than 1 TB treatment course.[79] Equally, drug resistance should be suspected in residents of or travelers to countries or locations known to have a high prevalence of DR-TB.[9]

DR-TB is categorized as either INH monoresistant, RIF monoresistant, polyresistant, or MDR (resistant to both INH and RIF).[9] Every effort should be made to achieve microbiological confirmation where drug resistance is suspected; however, where microbiological confirmation and drug susceptibility testing are unavailable from the child, treatment should be based on results from the likely source case.[91] INH monoresistant TB could be treated by the addition of EMB for the full duration of treatment or replacement of INH with a quinolone (moxifloxacin or levofloxacin). RIF-resistant and MDR-TB are generally managed in a similar way, but if RIF monoresistance is confirmed, then INH can still be counted as an active drug.

DR-TB and MDR-TB treatment requires the use of at least 4 active drugs.[92] A recent WHO review of emerging clinical trial data reprioritized second-line TB drugs into 3 groups (Table 3), encouraging injectable-free regimens, which is a high priority in children who may experience ototoxicity at a critical time of language development.[80,81,93,94] To design an adequate regimen, drugs are added sequentially from group A (moxifloxacin or levofloxacin, bedaquiline, and linezolid) and group B (cycloserine/terizidone, clofazimine), with drugs in group C drugs used as a last resort.[92,94] The usual treatment duration is 18 to 24 months, but shorter durations have been suggested for children with likely paucibacillary disease.[95,96] Revised WHO guidelines still endorse the use of injectables in the short course (9 months) MDR-TB regimen, where injectables are used for 4 to 6 months in children without HIV infection.[92] For MDR-TBM high level penetration of drugs into the CNS is a key consideration.[92] Drugs with good CNS penetration include fluoroquinolones, ethionamide, prothionamide, cycloserine, terizidone, linezolid, PZA, and high-dose INH (unless high level

Table 3
Overview of medicines used in the treatment of MDR-TB in children, using the new WHO grouping

Drug	Recommended Dose[a]	Adverse Effects
WHO Group A		
Levofloxacin Moxifloxacin	15–20 mg/kg/d (max 750 mg) 10–15 mg/kg/d (max 400 mg)	Sleep disturbance, GI disturbance, arthritis, tendonitis, raised ICP, QTc prolongation, peripheral neuropathy
Linezolid	≤15 kg 15 mg/kg/d >15 kg 10–12 mg/kg/d (max 600 mg/d)	Diarrhea, nausea, headaches, myelosuppression, neurotoxicity (peripheral and optic neuritis), pancreatitis, lactic acidosis
Bedaquiline	>6 y and 15–30 kg: 200 mg/d for 2 wk then 100 mg/d 3×/wk ≥30 kg: adult dose - 400 mg/d for 2 wk then 200 mg/d 3 ×/wk	Headache, nausea, liver dysfunction, QTc prolongation More data awaited on optimal dosing in younger children
WHO Group B		
Cycloserine/ Terizidone	15–20 mg/kg/d (max 1000 mg)	Psychological and neurologic effects
Clofazimine	2-5 mg/kg/d (max 300 mg) Only 50 mg and 100 mg gel capsules available: alternate day dosing may be required in young children	Skin discoloration, abdominal pain, QTc prolongation
WHO Group C[c]		
Delamanid	>6 y (25–34 kg) 50 mg twice daily ≥35 kg: 100 mg twice daily	Nausea, vomiting, dizziness, paresthesia, anxiety, QTc prolongation More data awaited on optimal dosing in younger children
Meropenem[b] Amoxicillin-clavulanate[b]	20–40 mg/kg/dose every 8 h (IV) 80 mg/kg/d of amoxicillin component in 3 divided doses	GI disturbance, hypersensitivity reactions, seizures, liver and renal dysfunction
Ethionamide/ prothionamide	15–20 mg/kg/d (max 1000 mg)	GI disturbance, metallic taste, hypothyroidism
p-aminosalicylic acid (PAS)	150–200 mg/kg/d (once or twice daily – max 8g)	GI intolerance, hypothyroidism, hepatitis
Injectables (IV or IM)		
Amikacin Streptomycin	15–25 mg/kg/d or 3 ×/wk 20–40 mg/kg/d or 3 ×/wk	Ototoxicity (irreversible), nephrotoxicity Regular audiology and renal function review during treatment; ideally with TDM

Abbreviations: GI, gastrointestinal; HIV, human immunodeficiency virus; ICP, intracranial pressure; IM, intramuscular; IV, intravenous; MDR-TB, multidrug-resistant tuberculosis; QTc, corrected QT interval; TDM, therapeutic dose monitoring; WHO, World Health Organization.
[a] Unless stated otherwise, use adult doses for children greater than 30 kg.
[b] To be used in combination, counting as a single active drug.
[c] Ethambutol and pyrazinamide also included, but already covered in **Table 2**.
Adapted from World Health Organization. Rapid communication: key changes to treatment of multidrug- and rifampicin-resistant tuberculosis (MDR/RR-TB). 2018; with permission.

resistance or *KatG* mutation). Para-amino salicylic acid, EMB, and the injectables do not penetrate the CNS well and there are few data for clofazimine, delamanid, and bedaquiline, but adequate CNS penetration is unlikely given that bedaquiline is highly protein bound. Comprehensive new WHO recommendations (awaited) will complement a recent overview of using new and repurposed drugs for MDR-TB treatment in children.[97]

Adverse Effects and Treatment Monitoring

Adverse effects are rare in young children treated with first-line TB drugs. Transient alteration of liver function tests is common, such that routine monitoring is not required.[26] Children usually also tolerate second-line drugs well, but more vigilant monitoring is important to identify adverse events early; a proposed monitoring schedule has been published elsewhere.[96]

Gastrointestinal symptoms such as nausea, vomiting, and epigastric pain may be addressed initially by split dosing. Clinical jaundice or hepatitis (elevated transaminases [alanine aminotransferase/aspartate aminotransferase] >5× the upper limit of normal or conjugated bilirubin >2× the upper limit of normal) requires cessation of all potentially implicated medications, with sequential reintroduction of individual drugs. Mild, itchy rash without mucous membrane involvement or systemic symptoms can be managed symptomatically, but persistent, generalized rash or mucous membrane involvement is suggestive of Stevens Johnson syndrome and requires ceasing potentially implicated medications. INH-associated neuropathy can be prevented by supplementary administration of pyridoxine (vitamin B_6) that should be given routinely to all children who are HIV infected, malnourished, exclusively breast fed, or being treated with terizidone, cycloserine, or high-dose INH.[26] Despite concern regarding the osteoarticular adverse effects of fluoroquinolones these have not been observed in practice.[98]

Immune-reconstitution inflammatory syndrome (IRIS) can present as unmasking or paradoxic reactions. Unmaking IRIS typically occurs in severely immune compromised HIV-infected children who are initiated on antiretroviral therapy where immune reconstitution unmasks occult sites of disease. Paradoxic IRIS may also occur after antiretroviral therapy initiation in a child recently diagnosed with TB, but is most commonly observed in HIV-uninfected children with superficial lymph node disease. IRIS does not indicate treatment failure and normal treatment should be continued, although severe IRIS may require adjunctive corticosteroids.[79]

SUMMARY

TB contributes significantly to childhood morbidity and mortality globally. BCG provides limited protection against severe forms of disease in young children, and given their vulnerability preventive therapy is advised with recent TB exposure or documented infection. TB in young children can present with acute onset or nonspecific signs and symptoms. Although the diagnosis can be challenging, an accurate presumptive diagnosis can be achieved in most cases. Immune-based testing indicates infection, but it does not

differentiate infection from disease and has insufficient sensitivity to reliably exclude TB disease. Treatment outcomes in children are usually excellent, even in those infected with MDR-TB. Diagnostic and treatment access, as well as the availability of child-friendly formulations remain an issue.

REFERENCES

1. Dodd PJ, Gardiner E, Coghlan R, et al. Burden of childhood tuberculosis in 22 high-burden countries: a mathematical modelling study. Lancet Glob Health 2014;2(8):e453–9.
2. Newton SM, Brent AJ, Anderson S, et al. Paediatric tuberculosis. Lancet Infect Dis 2008;8(8):498–510.
3. Marais BJ, Obihara CC, Warren RM, et al. The burden of childhood tuberculosis: a public health perspective. Int J Tuberc Lung Dis 2005;9(12):1305–13.
4. Marais BJ, Gupta A, Starke JR, et al. Tuberculosis in women and children. Lancet 2010;375(9731): 2057–9.
5. World Health Organization. Global tuberculosis report. Geneva (Switzerland): World Health Organization; 2016.
6. Jaganath D, Zalwango S, Okware B, et al. Contact investigation for active tuberculosis among child contacts in Uganda. Clin Infect Dis 2013;57(12): 1685–92.
7. Marais BJ, Gie RP, Schaaf HS, et al. The natural history of childhood intra-thoracic tuberculosis: a critical review of literature from the pre-chemotherapy era. Int J Tuberc Lung Dis 2004;8(4):392–402.
8. Yuen CM, Kammerer JS, Marks K, et al. Recent transmission of tuberculosis - United States, 2011-2014. PLoS One 2016;11(4):e0153728.
9. Dodd PJ, Sismanidis C, Seddon JA. Global burden of drug-resistant tuberculosis in children: a mathematical modelling study. Lancet Infect Dis 2016; 16(10):1193–201.
10. Jenkins HE, Tolman AW, Yuen CM, et al. Incidence of multidrug-resistant tuberculosis disease in children: systematic review and global estimates. Lancet 2014;383(9928):1572–9.
11. Dharmadhikari AS, Mphahlele M, Venter K, et al. Rapid impact of effective treatment on transmission of multidrug-resistant tuberculosis. Int J Tuberc Lung Dis 2014;18(9):1019–25.
12. van Cutsem G, Isaakidis P, Farley J, et al. Infection control for drug-resistant tuberculosis: early diagnosis and treatment is the key. Clin Infect Dis 2016;62(Suppl 3):S238–43.
13. Ho J, Fox GJ, Marais BJ. Passive case finding for tuberculosis is not enough. Int J Mycobacteriol 2016;5(4):374–8.
14. Raviglione M, Marais B, Floyd K, et al. Scaling up interventions to achieve global tuberculosis control:

progress and new developments. Lancet 2012; 379(9829):1902–13.

15. Jensen PA, Lambert LA, Iademarco MF, et al. Guidelines for preventing the transmission of Mycobacterium tuberculosis in health-care settings, 2005. MMWR Recomm Rep 2005;54(RR-17):1–141.

16. Mangtani P, Abubakar I, Ariti C, et al. Protection by BCG vaccine against tuberculosis: a systematic review of randomized controlled trials. Clin Infect Dis 2014;58(4):470–80.

17. Rodrigues LC, Diwan VK, Wheeler JG. Protective effect of BCG against tuberculous meningitis and miliary tuberculosis: a meta-analysis. Int J Epidemiol 1993;22(6):1154–8.

18. Trunz BB, Fine P, Dye C. Effect of BCG vaccination on childhood tuberculous meningitis and miliary tuberculosis worldwide: a meta-analysis and assessment of cost-effectiveness. Lancet 2006; 367(9517):1173–80.

19. Fine PE. Variation in protection by BCG: implications of and for heterologous immunity. Lancet 1995; 346(8986):1339–45.

20. Hesseling AC, Johnson LF, Jaspan H, et al. Disseminated bacille Calmette-Guerin disease in HIV-infected South African infants. Bull World Health Organ 2009;87(7):505–11.

21. Van-Dunem JC, Rodrigues LC, Alencar LC, et al. Effectiveness of the first dose of BCG against tuberculosis among HIV-infected, predominantly immunodeficient children. Biomed Res Int 2015;2015: 275029.

22. Revised BCG vaccination guidelines for infants at risk for HIV infection. Wkly Epidemiol Rec 2007; 82(21):193–6.

23. Marais BJ, Seddon JA, Detjen AK, et al. Interrupted BCG vaccination is a major threat to global child health. Lancet Respir Med 2016;4(4):251–3.

24. Al Yazidi LS, Marais BJ, Wickens M, et al. Overview of paediatric tuberculosis cases treated in the Sydney Children's Hospitals Network, Australia. Public Health Res Pract 2019;29(2) [pii:282318076].

25. Britton PN, Yeung V, Lowbridge C, et al. Spectrum of disease in children treated for tuberculosis at a Tertiary Children's Hospital in Australia. J Pediatric Infect Dis Soc 2013;2(3):224–31.

26. WHO. Guidance for national tuberculosis programmes on the management of tuberculosis in children. Geneva (Switzerland): WHO; 2014.

27. Rangaka MX, Cavalcante SC, Marais BJ, et al. Controlling the seedbeds of tuberculosis: diagnosis and treatment of tuberculosis infection. Lancet 2015; 386(10010):2344–53.

28. WHO. Latent tuberculosis infection: updated and consolidated guidelines for programmatic management. Geneva (Switzerland): WHO; 2018.

29. Hill PC, Rutherford ME, Audas R, et al. Closing the policy-practice gap in the management of child contacts of tuberculosis cases in developing countries. PLoS Med 2011;8(10):e1001105.

30. Churchyard GJ, Fielding KL, Grant AD. A trial of mass isoniazid preventive therapy for tuberculosis control. N Engl J Med 2014;370(17):1662–3.

31. Trauer JM, Moyo N, Tay EL, et al. Risk of active tuberculosis in the five years following infection . . . 15%? Chest 2016;149(2):516–25.

32. Zar HJ, Cotton MF, Strauss S, et al. Effect of isoniazid prophylaxis on mortality and incidence of tuberculosis in children with HIV: randomised controlled trial. BMJ 2007;334(7585):136.

33. Diallo T, Adjobimey M, Ruslami R, et al. Safety and side effects of rifampin versus isoniazid in children. N Engl J Med 2018;379(5):454–63.

34. Getahun H, Matteelli A, Abubakar I, et al. Management of latent Mycobacterium tuberculosis infection: WHO guidelines for low tuberculosis burden countries. Eur Respir J 2015;46(6):1563–76.

35. Triasih R, Robertson CF, Duke T, et al. A prospective evaluation of the symptom-based screening approach to the management of children who are contacts of tuberculosis cases. Clin Infect Dis 2015;60(1):12–8.

36. Marais BJ, Ayles H, Graham SM, et al. Screening and preventive therapy for tuberculosis. Clin Chest Med 2009;30(4):827–46, x.

37. Targeted tuberculin testing and treatment of latent tuberculosis infection. American Thoracic Society. MMWR Recomm Rep 2000;49(RR-6):1–51.

38. Migliori GB, Zellweger JP, Abubakar I, et al. European Union standards for tuberculosis care. Eur Respir J 2012;39(4):807–19.

39. Marais BJ, Gie RP, Schaaf HS, et al. The spectrum of disease in children treated for tuberculosis in a highly endemic area. Int J Tuberc Lung Dis 2006;10(7): 732–8.

40. Wiseman CA, Gie RP, Starke JR, et al. A proposed comprehensive classification of tuberculosis disease severity in children. Pediatr Infect Dis J 2012; 31(4):347–52.

41. Schaaf HS, Michaelis IA, Richardson M, et al. Adult-to-child transmission of tuberculosis: household or community contact? Int J Tuberc Lung Dis 2003; 7(5):426–31.

42. Marais BJ, Gie RP, Hesseling AC, et al. A refined symptom-based approach to diagnose pulmonary tuberculosis in children. Pediatrics 2006;118(5): e1350–9.

43. Mohapatra PR, Janmeja AK. Tuberculous lymphadenitis. J Assoc Physicians India 2009;57:585–90.

44. Marais BJ, Gie RP, Schaaf HS, et al. A proposed radiological classification of childhood intrathoracic tuberculosis. Pediatr Radiol 2004;34(11): 886–94.

45. Andronikou S, Van der Merwe D, Goussard P, et al. Usefulness of lateral radiographs for

detecting tuberculous lymphadenopathy in children–confirmation using sagittal CT reconstruction with multiplanar cross-referencing. South Afr J Radiol 2012;16:87–92.

46. Goussard P, Gie R. The role of bronchoscopy in the diagnosis and management of pediatric pulmonary tuberculosis. Expert Rev Respir Med 2014;8(1): 101–9.

47. Wessels G, Schaaf HS, Beyers N, et al. Haematological abnormalities in children with tuberculosis. J Trop Pediatr 1999;45(5):307–10.

48. Porcel JM, Light RW. Pleural effusions. Dis Mon 2013;59(2):29–57.

49. Marais S, Thwaites G, Schoeman JF, et al. Tuberculous meningitis: a uniform case definition for use in clinical research. Lancet Infect Dis 2010;10(11): 803–12.

50. Tuon FF, Litvoc MN, Lopes MI. Adenosine deaminase and tuberculous pericarditis–a systematic review with meta-analysis. Acta Trop 2006;99(1):67–74.

51. Pormohammad A, Riahi SM, Nasiri MJ, et al. Diagnostic test accuracy of adenosine deaminase for tuberculous meningitis: a systematic review and meta-analysis. J Infect 2017;74(6):545–54.

52. Wei JL, Bond J, Sykes KJ, et al. Treatment outcomes for nontuberculous mycobacterial cervicofacial lymphadenitis in children based on the type of surgical intervention. Otolaryngol Head Neck Surg 2008; 138(5):566–71.

53. Seddon JA, Paton J, Nademi Z, et al. The impact of BCG vaccination on tuberculin skin test responses in children is age dependent: evidence to be considered when screening children for tuberculosis infection. Thorax 2016;71(10):932–9.

54. Turnbull L, Bell C, Child F. Tuberculosis (NICE clinical guideline 33). Arch Dis Child Educ Pract Ed 2017;102(3):136–42.

55. Abubakar I, Drobniewski F, Southern J, et al. Prognostic value of interferon-gamma release assays and tuberculin skin test in predicting the development of active tuberculosis (UK PREDICT TB): a prospective cohort study. Lancet Infect Dis 2018; 18(10):1077–87.

56. Machingaidze S, Wiysonge CS, Gonzalez-Angulo Y, et al. The utility of an interferon gamma release assay for diagnosis of latent tuberculosis infection and disease in children: a systematic review and meta-analysis. Pediatr Infect Dis J 2011;30(8): 694–700.

57. Starke JR, Committee On Infectious Diseases. Interferon-gamma release assays for diagnosis of tuberculosis infection and disease in children. Pediatrics 2014;134(6):e1763–73.

58. Mack U, Migliori GB, Sester M, et al. LTBI: latent tuberculosis infection or lasting immune responses to M. tuberculosis? A TBNET consensus statement. Eur Respir J 2009;33(5):956–73.

59. WHO. Guidelines on the management of latent tuberculosis infection. Geneva (Switzerland): WHO; 2015.

60. Lalvani A, Millington KA. T cell-based diagnosis of childhood tuberculosis infection. Curr Opin Infect Dis 2007;20(3):264–71.

61. Rayment JH, Guthrie JL, Lam K, et al. Culture-positive pediatric tuberculosis in Toronto, Ontario: sources of infection and relationship of birthplace and mycobacterial lineage to phenotype. Pediatr Infect Dis J 2016;35(1):13–8.

62. Wobudeya E, Lukoye D, Lubega IR, et al. Epidemiology of tuberculosis in children in Kampala district, Uganda, 2009-2010; a retrospective cross-sectional study. BMC Public Health 2015;15:967.

63. Mpagama SG, Mtabho C, Mwaigwisya S, et al. Comparison of overnight pooled and standard sputum collection method for patients with suspected pulmonary tuberculosis in northern Tanzania. Tuberc Res Treat 2012;2012:128057.

64. Singh S, Singh A, Prajapati S, et al. Xpert MTB/RIF assay can be used on archived gastric aspirate and induced sputum samples for sensitive diagnosis of paediatric tuberculosis. BMC Microbiol 2015;15:191.

65. Zar HJ, Hanslo D, Apolles P, et al. Induced sputum versus gastric lavage for microbiological confirmation of pulmonary tuberculosis in infants and young children: a prospective study. Lancet 2005; 365(9454):130–4.

66. Chow F, Espiritu N, Gilman RH, et al. La cuerda dulce–a tolerability and acceptability study of a novel approach to specimen collection for diagnosis of paediatric pulmonary tuberculosis. BMC Infect Dis 2006;6:67.

67. Walters E, Gie RP, Hesseling AC, et al. Rapid diagnosis of pediatric intrathoracic tuberculosis from stool samples using the Xpert MTB/RIF Assay: a pilot study. Pediatr Infect Dis J 2012;31(12):1316.

68. Somu N, Swaminathan S, Paramasivan CN, et al. Value of bronchoalveolar lavage and gastric lavage in the diagnosis of pulmonary tuberculosis in children. Tuber Lung Dis 1995;76(4):295–9.

69. Denkinger CM, Schumacher SG, Boehme CC, et al. Xpert MTB/RIF assay for the diagnosis of extrapulmonary tuberculosis: a systematic review and meta-analysis. Eur Respir J 2014;44(2):435–46.

70. Fischer GB, Andrade CF, Lima JB. Pleural tuberculosis in children. Paediatr Respir Rev 2011;12(1): 27–30.

71. Bahr NC, Nuwagira E, Evans EE, et al. Diagnostic accuracy of Xpert MTB/RIF Ultra for tuberculous meningitis in HIV-infected adults: a prospective cohort study. Lancet Infect Dis 2018;18(1):68–75.

72. WHO. Automated real-time nucleic acid amplification technology for rapid and simultaneous detection of tuberculosis and rifampicin resistance: Xpert

MTB/RIF assay for the diagnosis of pulmonary and extrapulmonary TB in adults and children: policy update. Geneva (Switzerland): WHO; 2013.

73. Roya-Pabon CL, Perez-Velez CM. Tuberculosis exposure, infection and disease in children: a systematic diagnostic approach. Pneumonia (Nathan) 2016;8:23.

74. Bates M, O'Grady J, Maeurer M, et al. Assessment of the Xpert MTB/RIF assay for diagnosis of tuberculosis with gastric lavage aspirates in children in sub-Saharan Africa: a prospective descriptive study. Lancet Infect Dis 2013;13(1):36–42.

75. Johnston JC, Campbell JR, Menzies D. Effect of intermittency on treatment outcomes in pulmonary tuberculosis: an updated systematic review and metaanalysis. Clin Infect Dis 2017;64(9):1211–20.

76. Manson AL, Cohen KA, Abeel T, et al. Genomic analysis of globally diverse Mycobacterium tuberculosis strains provides insights into the emergence and spread of multidrug resistance. Nat Genet 2017; 49(3):395–402.

77. Sanchez-Padilla E, Merker M, Beckert P, et al. Detection of drug-resistant tuberculosis by Xpert MTB/RIF in Swaziland. N Engl J Med 2015;372(12): 1181–2.

78. World Health Organization. Molecular line probe assays for rapid screening of patients at risk of multidrug-resistant tuberculosis (MDR-TB). Geneva (Switzerland): World Health Organization; 2008.

79. Perez-Velez CM, Marais BJ. Tuberculosis in children. N Engl J Med 2012;367(4):348–61.

80. Outhred AC, Britton PN, Marais BJ. Drug-Resistant tuberculosis - primary transmission and management. J Infect 2017;74(Suppl 1):S128–35.

81. Schaaf HS, Marais BJ, Carvalho I, et al. Challenges in childhood tuberculosis. In: Migliori GB, Bothamley G, Duarte R, et al, editors. Tuberculosis. United Kingdom: European Respiratory Society; 2018.

82. M'Imunya JM, Kredo T, Volmink J. Patient education and counselling for promoting adherence to treatment for tuberculosis. Cochrane Database Syst Rev 2012;(5):CD006591.

83. Nahid P, Dorman SE, Alipanah N, et al. Official American Thoracic Society/Centers for Disease Control and Prevention/Infectious Diseases Society of America Clinical Practice Guidelines: treatment of drug-susceptible tuberculosis. Clin Infect Dis 2016; 63(7):e147–95.

84. TB alliance. Child-friendly medicines. Available at: https://www.tballiance.org/child-friendly-medicines. Accessed December 12, 2018.

85. Bose A, Kalita S, Rose W, et al. Intermittent versus daily therapy for treating tuberculosis in children. Cochrane Database Syst Rev 2014;(1):CD007953.

86. Thwaites G, Fisher M, Hemingway C, et al. British Infection Society guidelines for the diagnosis and treatment of tuberculosis of the central nervous system in adults and children. J Infect 2009;59(3): 167–87.

87. van Toorn R, Schaaf HS, Laubscher JA, et al. Short intensified treatment in children with drug-susceptible tuberculous meningitis. Pediatr Infect Dis J 2014;33(3):248–52.

88. Donald PR. Chemotherapy for tuberculous meningitis. N Engl J Med 2016;374(2):179–81.

89. Jullien S, Ryan H, Modi M, et al. Six months therapy for tuberculous meningitis. Cochrane Database Syst Rev 2016;(9):CD012091.

90. Prasad K, Singh MB, Ryan H. Corticosteroids for managing tuberculous meningitis. Cochrane Database Syst Rev 2016;(4):CD002244.

91. Shah NS, Yuen CM, Heo M, et al. Yield of contact investigations in households of patients with drug-resistant tuberculosis: systematic review and meta-analysis. Clin Infect Dis 2014;58(3):381–91.

92. WHO. WHO treatment guidelines for drug-resistant tuberculosis, 2016 update 2016.

93. Seddon JA, Schaaf HS, Marais BJ, et al. Time to act on injectable-free regimens for children with multidrug-resistant tuberculosis. Lancet Respir Med 2018;6(9):662–4.

94. WHO. Rapid communication: key changes to treatment of multidrug- and rifampicin-resistant tuberculosis. (MDR/RR-TB); 2018.

95. Schaaf HS, Marais BJ. Management of multidrug-resistant tuberculosis in children: a survival guide for paediatricians. Paediatr Respir Rev 2011;12(1): 31–8.

96. Seddon JA, Furin JJ, Gale M, et al. Caring for children with drug-resistant tuberculosis: practice-based recommendations. Am J Respir Crit Care Med 2012;186(10):953–64.

97. Harausz EP, Garcia-Prats AJ, Seddon JA, et al. New and repurposed drugs for pediatric multidrug-resistant tuberculosis. practice-based recommendations. Am J Respir Crit Care Med 2017;195(10): 1300–10.

98. Garcia-Prats AJ, Draper HR, Finlayson H, et al. Clinical and cardiac safety of long-term levofloxacin in children treated for multidrug-resistant tuberculosis. Clin Infect Dis 2018;67(11):1777–80.

New Drugs for the Treatment of Tuberculosis

Elisa H. Ignatius, MD, MSc[a], Kelly E. Dooley, MD, PhD[b],*

KEYWORDS

• Tuberculosis • Bedaquiline • Delamanid • Pretomanid • New drugs • Pharmacology

KEY POINTS

- Treatment success rates for drug-susceptible tuberculosis are too low, and prognosis for drug-resistant TB remains poor.
- Though shorter 9- to 12-month regimens are available for the treatment of MDR-TB, therapy is complex and often toxic.
- The diarylquinoline, bedaquiline (BDQ), and the nitroimidazoles delamanid and pretomanid, have excellent preclinical and clinical data to support their use for MDR or XDR-TB. Multiple trials are centered on use of these drugs to produce well-tolerated, all-oral, short-course regimens.
- Further study of new drugs is urgently needed among children, pregnant women, and people living with HIV to guide clinicians.
- The pipeline now contains numerous new chemical entities from 16 drug classes with encouraging results from late preclinical or early clinical testing, the "third wave" of TB drug development.

INTRODUCTION

In 2014, tuberculosis (TB) surpassed HIV as the leading infectious cause of death. According to the World Health Organization (WHO), there were 10 million incident cases of TB in 2017 with 1.3 million deaths.[1] Treatment success was 82%, a number that seems to be decreasing. This is alarming given that small changes in treatment efficacy meaningfully affect population-level incidence and mortality.[2] The first-line regimen, developed in the 1950s to 1970s, remains lengthy (≥6 months) and is unforgiving to minor lapses in adherence.[3] Meanwhile, in 2017, 458,000 people developed multidrug-resistant (MDR) TB,

Mycobacterium tuberculosis (*M.tb.*) resistant to isoniazid and rifampicin. Despite efforts to extend access to treatment, the prognosis for patients with MDR-TB remains poor, with only 55% treatment success.[1] Treatment outcomes for patients with extensively drug-resistant (XDR) TB (MDR-TB that is also resistant to fluoroquinolones and injectable agents) are exceptionally poor, and now totally drug-resistant (TDR)-TB is documented, ushering us back to the preantibiotic era.[4] In a study of patients in South Africa with "programmatically incurable tuberculosis," many were discharged to the community once treatment options were exhausted, and community-level transmission occurred. Despite treatment

Disclosure Statement: E.H. Ignatius has no conflicts of interest to report. K.E. Dooley is principal investigator or protocol chair for trials involving BDQ, delamanid, pretomanid, rifapentine, levofloxacin, high-dose isoniazid, and meropenem. Support and funding for these trials are provided by the NIH or FDA. She receives no salary support from drug companies for these studies. This work was supported by the National Institutes of Health T32-AI007291-27 to E.H. Ignatius. The content is solely the responsibility of the authors and does not necessarily represent the official views of the National Institutes of Health. K.E. Dooley received no support for her work on this article.

[a] Department of Medicine, Johns Hopkins University School of Medicine, 1830 Building Room 450B, 1830 East Monument Street, Baltimore, MD 21287, USA; [b] Department of Medicine, Center for Tuberculosis Research, Johns Hopkins University School of Medicine, 600 North Wolfe Street, Osler 527, Baltimore, MD, USA
* Corresponding author.
E-mail address: kdooley1@jhmi.edu

Clin Chest Med 40 (2019) 811–827
https://doi.org/10.1016/j.ccm.2019.08.001
0272-5231/19/© 2019 Elsevier Inc. All rights reserved.

chestmed.theclinics.com

failure, 90% of their sputum isolates were sensitive to newer drugs, namely linezolid, BDQ, and delamanid.[5]

There have been recent WHO updates to guidance for MDR-TB treatment.[6] A short-duration regimen, commonly referred to as the Bangladesh regimen, yielded promising results for a 9- to 12-month course,[7] and subsequent cohort studies and a phase 3 clinical trial, STREAM, confirmed these impressive results.[8] This "short-course" MDR-TB regimen still requires use of 7 drugs and is offered as a complete regimen, with no allowance for substitutions or deletions. Thus, the application of this regimen in some settings may be limited by drug-resistance patterns.[9]

Fortunately, the second wave of antituberculosis drug development, which included the diarylquinoline, BDQ, and 2 nitroimidazoles, delamanid and pretomanid, offers the potential for simple, shorter, all-oral regimens for MDR- and XDR-TB treatment. In vitro, animal, and early clinical experience with these 3 compounds has been promising, and trials are ongoing to determine the best multidrug combinations, including among children and persons living with HIV (PLWH). Emerging results from the Otsuka phase 3 randomized controlled trial (RCT) of delamanid, the short-course MDR-TB regimen (STREAM Stage 1), and pediatric pharmacokinetic (PK) and safety studies of BDQ and delamanid, led the WHO to release a rapid communication in August 2018 with updated guidance (**Table 1**).[10] Standard-duration treatment of MDR-TB now should include fluoroquinolone, BDQ, and linezolid plus clofazimine or cycloserine, with additional drugs such as delamanid used to comprise a 4- to 5-drug regimen.

This article outlines the history, mechanisms of action and resistance, preclinical studies, pharmacology, clinical evaluation, and treatment niche for new drugs for TB treatment that are licensed or in late clinical testing: BDQ, delamanid, and pretomanid. Also provided is a short summary of promising new chemical entities in the "third wave" of mycobacterial drug development, those that are in earlier phases of clinical testing but show great promise for shorter or less toxic regimens.

NEW DRUGS IN CLINICAL USE OR LATE-PHASE CLINICAL TESTING
BDQ

BDQ is a diarylquinoline that blocks the proton pump of adenosine triphosphate (ATP) synthase.

Table 1
Standard-duration therapy for MDR-TB recommended by the WHO

Group	Drug
Group A: Include all 3	Levofloxacin (Lfx) OR moxifloxacin (Mfx, M) Bedaquiline (BDQ, B) Linezolid (LZD)
Group B: Add one or both medicines	Clofazamine (CFZ) Cycloserine (Cs) OR terizidone (Trd)
Group C: To complete regimen OR Group A or B cannot be used	Ethambutol (Emb, E) Delamanid (DLM, D) Pyrazinamide (PZA, or Z) Imipenem-cilastatin (Ipm/Cln) OR meropenem (Mpm)[a] Amikacin (Am) OR streptomycin (S) Ethionamide (Eto) OR prothionamide (Pto) p-Aminosalicylic acid (PAS)

[a] With amoxicillin-clavulanic acid.
From World Health Organization (WHO). WHO Technical report on critical concentrations for TB drug susceptibility testing of medicines used in the treatment of drug-resistant TB. Geneva; 2019. Available at: https://apps.who.int/iris/bitstream/handle/10665/311389/9789241550529-eng.pdf?ua=1

It was granted approval for MDR-TB at 400 mg daily for 14 days followed by 200 mg thrice weekly for 22 weeks by the US Food and Drug Administration (FDA) in 2012 and by the European Medicines Agency (EMA) in 2013, making it the first drug approved for the treatment of TB in 40 years. Shortly thereafter, the WHO released interim guidance that BDQ could be used in combination with second-line drugs to treat pulmonary MDR-TB.[11]

Preclinical data
BDQ is bactericidal against M.tb. and bacteriostatic against other nontuberculous mycobacteria.[12,13] In mice, BDQ has sterilizing activity superior to that of rifampicin and shortens treatment duration required for cure in multidrug regimens.[14,15] BDQ-pyrazinamide (BZ) has superior activity to rifampin-pyrazinamide (RZ).[16,17] Relapse rates after 3 months of BDQ-pyrazinamide plusrifapentine (BZP) or moxifloxacin (BZM) were similar to 6 months of standard treatment.[18] Pyrazinamide-free regimens, BPM or B-pretomanid (Pa)-M (BPaM), given for

4 months showed lower relapse rate than standard 6-month treatment.[16] BPaMZ cured mice in 2 months.[19]

Clinical pharmacology
BDQ is well absorbed, and food increases bioavailability 2-fold.[20] BDQ is highly protein bound (99.9%) and has a large volume of distribution (V_d), greater than 10,000 L.[21] BDQ is primarily metabolized by cytochrome P450 (CYP) 3A4, forming a metabolically active M2 metabolite. The terminal half-life of BDQ and M2 is long, ~160 days.[22] BDQ's bactericidal activity is concentration dependent.[23] BDQ exposures are lower in patients of Black race or with low albumin.[24,25] Rifampicin and rifapentine reduce BDQ concentrations substantially (70%–80%),[26] as does EFV (50%).[27] BDQ can be given with nevirapine without dose adjustment. Ritonavir-boosted lopinavir decreases BDQ clearance by 75%, so coadministration requires caution and ECG monitoring.[28]

Resistance
Spontaneous resistance mutations to BDQ occur at rates comparable with rifampicin with no loss of fitness.[29] Given BDQ's unique target, cross-resistance was not anticipated, but a study of clofazimine-resistant isolates found coexisting BDQ resistance via upregulation of the efflux pump MmpS5-MmpL5, owing to mutations in the transcriptional regulatory Rv0678.[30] Clinical and murine studies have implicated Rv0678 and Rv2535c.[31,32] Although BDQ resistance generally confers cross-resistance to clofazimine, the opposite is not universally true.[33] Critical concentrations of 0.25 µg/mL on 7H11 and 1 µg/mL on MGIT have been proposed.[34]

Clinical data
In humans, BDQ monotherapy has delayed early bactericidal activity (EBA), likely because of its mechanism of shifting ATP use to alternative pathways such as glycolysis, leading to eventual (not immediate) cell death.[35–37] In a phase 2b RCT among 160 patients with pulmonary MDR-TB receiving multidrug background regimen (MBR), time to culture conversion was 83 days with BDQ versus 125 days with placebo. Twenty-four-week culture conversion was higher (79% vs 58%), as was cure (58% vs 32%). The BDQ arm had greater QTc prolongation and mortality, although deaths were late and of variable causes.[38] A subsequent single-arm trial of 233 patients confirmed the efficacy of 24 weeks of BDQ.[39] Multiple trials involving BDQ as part of all-oral or treatment-shortening regimens are currently under way in both drug-sensitive and drug-resistant TB (**Table 2**).

Reassuringly, large observational cohort studies, including a meta-analysis of 12,030 patients with MDR-TB and studies among PLWH, have shown that BDQ decreases rather than increases mortality.[6,40,41] Although QT prolongation of 15 to 20 milliseconds is common, there have been no reports of clinically important cardiac toxicity, even with therapy up to 12 months.[42,43] Although most data are for BDQ added to MBR, it also confers benefit when substituted for injectables.[44]

Delamanid

Delamanid (OPC-67683, DLM) is a nitroimidazole that inhibits synthesis of ketomycolate, a cell wall lipid that constitutes one-third of *M.tb*'s dry weight.[45] Delamanid was approved by EMA in 2014 at a dose of 100 mg twice daily for 6 months and is recommended by WHO for MDR-TB in certain circumstances. It is approved in Europe but is not yet FDA approved.

Preclinical data
DLM has an extremely low minimal inhibitory concentration (MIC) against *M.tb*. (0.006–0.024 µg/mL) and displays activity against replicating and dormant bacilli.[46] Animal studies are limited, although a guinea pig model of cavitary disease demonstrated activity.[47] In a mouse model, DLM-RZ had similar treatment efficacy at 4 months as RZHE for 6 months.[46]

Clinical pharmacology
Delamanid's absorption is enhanced by food and may be reduced by concomitant dosing with other medications.[48] It displays less-than-proportional PK.[49] Delamanid is catalyzed to DM-6705 by a pathway that involves albumin.[50] DLM is not a substrate, inhibitor, or inducer of CYP enzymes. Whereas the half-life of the parent drug is 38 hours, DM-6705 has a terminal half-life of 121 to 322 hours.[51] There were no clinically significant interactions when DLM was coadministered with efavirenz, lopinavir/ritonavir, or tenofovir.[48]

Resistance
Both delamanid and pretomanid (see later discussion) require activation involving coenzyme F_{420}. Resistance mutations have been identified in *fbiA*, *fbiB*, and *fbiC* (involved in F_{420} biosynthesis) and *fgd1* and *ddn* (prodrug activation). The F_{420} cofactor is not present in mammalian cells, explaining the narrow spectrum of activity.[52] There are limited data on treatment-induced resistance, but case reports describe emergence of *fgd1*, *fbiA*, *fbiB*, and *fbiC* mutants.[33,53] A break point of

Table 2
Recent, ongoing, or upcoming trials involving BDQ, delamanid, or pretomanid

Trial	Status	Population	Sample	Description
Diarylquinoline				
BDQ				
Janssen C211 (NCT02354014)	Phase 1–2 Enrolling	India, Philippines, Russian Federation, South Africa	60	Pediatric/adolescent PK, safety, tolerability of BDQ + background regimen
IMPAACT P1108 (NCT02906007)	Phase 1–2 Enrolling	Haiti, India, South Africa	72	Pediatric PK, safety, tolerability of 24 wk BDQ + BR for MDR-TB in HIV-infected/uninfected children
STREAM stage 2 (NCT02409290)	Phase 3 Enrolling	China, Ethiopia, Georgia, India, Indonesia, Republic of Moldova, Mongolia, South Africa, Uganda, Vietnam	1155	Locally used WHO approved MDR regimen OR 40 wk (Bangladesh): MXF-CFZ-EMB-PZA + INH-PTO-KAN (1st 16 wk) OR 40 wk (all-oral): CFZ-EMB-PZA-LFX-BDQ + INH-PTO (1st 16 wk) OR 28 wk CFZ-PZA-LFX-BDQ + INH-KAN (1st 8 wk)
TRUNCATE-TB (NCT03474198)	Phase 3 Enrolling	Philippines, Singapore, Thailand	900	Multiarm, multistage (MAMS) trial of ultrashort regimens in drug-sensitive TB: 8 wk RHZE, then 16 wk RH OR 8–12 wk RHZE-Lzd OR 8–12 wk RHZE-CFZ OR 8–12 wk RPT-HZ-LZD-LFX OR 8–12 wk HZE-LZD-BDQ
NExT (NCT02454205)	Phase 3 Terminated	South Africa	300	6–8 mo KAN-MXF-PZA-ETH-TRD, then 18 mo MXF-PZA-ETH-TRD OR 6–9 mo LZD-BDQ-LFX-PZA-TRD-ETH/INH
Nitroimidazoles				
Delamanid				
Otsuka 213 (NCT01424670)	Phase 3 Complete	Estonia, Latvia, Lithuania, Moldova, Peru, Philippines, South Africa	511	DLM or placebo × 6 mo + BR × 18–24 mo
Otsuka 232 (NCT01856634)	Phase 1 Complete	Philippines, South Africa	37	Pediatric PK, safety of DLM + BR for 10 d DLM 100 or 50 mg; pediatric formulation DLM 25, 10, or 5 mg; or optimized BR
Otsuka 233 (NCT01859923)	Phase 2 Complete	Philippines, South Africa	37	Pediatric 6-mo tolerability, PK/PD, efficacy various doses DLM + BR (follow-up 232)

(continued on next page)

Table 2
(continued)

Trial	Status	Population	Sample	Description
MDR-END (NCT02619994)	Phase 2 Enrolling	Republic of Korea	238	9–12 mo DLM-LZD-LFX-PZA vs 20–24 mo MDR-TB standard of care
IMPAACT 2005 (NCT03141060)	Phase 1–2 Enrolling	Botswana, India, South Africa, Tanzania	48	PK, safety, tolerability of DLM + BR for HIV-infected/noninfected children with MDR-TB 24 wk DLM + BR continued
ACTG A5356	Phase 2a In development	ACTG sites globally	120	24 wk DLM-LZD 600 mg daily + BR *OR* 24 wk DLM-LIN 600 + BR *OR* 24 wk DLM-LZD 1200 every other day
ACTG 5300/IMPAACT 2003 (PHOENIx)	Phase 3 Enrolling			Treatment of adult and child contacts of MDR cases: 26 wk DLM *OR* 26 wk INH
Pretomanid				
NC-006 STAND (NCT02342886)	Phase 3 Terminated	Georgia, Kenya, Malaysia, Philippines, South Africa, Tanzania, Uganda, Zambia	1500	24 wk PaMZ (MDR or DS-TB) *OR* 17 wk PaMZ (DS-TB) *OR* 24 wk RHZE (DS-TB)
APT (NCT02256696)	Phase 2 Enrolling	South Africa	183	8 wk Pa-rifabutin-INH-PZA, then 4 wk Pa-Rb-INH *OR* 8 wk Pa-RIF-INH-PZA, then 4 wk Pa-RIF-INH *OR* 8 wk Pa-Rb-INH-PZA, then 4 wk Pa-Rb-INH *OR* 8 wk RHZE, then 4 wk RH
Combinations of new drugs				
NixTB (NCT02333799)	Phase 3 Complete	South Africa	109	6–9 mo BPaLzd for XDR-TB and nonresponsive MDR-TB
DELIBERATE (ACTG 5343) (NCT02583048)	Phase 2 Complete	Peru, South Africa	84	Cardiac (QT) safety of BDQ vs DLM vs BDQ plus DLM, with BR in MDR-TB $\times$ 24 wk
NC-005 (NCT02193776)	Phase 2b Complete	South Africa, Tanzania, Uganda	240	Drug-sensitive: 8 wk BPaZ (with or without BDQ loading dose) *OR* 4HRZE/2RH Drug-resistant: 8 wk B-Pa-MXF-PZA
TB-PRACTECAL (NCT02589782)	Phase 2–3 Enrolling	Belarus, South Africa, Uzbekistan	630	Short-course treatment, adaptive design 24 wk BDQ-Pa-LZD-MXF *OR* 24 wk BDQ-Pa-LZD-CFZ *OR* 24 wk BDQ-Pa-LZD *OR* local standard of care

(continued on next page)

Table 2
(continued)

Trial	Status	Population	Sample	Description
endTB (NCT02754765)	Phase 3 Enrolling	Georgia, Kazakhstan, Kyrgyzstan, Lesotho, Peru, South Africa	750	Adaptive design 39 wk BDQ-LZD-MXF-PZA *OR* 39 wk BDQ-LZD-CFZ-LFX-PZA *OR* 39 wk BQD-DLM-LZD-LFX-PZA *OR* 39 wk DLM-LZD-CFZ-LFX-PZA *OR* 39 wk DLM-CFZ-MXF-PZA *OR* 86 wk local standard of care
ZeNiX (NCT03086486)	Phase 3 Enrolling	Georgia, Republic of Moldova, Russian Federation, South Africa	180	26 wk tx for XDR or nonresponsive MDR-TB, duration/dose Lzd LZD 1200 mg × 26 wk-Pa-BDQ *OR* LZD 1200 mg × 9 wk-Pa-BDQ *OR* LZD 600 mg × 26 wk-Pa-BDQ *OR* LZD 600 mg × 9 wk-Pa-BDQ
SimpliciTB (NCT03338621)	Phase 2–3 Enrolling	Georgia	450	Drug-sensitive: 17 wk BDQ-Pa-MXF-PZA *OR* 26 wk standard (2HRZE/4HR) Drug-resistant: 26 wk BDQ-Pa-MXF-PZA
IMPAACT 2020	Phase 2 In development	IMPAACT international sites	148	Children with MDR-TB 8 wk LZD + 24 wk BDQ-DMN-LFX/FLO
BEAT TB	Phase 3 In development			BDQ-DLM-LZD-CF-LFX for 6 mo treatment of MDR-TB

Abbreviations: BR, background regimen; CFZ, clofazimine; DLM/D, delamanid; DS, drug-sensitive; EMB, ethambutol; ETH, ethionamide; INH, isoniazid; KAN, kanamycin; LFX, levofloxacin; LZD/L, linezolid; MXF, moxifloxacin; Pa, pretomanid; PTO, prothionamide; PZA, pyrazinamide; Rb, rifabutin; RIF, rifampin; TRD, terizidone.

0.016 μg/mL on 7H11 and 0.06 μg/mL on MGIT is proposed.[34]

Clinical data

Phase 2a EBA trials demonstrated measurable but overlapping activity of different doses of delamanid.[51] In a phase 2b RCT in 481 patients with MDR-TB receiving MBR, delamanid 100 mg or 200 mg twice daily given for 8 weeks had higher culture conversion at 2 months (45% and 42%) than placebo (30%).[49] Modest QT prolongation was seen. In a nonrandomized follow-on study, longer delamanid use was associated with favorable outcomes (74.5% vs 55%) and decreased mortality (1.0% vs 8.3%).[54] In the phase 3 RCT of delamanid versus placebo added to MBR, overall treatment success at 30 months was high in both arms (>80%), so a statistically significant difference was not detected.[55] Nonetheless, given the measurable activity of the drug in the phase 2 program coupled with the drug's excellent safety profile, the WHO includes DLM among drugs that can be used for MDR-TB. Simplified regimens including delamanid are under study (see **Table 2**). Though marketed for use for 6 months, it has been well tolerated for up to 20 months.[56,57]

Pretomanid

Like delamanid, pretomanid (Pa) (PA-824) is a nitroimidazole that inhibits mycolic acid synthesis in actively multiplying bacilli. In addition, when it is activated by the *M.tb*.-specific F420-dependent nitroreductase, toxic reactive nitrogen species are released, killing nonreplicating bacilli.[58,59] A new drug application to the FDA was approved in 2019.

Preclinical data

Pretomanid's MIC against *M.tb.* is between 0.015 and 0.25 μg/mL for drug-sensitive strains and 0.03 to 0.53 μg/mL for drug-resistant strains.[60] Pretomanid is active against "persisters"[61] and under oxygen-poor conditions.[60] Mouse models have revealed time above MIC to be the PK driver for nitroimidazoles.[62] PaMZ in mice reduced treatment time by 1 to 2 months compared with standard therapy,[63] and the addition of BDQ (BPaMZ) cured mice in 2 months.[19]

Clinical pharmacology

Pretomanid has a half-life of 16 to 20 hours, is 94% protein bound, and has a large V_d[64,65]; PK is dose proportional up to 200 mg, then less-than-dose-proportional. CYP3A is responsible for 20% of its metabolism.[66] In a healthy volunteer trial, efavirenz and rifampicin decreased pretomanid trough concentrations by 46% and 85% and exposures (area under the curve) by 35% and 66%, respectively, raising concerns for coadministration.[66] Lopinavir/ritonavir did not affect pretomanid exposures meaningfully.

Resistance

Like delamanid, resistance to pretomanid can be related to prodrug activation (*fgd1*, *ddn*) or the F420 biosynthetic pathway (*fbiA*, *fbiB*, *fbiC*).[52] Resistance is present in 1 in 10^5 organisms pretreatment. Mutations in *Rv2983* in mouse models disrupt F420 biosynthesis, a newly identified mechanism of resistance yet to be identified in clinical samples.[67]

Clinical data

In the first EBA study of pretomanid, doses of 200 to 1200 mg produced similar, measurable activity.[68] In a second EBA, 50 mg was less active than 100 to 200 mg. Pretomanid causes dose-dependent increases in creatinine and modest QT prolongation.[69] In an EBA study of multidrug regimens, BPaZ had the highest microbiological activity, and 3 patients receiving regimens containing DPa had grade 3 or 4 transaminase elevations.[70] An 8-week study of PaMZ in drug-sensitive TB showed higher 8-week culture conversion (66%–71%) than HRZE (38%).[71] A phase 3 RCT (STAND) opened in 2015 to investigate PaMZ, but was put on temporary clinical hold to investigate cases of fatal hepatitis. In the meantime, a different trial showed exceptionally high culture conversion rates in patients with MDR-TB receiving BPaMZ,[72] and for this reason the SimpliciTB phase 3 RCT was launched to explore this regimen. Remarkably, in patients with XDR-TB, thought nearly untreatable, a regimen of BDQ-pretomanid-linezolid (BPaLz) tested in the NixTB trial showed favorable outcomes in ~90% of patients. Duration-dependent myelosuppression and neuropathy from linezolid are common; therefore, ZeNix was started to evaluate optimal linezolid dose and duration in BPaLZ regimens.[73]

PRACTICAL ASPECTS OF TREATMENT WITH NEW DRUGS
Coadministration

There is mounting evidence to support concurrent use of BDQ and a nitroimidazole, despite initial concerns for QT prolongation risk. Medecins Sans Frontières has endorsed judicious use of BDQ and delamanid since 2016 and has reported excellent outcomes (74% conversion by 6 months) and infrequent QT prolongation in a small cohort.[74] Other small series have reported similar efficacy results,[75–77] with episodes of QTc interval greater than 500 milliseconds generally occurring only with concurrent moxifloxacin or clofazimine.[42] Interim results from DELIBERATE, an AIDS Clinical Trials Group RCT, suggest no more than additive QT prolongation when BDQ and delamanid are combined. If BDQ and delamanid will be coadministered, considerations include: (1) repletion of K^+ and Mg^{2+} electrolytes; (2) measuring QTcF at baseline and serially; and (3) close attention to companion drugs (fluoroquinolones, clofazimine, ritonavir, methadone, and aminoglycosides all prolong QT). Pretomanid has a modest effect on the QT interval, and with moxifloxacin did not cause QTc greater than 500 milliseconds.[71] QTcF was prolonged by ~20 milliseconds in patients receiving BPaZ or BPaMZ, which is only clinically significant if baseline QTcF is high.[78] Although the WHO recommends BDQ in the standard (18–24 months) duration regimen, it is licensed only for 24 weeks; guidance regarding prolonged use is awaited.

Extrapulmonary Tuberculosis

There are no data for pleural or pericardial TB and only limited data for central nervous system (CNS) TB. In one patient with MDR-TB meningitis (TBM), BDQ levels in cerebrospinal fluid (CSF) were undetectable, but collection conditions were not optimized for measurement of this highly lipophilic drug.[79,80] A study in rats using radiolabeled delamanid showed lasting distribution into the brain.[81] Recent work in a rabbit model of TBM showed high brain but low CSF levels. Three patients with XDR-TBM, which is generally fatal, who were treated with delamanid containing

Table 3
New chemical entities in development for treatment of tuberculosis

Name	Developer	Supporting Data	Preclinical/Clinical	Trial Objectives	Trial Design
[a]Ethylenediamine: targets Mmpl3 involved in mycolate transport and processing, disrupting incorporation into cell wall					
SQ109	Sequella, Inc	Phase 2 EBA/safety with gastrointestinal upset, no QT prolongation, significant decline in exposure when administered at 150 mg with rifampin (overcome at 300 mg SQ109)	SQ109 EBA NCT01218217 (2a, published)	EBA, safety, tolerability, PK of several doses with/ without RIF	14 d: SQ109 75, 150, 300 as monotherapy OR SQ109 15, 300 + RIF OR RIF monotherapy
		Decreases RIF MIC; No EBA as monotherapy or additive to others; No difference in culture conversion rate	MAMS-TB, NCT01785186 (2b, published)	MAMS trial to evaluate 4 regimens	14 wk $INH-RIF_{35}-PZA-EMB$ OR $INH-RIF_{10}-PZA-Q_{300}$ OR $INH-RIF_{20}-PZA-Q_{300}$ OR $INH-RIF_{20}-PZA-MXF$ OR $INH-RIF_{10}-PZA-EMB$
		Patient with INH resistance on RHZ-SQ109 developed RIF/PZA resistance	(2b–3, complete)	Additive for MDR-TB in Russia	HRZE-SQ109 OR HRZE-placebo
Imidazopyridine amide: inhibits qcrB subunit of cytochrome bc_1 complex					
Q203, Telacebec	Qurient Co. Ltd./LLC "Infectex"	Mouse models demonstrate efficacy with once daily doses <1 mg/kg; active intracellularly and extracellularly, no CYPp450 inhibition in vitro	NCT02530710 (1a, complete)	Safety, tolerability, PK of single doses in healthy adults	Doses of 10, 20, 50, 100, 150, 200, 400, 800 mg/kg
			NCT02858973 (1b, complete)	Safety, tolerability, PK of multiple doses in adults	Q203 vs placebo
			NCT03563599 (2, enrolling)	EBA of Q203 vs RHZE	Mid, high, low doses of Q203

aOxaborole: Inhibits leucyl-tRNA synthetase (LeuRS), protein synthesis inhibitor

Drug	Sponsor	Characteristics	Trial (phase, status)	Study	Dosing
GSK 070, GSK3036656	GlaxoSmithKline	Good oral bioavailability, low protein binding, activity comparable with INH in mice; Active at lower doses and wider intervals (48 h) than linezolid	NCT03557281 (2, pending)	EBA, safety, tolerability in 4 sequential cohorts with DS-TB	2 wk GSK3036656 or RHZE daily or RHZE
			NCT03075410 (1, complete)	Safety, tolerability, PK of single ascending and repeat doses in health adults	Single dose at 5, 25, or 100 mg Daily dosing

Oxazolidinone: protein synthesis inhibitor, binds bacterial 23s rRNA of 50S subunit to prevent formation of 70S initiation complex

Drug	Sponsor	Characteristics	Trial (phase, status)	Study	Dosing
Sutezolid, PNU-100480	Sequella, Inc, TB Alliance	In mice, shortens standard treatment by 1 mo, activity superior to linezolid Safety and tolerability up to 1000 mg in humans Highly active primary metabolite (PNU-101603) at higher concentration than parent Phase 2 data: synergy with PZA, t_{max} 1–2 h (fasting), 3 h (fed), half-life 3.4 h, 600 mg BID consistently higher than MIC (1200 mg was not) No heme/neuro AE, 14% patients with ALT elevation	NCT01225640 (2, complete)	EBA and whole blood activity	STZ 600 mg BID, 1200 mg daily or RHZE
			SUDOCU (2, proposed)	Sutezolid EBA and dose finding study	BDQ-DLM-MXF *PLUS* STZ 0 mg 600 mg daily, 1200 mg daily, 600 mg twice daily, OR 800 mg twice daily
			STEP (2c, proposed)	Safety, efficacy, exposure-response of rifampin doses, STZ	4 mo R_{high}HZE *OR* 4 mo R_{high}HZ$_{high}$E *OR* 4–6 mo STZ-BDM *OR* 6 mo HRZE
			NCT03237182 (4, enrolling)	Gene-derived individualized drug-resistant TB regimens, including sutezolid	
Delpazolid, LCB01-0371	LegoChem Biosciences, Inc	Phase 1: tolerated to 1200 mg twice daily (though decline in heme values for daily doses >800 mg), rapid PO absorption, 100% oral bioavailability, t_{max} 0.5–1 hr, half-life 1.3–2.1 h, plasma binding 37%	NCT02836483 (2, enrolling)	EBA, safety, and PK	800 mg daily, 400 mg twice daily, 800 mg twice daily, LZD 600 mg twice daily

(continued on next page)

Table 3 *(continued)*

Name	Developer	Supporting Data	Preclinical/Clinical	Trial Objectives	Trial Design
Contezolid, MRX-4	MicuRx Pharmaceuticals, Inc	Broad gram-positive activity, comparable with linezolid; MRX-1 in phase 3 trials in China for skin/soft tissue, MRX-4 (prodrug of MRX-1) being studied in USA	NCT03033329 (1, complete)	Safety, tolerability, PK with dose escalation (IV), crossover to PO	• Single IV dose 150–1800 mg • BID IV dosing for 10 d: 600, 900, 1200, 1500 mg
TBI-223	TB Alliance, Institute of Materia Medica	Lower activity on mammalian mitochondrial protein synthesis; hepatocyte stability across 5 animal species, no evidence *in vitro* of CYP induction, half-life 3 h in mice, 8 h in rats; success in mice with BPa-TBI223 (replace linezolid); no hematologic/marrow toxicity in 14 and 28 d rat toxicity studies	NCT03758612 (1, pending)	Single and multiple ascending dose trial	
^aDprE1 inhibitors: covalent (benzothiazinone): inhibits decaprenyl-phosphoribose epimerase (DprE1) involved in cell wall arabinan biosynthesis					
BTZ043	University of Munich, Hans-Knöll Institute, Jena, German Center for Infection Research (DZIF)	Superior to INH at 2 mo in mice (6 mo pending) No antagonism with existing drugs, apparent synergy *in vivo* with BDQ-RIF Low-level CYP450 interaction	NCT03590600 (1, enrolling)	Ascending dose study	BTZ043 125, 250, 500, 1000, 2000 mg or placebo

Drug	Sponsor	Activity	Trial (phase, status)	Objective	Doses
Macozinone, MCZ, PBTZ169	iM4TB-Innovative Medicines for Tuberculosis, Bill & Melinda Gates Foundation, Nearmedic Plus LLC	Highly active against replicating bacteria; no antagonism with RHZE, synergy in vitro with BDQ, CFZ, DLM, sutezolid; Prior formulation with good tolerability, bactericidal activity against DS-TB at 640 mg	NCT03776500 (1, pending)	Safety, tolerability, PK at multiple ascending doses	150 mg BID OR 300 mg BID OR 600 mg daily OR 600 mg BID
[a]DprE1 inhibitor: non-covalent (OPC-167832: carbostyril, TBA-7371: azaindole): see above					
OPC-167832	Otsuka Pharmaceutical Development & Commercialization, Inc	Activity against replicating and dormant intracellular bacilli; active in acute and chronic murine models; no antagonism with other TB drugs; additive effect with DLM exceeding RHZE	NCT03678688 (1–2, enrolling)	Safety, tolerability, PK, efficacy of multiple oral doses in DS-TB	Stage 1: 14 d of OPC-167832 10 mg OR 30 mg OR 90 mg OR 270 mg OR RHZE. Stage 2: 14 d of OPC-167832$_{Low}$DLM$_{200}$ OR OPC-167832$_{High}$DLM$_{200}$ OR DLM200
TBA-7371	TB Alliance	Efficacy in vitro and in mice Phase 1 trial complete on food effect, optimal dose, DDI, PK, PD as single dose or multiple doses	NCT03199339 (1, complete)	Safety, tolerability of single and multiple doses among healthy adults	Single doses of 100, 250, 500 1000, 1500 mg; Multiple doses of 100, 200, 400; DDI with midazolam, bupropion
Riminophenazine: Same class as CFZ					
TBI-166	Institute of Materia Medica, CAMS & PUMC	Excellent in vivo, shorter half-life, less lipophilicity, less potential for skin discoloration and other toxicities of CFZ	Unknown name (1, enrolling)	Safety, tolerability among patients in China	

Abbreviations: EBA, early bactericidal activity; RIF or R, rifampin/rifampicin; MIC, minimal inhibitory concentration; PZA or Z, pyrazinamide; PK, pharmacokinetics; INH or H, isoniazid; EMB or E, ethambutol; Q, SQ109; STZ, sutezolid; BDQ or B, bedaquiline; DLM or D, delamanid; MXF or M, moxifloxacin; LZD, linezolid; PO, per oral; Pa, pretomanid; CYP, cytochrome p450; d, day; mg, milligram; DDI, drug-drug interaction; BID, twice daily; PD, pharmacodynamic; CFZ, clofazamine.

[a] Denotes novel class.

Adapted from Working Group on New TB Drugs (https://www.newtbdrugs.org/pipeline/clinical) as of January 2019.

regimens displayed marked clinical improvement despite very low delamanid CSF/plasma ratios.[82] In rats, pretomanid seems to cross the blood-brain barrier and penetrate into the brain, although clinical correlation is needed.[83]

Children and Pregnant Women

Initial results from Otsuka trials 232/233 demonstrated acceptable PK and safety of delamanid in HIV-uninfected children ≥3 years old; therefore, the WHO now recommends DLM for that age group. The WHO recommends BDQ in children with MDR-TB aged 6 to 17 years.[84] Trials are ongoing to optimize pediatric dosing (BDQ: Janssen C211, IMPAACT P1008; delamanid: Otsuka 233, 234, IMPAACT 2005). There is not yet a pediatric formulation of BDQ, but suspension or crushing gives similar bioavailability to whole tablets.[85] Dispersible formulations of BDQ and delamanid are in development. Safety and efficacy of these drugs in children seem similar to those in adults, although data are limited.[86–88] The pediatric investigation plan for pretomanid is progressing. There exist little data about use of these drugs in pregnancy[89]; given that these drugs are life-saving in MDR-TB, PK and safety studies in this population are needed.

THE DRUG DEVELOPMENT PIPELINE

The "third wave" of TB drug development is now here (**Table 3**). Some compounds are from drug classes already in clinical use for TB but have been redesigned to optimize bioavailability, potency, safety, or activity against resistant strains (fluoroquinolones, diarylquinolines, riminophenazines, carbapenems, oxazolidinones, nitroimidazoles). Many are from new classes with novel mechanisms of action (eg, inhibitors of DprE1, leucyl-tRNA synthetase, cholesterol catabolism). Many of these compounds are now in phase 1 or phase 2 trials.[90–117]

SUMMARY

BDQ is proven to reduce mortality in MDR-TB, and it is recommended for use as a first-line agent for patients with MDR-TB. Best practices for ECG monitoring, dosing in children, and HIV cotreatment are emerging. Delamanid, despite disappointing phase 3 results, has a role as a companion drug in all-oral regimens for MDR-TB. It is well tolerated, and rational dosing recommendations and formulations for children are coming soon. Pretomanid, in combination with linezolid and BDQ, displayed exceptional efficacy among patients with XDR-TB, and it is now approved for use in combination with LZD and BDQ in patients with highly resistant TB. In addition, nitroimidazoles may have brain penetration that allows for use in CNS TB, but clinical data are lacking. Now that the WHO has listed BDQ and delamanid among the options for MDR-TB in the newest guidelines, access to these drugs will improve. Lastly, the third wave of TB drug discovery offers exciting new compounds with numerous mechanisms of action that may expand the arsenal not only for MDR-TB but for ultrashort combination regimens for drug-sensitive TB.

REFERENCES

1. World Health Organization (WHO). Global tuberculosis report 2018. WHO; 2018. Geneva (Switzerland).
2. Kendall EA, Shrestha S, Cohen T, et al. Priority-setting for novel drug regimens to treat tuberculosis: an epidemiologic model. PLoS Med 2017; 14(1):e1002202.
3. Imperial MZ, Nahid P, Phillips PPJ, et al. A patient-level pooled analysis of treatment-shortening regimens for drug-susceptible pulmonary tuberculosis. Nat Med 2018;24(11):1708–15.
4. Slomski A. South Africa warns of emergence of "totally" drug-resistant tuberculosis. JAMA 2013; 309(11):1097–8.
5. Dheda K, Limberis JD, Pietersen E, et al. Outcomes, infectiousness, and transmission dynamics of patients with extensively drug-resistant tuberculosis and home-discharged patients with programmatically incurable tuberculosis: a prospective cohort study. Lancet Respir Med 2017; 5(4):269–81.
6. Ahmad N, Ahuja SD, Akkerman OW, et al. Treatment correlates of successful outcomes in pulmonary multidrug-resistant tuberculosis: an individual patient data meta-analysis. Lancet 2018; 392(10150):821–34.
7. Van Deun A, Maug AKJ, Salim MAH, et al. Short, highly effective, and inexpensive standardized treatment of multidrug-resistant tuberculosis. Am J Respir Crit Care Med 2010;182(5):684–92.
8. Trébucq A, Schwoebel V, Kashongwe Z, et al. Treatment outcome with a short multidrug-resistant tuberculosis regimen in nine African countries. Int J Tuberc Lung Dis 2018;22(1):17–25.
9. Sotgiu G, Tiberi S, D'Ambrosio L, et al. Faster for less: the new "shorter" regimen for multidrug-resistant tuberculosis. Eur Respir J 2016;48(5): 1503–7.
10. World Health Organization. Rapid communication : key changes to treatment of multidrug- and rifampicin-resistant tuberculosis (MDR/RR-TB). Geneva (Switzerland): WHO; 2018.

11. World Health Organization (WHO). The use of bedaquiline in the treatment of multidrug-resistant tuberculosis: interim policy guidance. Geneva (Switzerland): World Health Organization; 2013.

12. Andries K, Verhasselt P, Guillemont J, et al. A diarylquinoline drug active on the ATP synthase of Mycobacterium tuberculosis. Science 2005; 307(5707):223–7.

13. Lounis N, Gevers T, Van Den Berg J, et al. ATP synthase inhibition of Mycobacterium avium is not bactericidal. Antimicrob Agents Chemother 2009; 53(11):4927–9.

14. Zhang T, Li SY, Williams KN, et al. Short-course chemotherapy with TMC207 and rifapentine in a murine model of latent tuberculosis infection. Am J Respir Crit Care Med 2011;184(6):732–7.

15. Shang S, Shanley CA, Caraway ML, et al. Activities of TMC207, rifampin, and pyrazinamide against Mycobacterium tuberculosis infection in Guinea pigs. Antimicrob Agents Chemother 2011;55(1): 124–31.

16. Tasneen R, Li SY, Peloquin CA, et al. Sterilizing activity of novel TMC207- and PA-824-containing regimens in a murine model of tuberculosis. Antimicrob Agents Chemother 2011;55(12):5485–92.

17. Ibrahim M, Andries K, Lounis N, et al. Synergistic activity of R207910 combined with pyrazinamide against murine tuberculosis. Antimicrob Agents Chemother 2007;51(3):1011–5.

18. Andries K, Gevers T, Lounis N. Bactericidal potencies of new regimens are not predictive of their sterilizing potencies in a murine model of tuberculosis. Antimicrob Agents Chemother 2010;54(11): 4540–4.

19. Li S-Y, Tasneen R, Tyagi S, et al. Bactericidal and sterilizing activity of a novel regimen with bedaquiline, pretomanid, moxifloxacin, and pyrazinamide in a murine model of tuberculosis. Antimicrob Agents Chemother 2017;61(9):1–8.

20. FDA. SIRTURO® (bedaquiline) tablets, for oral use highlights of prescribing information 2012. Available at: https://www.sirturo.com/sites/default/files/pdf/sirturo-pi.pdf. Accessed January 13, 2019.

21. van Heeswijk RPG, Dannemann B, Hoetelmans RMW. Bedaquiline: a review of human pharmacokinetics and drug-drug interactions. J Antimicrob Chemother 2014;69(9):2310–8.

22. Diacon AH, Donald PR, Pym A, et al. Randomized pilot trial of eight weeks of bedaquiline (TMC207) treatment for multidrug-resistant tuberculosis: long-term outcome, tolerability, and effect on emergence of drug resistance. Antimicrob Agents Chemother 2012;56(6):3271–6.

23. Rouan MC, Lounis N, Gevers T, et al. Pharmacokinetics and pharmacodynamics of TMC207 and its N-desmethyl metabolite in a murine model of tuberculosis. Antimicrob Agents Chemother 2012; 56(3):1444–51.

24. McLeay SC, Vis P, Van Heeswijk RPG, et al. Population pharmacokinetics of bedaquiline (TMC207), a novel antituberculosis drug. Antimicrob Agents Chemother 2014;58(9):5315–24.

25. Svensson EM, Dosne AG, Karlsson MO. Population pharmacokinetics of bedaquiline and metabolite M2 in patients with drug-resistant tuberculosis: the effect of time-varying weight and albumin. CPT Pharmacometrics Syst Pharmacol 2016; 5(12):682–91.

26. Svensson EM, Murray S, Karlsson MO, et al. Rifampicin and rifapentine significantly reduce concentrations of bedaquiline, a new anti-TB drug. J Antimicrob Chemother 2014;70(4): 1106–14.

27. Svensson EM, Aweeka F, Park JG, et al. Model-based estimates of the effects of efavirenz on bedaquiline pharmacokinetics and suggested dose adjustments for patients coinfected with HIV and tuberculosis. Antimicrob Agents Chemother 2013; 57(6):2780–7.

28. Brill MJE, Svensson EM, Pandie M, et al. Confirming model-predicted pharmacokinetic interactions between bedaquiline and lopinavir/ritonavir or nevirapine in patients with HIV and drug-resistant tuberculosis. Int J Antimicrob Agents 2017;49(2): 212–7.

29. Huitric E, Verhasselt P, Koul A, et al. Rates and mechanisms of resistance development in Mycobacterium tuberculosis to a novel diarylquinoline ATP synthase inhibitor. Antimicrob Agents Chemother 2010;54(3):1022–8.

30. Hartkoorn RC, Uplekar S, Cole ST. Cross-resistance between clofazimine and bedaquiline through upregulation of mmpl5 in mycobacterium tuberculosis. Antimicrob Agents Chemother 2014; 58(5):2979–81.

31. Almeida D, Ioerger T, Tyagi S, et al. Mutations in pepQ confer low-level resistance to bedaquiline and clofazimine in Mycobacterium tuberculosis. Antimicrob Agents Chemother 2016;60(8):4590–9.

32. Villellas C, Coeck N, Meehan CJ, et al. Unexpected high prevalence of resistance-associated Rv0678 variants in MDR-TB patients without documented prior use of clofazimine or bedaquiline. J Antimicrob Chemother 2017;72(3):684–90.

33. Bloemberg GV, Keller PM, Stucki D, et al. Acquired resistance to bedaquiline and delamanid in therapy for tuberculosis. N Engl J Med 2015;373(20): 1986–8.

34. World Health Organization (WHO). WHO technical report on critical concentrations for TB drug susceptibility testing of medicines used in the treatment of drug-resistant TB. Geneva (Switzerland): WHO; 2018. . Available at: http://

www.who.int/tb/publications/2018/WHO_technical_report_concentrations_TB_drug_susceptibility/en/.

35. Diacon AH, Dawson R, Von Groote-Bidlingmaier F, et al. 14-day bactericidal activity of PA-824, bedaquiline, pyrazinamide, and moxifloxacin combinations: a randomised trial. Lancet 2012;380(9846): 986–93.

36. Diacon AH, Dawson R, Von Groote-Bidlingmaier F, et al. Randomized dose-ranging study of the 14-day early bactericidal activity of bedaquiline (TMC207) in patients with sputum microscopy smear-positive pulmonary tuberculosis. Antimicrob Agents Chemother 2013;57(5):2199–203.

37. Koul A, Vranckx L, Dhar N, et al. Delayed bactericidal response of *Mycobacterium tuberculosis* to bedaquiline involves remodelling of bacterial metabolism. Nat Commun 2014;5:3369.

38. Diacon AH, Pym A, Grobusch MP, et al. Multidrug-resistant tuberculosis and culture conversion with bedaquiline. N Engl J Med 2014;371(8):723–32.

39. Pym AS, Diacon AH, Tang SJ, et al. Bedaquiline in the treatment of multidrug- and extensively drugresistant tuberculosis. Eur Respir J 2016;47(2): 564–74.

40. Schnippel K, Ndjeka N, Maartens G, et al. Effect of bedaquiline on mortality in South African patients with drug-resistant tuberculosis: a retrospective cohort study. Lancet Respir Med 2018;6(9): 699–706.

41. Ndjeka N, Schnippel K, Master I, et al. High treatment success rate for multidrug-resistant and extensively drug-resistant tuberculosis using a bedaquiline-containing treatment regimen. Eur Respir J 2018;52(6):1801528.

42. Guglielmetti L, Jaspard M, Le Dû D, et al. Long-term outcome and safety of prolonged bedaquiline treatment for multidrug-resistant tuberculosis. Eur Respir J 2017;49(3). https://doi.org/10.1183/13993003.01799-2016.

43. Borisov SE, Dheda K, Enwerem M, et al. Effectiveness and safety of bedaquiline-containing regimens in the treatment of MDR- and XDR-TB: a multicentre study. Eur Respir J 2017;49(5). https://doi.org/10.1183/13993003.00387-2017.

44. Zhao Y, Fox T, Manning K, et al. Improved treatment outcomes with bedaquiline when substituted for second-line injectable agents in multidrug resistant tuberculosis: a retrospective cohort study. Clin Infect Dis 2019;68(9):1522–9.

45. Stover CK, Warrener P, VanDevanter DR, et al. A small-molecule nitroimidazopyran drug candidate for the treatment of tuberculosis. Nature 2000;405(6789):962–6.

46. Matsumoto M, Hashizume H, Tomishige T, et al. OPC-67683, a nitro-dihydro-imidazooxazole derivative with promising action against tuberculosis in vitro and in mice. PLoS Med 2006;3(11):2131–44.

47. Chen X, Hashizume H, Tomishige T, et al. Delamanid kills dormant mycobacteria in vitro and in a Guinea pig model of tuberculosis. Antimicrob Agents Chemother 2017;61(6):1–11.

48. Mallikaarjun S, Wells C, Petersen C, et al. Delamanid coadministered with antiretroviral drugs or antituberculosis drugs shows no clinically relevant drug-drug interactions in healthy subjects. Antimicrob Agents Chemother 2016;60(10):5976–85.

49. Gler MT, Skripconoka V, Sanchez-Garavito E, et al. Delamanid for multidrug-resistant pulmonary tuberculosis. N Engl J Med 2012;366(23):2151–60.

50. Sasahara K, Shimokawa Y, Hirao Y, et al. Pharmacokinetics and metabolism of delamanid, a novel anti-tuberculosis drug, in animals and humans: importance of albumin metabolism in vivo. Drug Metab Dispos 2015;43(8):1267–76.

51. Diacon AH, Dawson R, Hanekom M, et al. Early bactericidal activity of delamanid (OPC-67683) in smear-positive pulmonary tuberculosis patients. Int J Tuberc Lung Dis 2011;15(7):949–54.

52. Haver HL, Chua A, Ghode P, et al. Mutations in genes for the F420biosynthetic pathway and a nitroreductase enzyme are the primary resistance determinants in spontaneous in vitro-selected PA-824-resistant mutants of *Mycobacterium tuberculosis*. Antimicrob Agents Chemother 2015;59(9): 5316–23.

53. Pang Y, Zong Z, Huo F, et al. In vitro drug susceptibility of bedaquiline, delamanid, linezolid, clofazimine, moxifloxacin, and gatifloxacin against extensively drug-resistant tuberculosis in Beijing, China. Antimicrob Agents Chemother 2017; 61(10):1–8.

54. Skripconoka V, Danilovits M, Pehme L, et al. Delamanid improves outcomes and reduces mortality in multidrug-resistant tuberculosis. Eur Respir J 2013;41(6):1393–400.

55. von Groote-Bidlingmaier F, Patientia R, Sanchez E, et al. Efficacy and safety of delamanid in combination with an optimised background regimen for treatment of multidrug-resistant tuberculosis: a multicentre, randomised, double-blind, placebo-controlled, parallel group phase 3 trial. Lancet Respir Med 2019;2600(18):1–12.

56. Kuksa L, Barkane L, Hittel N, et al. Final treatment outcomes of multidrug- and extensively drug-resistant tuberculosis patients in Latvia receiving delamanid-containing regimens. Eur Respir J 2017;50(5):1701105.

57. Chang K-C, Leung EC-C, Law W-S, et al. Early experience with delamanid-containing regimens in the treatment of complicated multidrug-resistant tuberculosis in Hong Kong. Eur Respir J 2018;51(6):2–5.

58. Dogra M, Palmer BD, Bashiri G, et al. Comparative bioactivation of the novel anti-tuberculosis agent

PA-824 in Mycobacteria and a subcellular fraction of human liver. Br J Pharmacol 2011;162(1): 226–36.

59. Baptista R, Fazakerley DM, Beckmann M, et al. Untargeted metabolomics reveals a new mode of action of pretomanid (PA-824). Sci Rep 2018;8(1): 5084.

60. Lenaerts AJ, Gruppo V, Marietta KS, et al. Preclinical testing of the nitroimidazopyran PA-824 for activity against *Mycobacterium tuberculosis* in a series of in vitro and in vivo models. Antimicrob Agents Chemother 2005;49(6): 2294–301.

61. Tyagi S, Nuermberger E, Yoshimatsu T, et al. Bactericidal activity of the nitroimidazopyran PA-824 in a murine model of tuberculosis. Antimicrob Agents Chemother 2005;49(6):2289–93.

62. Lakshminarayana SB, Boshoff HIM, Cherian J, et al. Pharmacokinetics-pharmacodynamics analysis of bicyclic 4-nitroimidazole analogs in a murine model of tuberculosis. PLoS One 2014;9(8). https:// doi.org/10.1371/journal.pone.0105222.

63. Nuermberger E, Tyagi S, Tasneen R, et al. Powerful bactericidal and sterilizing activity of a regimen containing PA-824, moxifloxacin, and pyrazinamide in a murine model of tuberculosis. Antimicrob Agents Chemother 2008;52(4):1522–4.

64. Hu Y, Coates ARM, Mitchison DA. Comparison of the sterilising activities of the nitroimidazopyran PA-824 and moxifloxacin against persisting *Mycobacterium tuberculosis*. Int J Tuberc Lung Dis 2008; 12(1):69–73. Available at: http://www.ncbi.nlm.nih. gov/pubmed/18173880.

65. Ginsberg AM, Laurenzi MW, Rouse DJ, et al. Safety, tolerability, and pharmacokinetics of PA-824 in healthy subjects. Antimicrob Agents Chemother 2009;53(9):3720–5.

66. Dooley KE, Luetkemeyer AF, Park JG, et al. Phase I safety, pharmacokinetics, and pharmacogenetics study of the antituberculosis drug PA-824 with concomitant lopinavir-ritonavir, efavirenz, or rifampin. Antimicrob Agents Chemother 2014; 58(9):5245–52.

67. Rifat D, Li S-Y, Ioerger T, et al. Mutations in Rv2983 as a novel determinant of resistance to nitroimidazole drugs in *Mycobacterium tuberculosis*. bioRxivorg 2018;457754. Available at: https://www. biorxiv.org/content/biorxiv/early/2018/10/31/457754. full.pdf.

68. Diacon AH, Dawson R, Hanekom M, et al. Early bactericidal activity and pharmacokinetics of PA-824 in smear-positive tuberculosis patients. Antimicrob Agents Chemother 2010;54(8):3402–7.

69. Diacon AH, Dawson R, Du Bois J, et al. Phase II dose-ranging trial of the early bactericidal activity of PA-824. Antimicrob Agents Chemother 2012; 56(6):3027–31.

70. Diacon AH, Dawson R, Von Groote-Bidlingmaier F, et al. Bactericidal activity of pyrazinamide and clofazimine alone and in combinations with pretomanid and bedaquiline. Am J Respir Crit Care Med 2015;191(8):943–53.

71. Dawson R, Diacon AH, Everitt D, et al. Efficiency and safety of the combination of moxifloxacin, pretomanid (PA-824), and pyrazinamide during the first 8 weeks of antituberculosis treatment: a phase 2b, open-label, partly randomised trial in patients with drug-susceptible or drug-resistant pul. Lancet 2015;385(9979):1738–47.

72. Clinical trial of BPaMZ regimen will replace phase 3 STAND trial. TB Alliance. 2016. Available at: https:// www.tballiance.org/news/clinical-trial-bpamz-regi men-will-replace-phase-3-stand-trial. Accessed January 13, 2019..

73. Conradie F, Diacon A, Howell P, et al. Sustained high rate of successful treatment outcomes: interim results of 75 patients in the Nix-TB clinical study of pretomanid, bedaquiline and linezolid. In: The Union 2018. The Hague. October 25, 2018.

74. Ferlazzo G, Mohr E, Laxmeshwar C, et al. Early safety and efficacy of the combination of bedaquiline and delamanid for the treatment of patients with drug-resistant tuberculosis in Armenia, India, and South Africa: a retrospective cohort study. Lancet Infect Dis 2018;18(5):536–44.

75. Maryandyshev A, Pontali E, Tiberi S, et al. Bedaquiline and delamanid combination treatment of 5 patients with pulmonary extensively drug-resistant tuberculosis. Emerg Infect Dis 2017;23(10): 1718–21.

76. Guglielmetti L, Barkane L, Le Du D, et al. Safety and efficacy of exposure to bedaquiline-delamanid in MDR-TB: a case series from France and Latvia. Eur Respir J 2018;51(3):1702550.

77. Tae Kim C, Kim T-O, Shin H-J, et al. Bedaquiline and delamanid for the treatment of multidrug-resistant tuberculosis: a multi-center cohort study in Korea. Eur Respir J 2018;51(3):1702467.

78. Dawson R, Harris K, Conradie A, et al. Efficacy of bedaquiline, pretomanid, moxifloxacin, & PZA (BPaMZ) against DS- & MDR-TB. In: CROI Conference. Seattle, Washington, February 13-16, 2017.

79. Akkerman OW, Odish OFF, Bolhuis MS, et al. Pharmacokinetics of bedaquiline in cerebrospinal fluid and serum in multidrug-resistant tuberculous meningitis. Clin Infect Dis 2015;62(4):523–4.

80. Verhaeghe T, Diels L, Dillen L. Quantitation of bedaquiline: points of attention. Clin Infect Dis 2016; 63(1):145–6.

81. Shibata M, Shimokawa Y, Sasahara K, et al. Absorption, distribution and excretion of the antituberculosis drug delamanid in rats: extensive tissue distribution suggests potential therapeutic

value for extrapulmonary tuberculosis. Biopharm Drug Dispos 2017;38(4):301–12.

82. Tucker EW, Pieterse L, Zimmerman MD, et al. Delamanid central nervous system pharmacokinetics in tuberculous meningitis in rabbits and humans. Antimicrob Agents Chemother 2019;63(10). pii: e00913-19.

83. Shobo A, Bratkowska D, Baijnath S, et al. Tissue distribution of pretomanid in rat brain via mass spectrometry imaging. Xenobiotica 2016;46(3):247–52.

84. World Health Organization (WHO). WHO treatment guidelines for multidrug- and rifampin-resistant tuberculosis: 2018 update. WHO; 2018. Geneva (Switzerland).

85. Svensson EM, du Bois J, Kitshoff R, et al. Relative bioavailability of bedaquiline tablets suspended in water: implications for dosing in children. Br J Clin Pharmacol 2018;84(10):2384–92.

86. Achar J, Hewison C, Cavalheiro AP, et al. Off-label use of bedaquiline in children and adolescents with multidrug-resistant tuberculosis. Emerg Infect Dis 2017;23(10):1711–3.

87. Schaaf HS, Thee S, van der Laan L, et al. Adverse effects of oral second-line antituberculosis drugs in children. Expert Opin Drug Saf 2016;15(10):1369–81.

88. Esposito S, Bosis S, Tadolini M, et al. Efficacy, safety, and tolerability of a 24-month treatment regimen including delamanid in a child with extensively drug-resistant tuberculosis. Medicine (Baltimore) 2016;95(46):e5347.

89. Jaspard M, Elefant-Amoura E, Melonio I, et al. Bedaquiline and linezolid for extensively drug-resistant tuberculosis in pregnant woman. Emerg Infect Dis 2017;23(10):153–5.

90. Clinical pipeline. Working group on new TB drugs. Available at: https://www.newtbdrugs.org/pipeline/clinical. Accessed January 15, 2019.

91. Takahashi Y, Igarashi M, Miyake T, et al. Novel semisynthetic antibiotics from caprazamycins A-G: Caprazene derivatives and their antibacterial activity. J Antibiot (Tokyo) 2013;66(3):171–8.

92. Kling A, Lukat P, Almeida DV, et al. Antibiotics. Targeting DnaN for tuberculosis therapy using novel griselimycins. Science 2015;348(6239):1106–12.

93. Ahmad Z, Minkowski A, Peloquin CA, et al. Activity of the fluoroquinolone DC-159a in the initial and continuation phases of treatment of murine tuberculosis. Antimicrob Agents Chemother 2011;55(4):1781–3.

94. Zhang T, Lu X, Tu Z, et al. Compound TB47 has strong activity against *Mycobacterium tuberculosis* both in vitro and in vivo. In: ASM Microbe. New Orleans, June 4, 2017.

95. Shoen C., Pucci M., M. DeStefano MC. Efficacy of SPR720 and SPR750 Gyrase inhibitors in a mouse *Mycobacterium tuberculosis* infection model. In: ASM Microbe. New Orleans, June 2, 2017.

96. Shionogi & Co. Ltd. Research and Development at Shionogi. Available at: http://www.shionogi.co.jp/en/ir/pdf/e_p180315.pdf.

97. GSK-286. Working group on new TB drugs. Available at: https://www.newtbdrugs.org/pipeline/compound/gsk-286. Accessed January 10, 2019.

98. Sutherland HS, Tong AST, Choi PJ, et al. Structure-activity relationships for analogs of the tuberculosis drug bedaquiline with the naphthalene unit replaced by bicyclic heterocycles. Bioorg Med Chem 2018;26(8):1797–809.

99. Our pipeline: TBAJ-876. TB alliance. Available at: https://www.tballiance.org/portfolio/compound/tbaj-876. Accessed January 10, 2019.

100. El-Gamal MI, Brahim I, Hisham N, et al. Recent updates of carbapenem antibiotics. Eur J Med Chem 2017;131:185–95.

101. Mdluli K., Cooper C., Yang T., et al. TBI-223: A safer oxazolidinone in pre-clinical development for tuberculosis. In: ASM Microbe. New Orleans, June 4, 2017. Available at: http://www.abstractsonline.com/pp8/#!/4358/presentation/6174.

102. Robertson GT, Scherman MS, Bruhn DF, et al. Spectinamides are effective partner agents for the treatment of tuberculosis in multiple mouse infection models. J Antimicrob Chemother 2017;72(3):770–7.

103. Lechartier B, Hartkoorn RC, Cole ST. In vitro combination studies of benzothiazinone lead compound BTZ043 against *Mycobacterium tuberculosis*. Antimicrob Agents Chemother 2012;56(11):5790–3.

104. Palencia A, Li X, Bu W, et al. Discovery of novel oral protein synthesis inhibitors of mycobacterium tuberculosis that target leucyl-tRNA synthetase. Antimicrob Agents Chemother 2016;60(10):6271–80.

105. Shoen C, DeStefano M, Hafkin B, et al. In vitro and in vivo activities of contezolid (MRX-I) against *Mycobacterium tuberculosis*. Antimicrob Agents Chemother 2018;62(8):1–11.

106. Lupien A, Vocat A, Foo CS-Y, et al. Optimized background regimen for treatment of active tuberculosis with the next-generation benzothiazinone macozinone (PBTZ169). Antimicrob Agents Chemother 2018;62(11):1–10.

107. Zhang D, Liu Y, Zhang C, et al. Synthesis and biological evaluation of novel 2-methoxypyridylamino-substituted riminophenazine derivatives as antituberculosis agents. Molecules 2014;19(4):4380–94.

108. Chatterji M, Shandil R, Manjunatha MR, et al. 1,4-azaindole, A potential drug candidate for treatment of tuberculosis. Antimicrob Agents Chemother 2014;58(9):5325–31.

109. Kang S, Kim RY, Seo MJ, et al. Lead optimization of a novel series of imidazo[1,2-a]pyridine amides leading to a clinical candidate (Q203) as a multi-

and extensively-drug- resistant anti-tuberculosis agent. J Med Chem 2014;57(12):5293–305.

110. Williams KN, Brickner SJ, Stover CK, et al. Addition of PNU-100480 to first-line drugs shortens the time needed to cure murine tuberculosis. Am J Respir Crit Care Med 2009;180(4):371–6.

111. Wallis RS, Jakubiec W, Kumar V, et al. Biomarker-assisted dose selection for safety and efficacy in early development of PNU-100480 for tuberculosis. Antimicrob Agents Chemother 2011;55(2): 567–74.

112. Wallis RS, Dawson R, Friedrich SO, et al. Mycobactericidal activity of sutezolid (PNU-100480) in sputum (EBA) and blood (WBA) of patients with pulmonary tuberculosis. PLoS One 2014;9(4). https://doi.org/10.1371/journal.pone.0094462.

113. Jeong JW, Jung SJ, Lee HH, et al. In vitro and in vivo activities of LCB01-0371, a new oxazolidinone. Antimicrob Agents Chemother 2010;54(12): 5359–62.

114. Choi Y, Lee SW, Kim A, et al. Safety, tolerability and pharmacokinetics of 21 day multiple oral administration of a new oxazolidinone antibiotic, LCB01-0371, in healthy male subjects. J Antimicrob Chemother 2018;73(1):183–90.

115. Tahlan K, Wilson R, Kastrinsky DB, et al. SQ109 targets MmpL3, a membrane transporter of trehalose monomycolate involved in mycolic acid donation to the cell wall core of Mycobacterium tuberculosis. Antimicrob Agents Chemother 2012;56(4): 1797–809.

116. Heinrich N, Dawson R, Bois J, et al. Early phase evaluation of SQ109 alone and in combination with rifampicin in pulmonary TB patients. J Antimicrob Chemother 2014;70(5):1558–66.

117. Boeree MJ, Heinrich N, Aarnoutse R, et al. High-dose rifampicin, moxifloxacin, and SQ109 for treating tuberculosis: a multi-arm, multi-stage randomised controlled trial. Lancet Infect Dis 2017; 17(1):39–49.

Diagnostic Tests for Latent Tuberculosis Infection

Michelle K. Haas, MD[a,b], Robert W. Belknap, MD[a,b],*

KEYWORDS

- Latent tuberculosis infection • LTBI • Tuberculin skin test • TST • Interferon-gamma release assay
- QuantiFERON • T-SPOT.TB

KEY POINTS

- Diagnostic tests for latent tuberculosis infection (LTBI) measure the host immune response and cannot differentiate a resolved infection from LTBI or active disease.
- The interferon-gamma release assays are more accurate in bacille Calmette-Guérin–vaccinated people, require a single visit, and results are easily retrieved electronically.
- The tuberculin skin test has logistical advantages under certain conditions, such as testing large groups in a field setting.
- Newer tests should focus on better predicting future risk for active tuberculosis.

INTRODUCTION
Brief Epidemiology

Tuberculosis (TB) is the leading cause of death from an infection globally, with an estimated 1.7 million TB-related deaths in 2016 and 10.4 million people with active TB.[1] In the United States there were 9093 individuals with active TB in 2017, a decrease from 2016 of only 1.8%.[2,3] An estimated 86% of individuals diagnosed with active TB in the United States each year have reactivation of latent TB infection (LTBI).[4] Globally, an estimated 1.7 billion people have LTBI,[5] including up to 13 million in the United States.[6,7] Ensuring individuals with LTBI have access to preventive treatment is important for decreasing the global TB burden and advancing toward TB elimination, particularly in low-TB-burden settings.[8–10]

Pathophysiology and Definition of Latent Tuberculosis Infection

Tuberculosis infection occurs primarily by inhaling droplet nuclei that contain viable *Mycobacterium tuberculosis* (Mtb). When these droplets reach the alveoli, the Mtb organisms begin to replicate and are transported via the pulmonary lymphatics to the mediastinal lymph nodes and eventually into the general circulation, where they spread throughout the body. In most individuals, eradication or containment is accomplished by the host immune response, with containment of the organism being associated with granuloma formation.

LTBI is defined by having a positive test for infection and no symptoms or radiographic/pathologic/microbiologic findings of active TB. This definition includes people with symptoms or radiographic abnormalities in whom active disease has been excluded using mycobacterial cultures. People living with human immunodeficiency virus (HIV) sometimes present with smear-negative, culture-positive active pulmonary TB despite a lack of symptoms and a normal chest radiograph.[11] TB and LTBI are now understood to encompass a spectrum rather than a dichotomy of different stages of infection. LTBI includes resolved infection with elimination of Mtb organisms, controlled

Disclosure: The authors have nothing to disclose.
[a] Denver Metro Tuberculosis Program, Denver Public Health, 605 Bannock Street, Denver, CO 80204, USA;
[b] Division of Infectious Diseases, Department of Medicine, University of Colorado-Denver Anschutz Medical Campus, 13001 E 17th Pl, Aurora, CO 80045, USA
* Corresponding author. Denver Metro Tuberculosis Program, Denver Public Health, 605 Bannock Street, Denver, CO 80204.
E-mail address: robert.belknap@dhha.org

Clin Chest Med 40 (2019) 829–837
https://doi.org/10.1016/j.ccm.2019.07.007
0272-5231/19/© 2019 Elsevier Inc. All rights reserved.

infection with nonreplicating but viable Mtb, and actively replicating Mtb organisms that manifest as subclinical active disease.[12]

Current tests for LTBI are unable to differentiate between different stages of infection. Importantly, none of them are sufficiently sensitive to definitively exclude active TB based on a negative result. They should never be used as the initial or definitive test for making decisions in someone who has suspected TB disease. Better understanding of the differences in the pathophysiology and immunology across the spectrum is necessary to develop better tools for identifying who to treat.

History of Diagnostic Tests for Identifying Latent Tuberculosis

Robert Koch was the first to identify the *M tuberculosis* bacillus as the cause of TB in 1882. Soon after this discovery, the first test developed to diagnose TB infection that was based on his findings was the tuberculin skin test (TST). This test was originally described by Clemens Von Pirquet[13] in 1909, in which he inoculated children with tuberculin by placing drops on the skin and then creating a superficial abrasion. He observed reactions that increased in prevalence in older children, reaching 70% by the age of 10 years. He noted that tuberculin reactions correlated with active disease but also derived that reactions occurred in individuals with latent infection.[14] This technique was eventually refined by Charles Mantoux as an intradermal injection.[15] The initial formulations of

tuberculin were prepared by incubating cultures of *M tuberculosis* at high temperatures for several hours then dissolving them in a glycerin-based solution. Florence Seibert later refined this process, leading to the modern version of purified protein derivative (PPD) that is in use today.

TST remained the only test for nearly 100 years until the interferon-gamma (IFN-γ) release assays (IGRAs) were developed. The 2 commercially available IGRAs are T-SPOT.TB (Oxford Immunotec, Abingdon, United Kingdom) and QuantiFERON (Qiagen, Hilden, Germany). Both the TST and the IGRAs are based on the immune response to TB and, as such, are indirect tests for TB infection, which presents challenges when identifying individuals at highest risk for progression to active TB who would benefit most from LTBI treatment. To minimize the risk and maximize the benefit of LTBI treatment, testing should be focused on people who have a risk for TB infection, risk of progression if infected, or both. A useful tool for estimating a person's lifetime risk for TB infection and progression is available online at www.tstin3d.com.[16]

TUBERCULIN SKIN TEST
Performing a Tuberculin Skin Test

The TST is an in vivo test that uses PPD to evaluate for TB infection. The Mantoux method of performing the test involves injecting PPD intradermally on the forearm and examining the area 48 to 72 hours later (**Fig. 1**). Individuals who have been

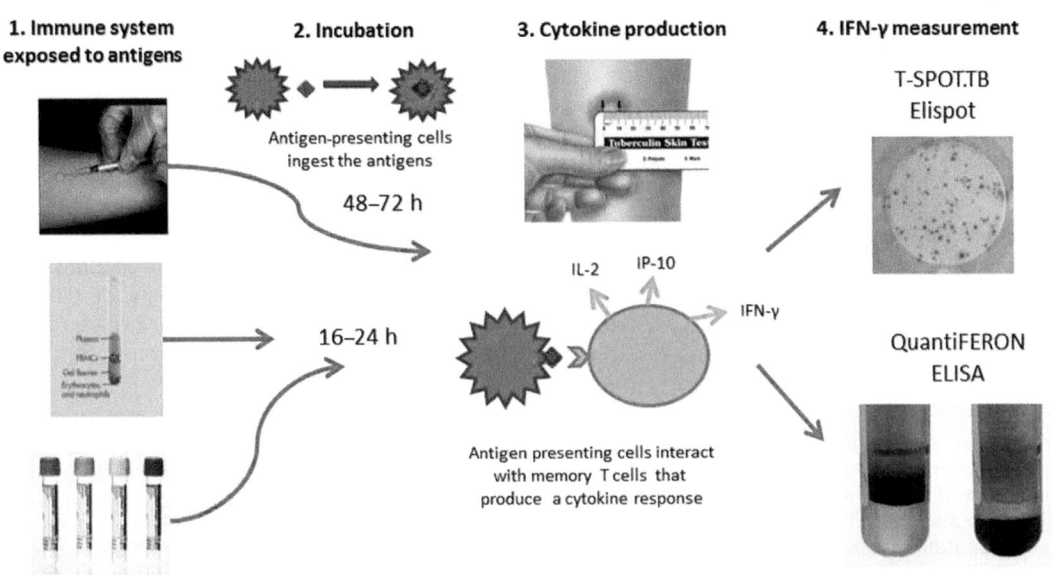

Fig. 1. Basic immunology of LTBI diagnostic tests. ELISA, enzyme-linked immunosorbent assay; IL-2, interleukin-2; IP-10, IFN-γ–induced protein 10.

sensitized to the antigens in PPD develop a delayed-type hypersensitivity reaction. Several cytokines, including IFN-γ, are released from T cells, causing induration and erythema at the injection site. The TST is read by measuring the induration in millimeters (and not erythema) perpendicular to the forearm.

Interpreting whether induration indicates TB infection requires knowledge of the individual's risk for TB exposure and risk of progression to active disease if infected. In the United States, cutoffs of 5, 10, or 15 mm are considered positive for infection depending on the patient's underlying risk factors and comorbid conditions.[17] The range of cutoffs reflect the imprecision of the test and attempts to balance the risks of underdiagnosing LTBI in patients at high risk for TB infection and progression to active TB disease and overdiagnosis in patients who are low risk for both acquisition of infection and progression to active TB.

Tuberculin Skin Test Advantages

For decades, the TST was the only available test to diagnose LTBI despite several well-documented limitations. The IGRAs have become the preferred test in many higher-risk populations but have not supplanted the TST entirely. The TST continues to be used because the material costs are low and its performance is comparable with IGRAs in people not vaccinated with bacille Calmette-Guérin (BCG). A logistical advantage of the TST is the ease of quickly testing a large number of people when follow-up 2 to 3 days after test placement can be ensured. **Table 1** summarizes the advantages and disadvantages of the TST compared with the IGRAs.

Tuberculin Skin Test Challenges

A major limitation is false-positive results in people who received BCG vaccine.[18] The antigens in PPD are contained in BCG and in many nontuberculous mycobacteria (NTM). BCG is used worldwide, particularly in countries where TB is endemic, to reduce TB morbidity and mortality in infants and young children. The vaccine is usually given shortly after birth, either as a 1-time dose or as a series during childhood, the latter of which may be associated with higher rates of false-positive results. The BCG vaccination schedule varies by country, and can be found at www.bcgatlas.com. The likelihood of a false-positive TST caused by BCG vaccination wanes with time but seems to persist in some individuals. As a result, the TST is less accurate for diagnosing LTBI in populations that are often at the highest risk for infection.

Because the TST relies on the host immune response, false-negative results can occur in patients who are most susceptible to TB infection. Among people living with HIV, false-negative tests are more common in patients with very low CD4 lymphocyte counts.[19,20] Similarly, TST may have reduced sensitivity for detecting LTBI in individuals

---

Table 1
Comparison of tuberculin skin test and interferon-gamma release assays

	TST	IGRA
Advantages	• Low cost for reagents • Easy to perform in field settings • Ability to test a large number of people quickly • Minimal test-retest variability in low-risk populations	• Single visit • Positive and negative controls built into the test • Objective results • Electronic laboratory reporting • More specific in BCG-vaccinated people
Disadvantages	• Requires 2 visits • Subjective results with inter-reader and intrareader variability • Low specificity in BCG-vaccinated people	• Higher cost for reagents • Requires transporting samples to a laboratory • More difficult in field settings (laboratory registration, drawing blood, labeling and transporting tubes to a laboratory)

Shared Challenges
• Limited sensitivity for active disease and inability to distinguish active TB from LTBI
• Low ability to predict short-term progression to active TB
• Reduced sensitivity in immunosuppressed populations
• Inability to differentiate a resolved infection from a new or ongoing infection

receiving tumor necrosis factor (TNF)-alpha inhibitors, corticosteroids, and other immunosuppressive regimens.[21–23] Testing for LTBI before immunosuppression should be done whenever possible, including solid organ transplant candidates in whom the risk of false-negative tests after transplant is high.[24] False-negative TSTs are also a concern in infants and young children, who are at higher risk for severe disease if infection is missed.[25]

False-negative TSTs can also occur in otherwise healthy people because of waning immunity from a remote TB infection. In this clinical scenario, an initial negative TST primes the immune system so that a subsequent test is positive. This response is called boosting and unless recognized can be misidentified as a new infection. Concern for boosting resulted in the 2-step TST approach for screening people who are required to get serial testing, such as health care workers.[26]

Other limitations with the TST include the need for a second in-person visit 2 to 3 days after the test is placed. This requirement can be a major barrier for patients and limits the days when the test can be done. Because reading a TST is subjective, variability in measurements is common between different readers.[27] Digit preference is also common, showing a natural tendency for people reading tests to round off results to the nearest cutoff.[28] This subjectivity in reading the test reduces the reproducibility and overall performance of the TST.

INTERFERON-GAMMA RELEASE ASSAYS

The IGRAs are in vitro tests for diagnosing LTBI that were developed to overcome many of the limitations associated with the TST.[29] T-SPOT.TB and QFT have many similarities, including:

- Using early secretory antigen target-6 (ESAT-6) and culture filtrate protein-10 (CFP-10) as TB-specific antigens to elicit a T-cell response
- Measuring IFN-γ produced by lymphocytes after incubation (see **Fig. 1**)
- Having negative and positive controls for internal test validation

ESAT-6 and CFP-10 were chosen because they are absent from BCG vaccine strains and most common NTM. False-positive results can occur from infection with *Mycobacterium leprae*, *Mycobacterium kansasii*, *Mycobacterium marinum*, *Mycobacterium szulgai*, and *Mycobacterium flavescens*.[30,31] The negative control (or nil) measures the amount of IFN-γ after incubation without antigens, whereas the positive control (or mitogen) uses phytohemagglutinin as a nonspecific stimulant. The controls are used to determine whether the test is interpretable. For example, if the IFN-γ level is too high in the nil control or too low in the positive control, then the result is not interpretable. These results are reported as indeterminate and do not give any information about the individual's risk for TB. Indeterminate test results occur for many reasons, some related to the individual being tested and others related to the variability that can occur before and after blood is drawn.[32,33] With quality control and standardized processes, the indeterminate rates can be minimized and should be less than 2% in most settings.

There is no gold standard test for diagnosing LTBI so the IGRAs were validated using surrogate markers for risk of infection. The sensitivities have been estimated from the positivity rates in people with culture-proven active TB, whereas specificity has been determined primarily from results in BCG-vaccinated populations at low risk for TB exposure. Most studies have used TST as the comparator, although some have compared the IGRAs with each other or newer-generation tests with the prior generation. Overall, T-SPOT.TB and QFT have shown a high concordance in populations with different TB risks. The main difference between them is the laboratory technique used to elicit an immune response. As such, the clinical decision about which test to use depends mainly on the cost and availability.

T-SPOT.TB

T-SPOT.TB uses an ELISpot (enzyme-linked immune absorbent spot) platform for diagnosing TB infection. The test involves collecting whole blood then isolating the peripheral blood mononuclear cells (PBMCs). After isolation, the PBMCs are washed, counted, and then added to microtiter wells containing antibodies to IFN-γ. ESAT-6, CFP-10, and phytohemagglutinin are added to separate wells and a fourth is used as the nil control. The plates are then incubated at 37°C for 16 to 20 hours. After incubation, the wells are washed, a second conjugated antibody is added, and the wells are incubated for another hour. The wells are washed again and a substrate is added that produces a visible spot where a T cell produced IFN-γ (see **Fig. 1**).

The number of spots in the TB antigen wells minus the spots counted in the nil well gives the quantitative result. If either the ESAT-6 or CFP-10 well minus nil are more than the cut point then the qualitative result is positive. T-SPOT.TB was developed in the United Kingdom and licensed in Europe using a cutoff of greater than or equal to 6 spots. In the United States, T-SPOT.TB includes a borderline zone so greater than or equal to 8 spots is positive, 5 to 7 is borderline, and less than or equal to 4 is negative. Often borderline tests are repeated because a second test produces a positive or negative result. In practice, the decision about what to do with an unexpected positive or borderline result often depends on the epidemiologic risk of the person being tested. Approaches include repeating the T-SPOT.TB, doing an alternative test (QFT or TST), using the international cut point, treating a borderline result as negative in people at low risk, or recommending LTBI treatment in those at high risk for infection and progression to active TB.

QuantiFERON

QFT is a whole-blood assay that uses an enzyme-linked immunosorbent assay (ELISA) to measure IFN-γ. The original test used PPD as the antigen but subsequent versions have used TB-specific antigens. The third-generation test, QFT Gold In-Tube (QFT-GIT), was the first to use specialized vacuum tubes with the peptides coated on the inside for the TB antigen and mitogen tubes. Blood can be drawn directly into the tubes or drawn into a lithium heparin tube and transferred later to the specialized tubes. The tubes must be gently shaken or inverted to combine the blood with the antigens on the inner surface. The tubes are then incubated at 37°C for 16 to 24 hours.

The QFT Gold Plus (QFT-Plus) is the fourth and most recent generation of the test. The main difference between QFT-Plus and QFT-GIT is the addition of a second TB antigen tube. The TB1 tube is similar to QFT-GIT and contains ESAT-6 and CFP-10 peptides that elicit a CD4 cell response. The TB2 tube contains shorter peptides that stimulate both CD4 and CD8 cells in people with TB infection. After incubation, the tubes are centrifuged and the IFN-γ levels in plasma are measured using an ELISA and reported as international units per milliliter (IU/mL). The quantitative results are calculated by subtracting the nil from TB1 and TB2. If the quantitative result from either tube is greater than or equal to 0.35 IU/mL then the qualitative result is reported as positive. The addition of the CD8 tube was intended to increase the test sensitivity. Comparisons of QFT-GIT and QFT-Plus in different populations show a high degree of correlation between the 2 tests but no definitive advantage of the QFT-Plus.[34–37]

Interferon-Gamma Release Assay Advantages

Because the IGRAs use ESAT-6 and CFP-10, they are more specific in individuals who have received BCG vaccination.[32] In an early meta-analysis, the IGRAs were as sensitive as or better than TST for diagnosing LTBI, with a much higher specificity. The pooled specificity for IGRA testing in BCG-vaccinated individuals was 96% compared with 59% for TST.[38] Thus IGRAs are preferred for use among individuals with prior BCG vaccination. The IGRAs also require a single blood draw, making them easy to perform in many clinical settings. As laboratory-based tests, the results are determined objectively and are easier to report and track compared with TST.

Interferon-Gamma Release Assay Challenges

Similar to the TST, IGRAs have decreased sensitivity in patients who are immunocompromised. In meta-analyses that rigorously evaluated the use of IGRAs in people with HIV, the sensitivities for T-SPOT.TB and QFT-GIT were lower than in HIV-negative patients.[39,40] Individuals receiving treatment with immunomodulating agents such as TNF-alpha antagonists also have higher false-negative[41,42] and indeterminate results.[43]

Both T-SPOT.TB and QuantiFERON have an inherent variability that is apparent when the tests are performed in people at low risk for infection and when multiple tests are done at the same time.[44–46] This variability manifests as false-positive and discordant positive-negative results, particularly in people whose quantitative results are close to the cut point. Recognition of this variability led the US Food and Drug Administration to require a borderline zone for T-SPOT.TB. Some experts have also suggested that QFT should include a borderline zone or risk-based cutoffs.[45] Because QFT-Plus has 2 antigen tubes, some investigators have suggested that both antigen tube results should be greater than the cutoff to be considered positive in low-risk individuals.[47] The 2017 US TB diagnostic guidelines recommend performing a confirmatory test for anyone with a positive result who is unlikely to be infected.[25]

Additional challenges using IGRAs compared with TST are the material costs of the tests and logistical challenges associated with laboratory-based tests. IGRAs require electronically registering patients, specimen collection, labeling, handling, and access to a laboratory that is capable of performing the test. Anecdotally, dizziness and vasovagal syncope are also more common with blood draws than with TST.

SPECIAL POPULATIONS

The IGRAs have been evaluated extensively in people living with HIV.[39,40] One meta-analysis found a pooled sensitivity for T.SPOT.TB of 72% compared with 60% for QFT-GIT in low-income countries compared with 94% and 67% respectively in high-income countries, although there was significant heterogeneity.[39] Most of the decreased sensitivity seems to be in patients with lower CD4 counts, particularly less than 100 cells/μL. Limited data are available that evaluate QFT-Plus in HIV-positive and HIV-negative individuals. A study of Zambian adults with active TB found no difference in QFT-Plus sensitivity by HIV status (85% in HIV positive and 80% in HIV negative).[48] A study of pregnant women in Ethiopia found 33% tested positive by QFT-Plus regardless of HIV-infection status.[49] Although IGRA performance may be reduced in people living with HIV, it seems to be more sensitive and specific compared with TST. Current guidelines recommend using an IGRA when available in people living with HIV without preferentially recommending one test rather than another.[50]

Both the TST and IGRAs have reduced sensitivity in HIV-negative patients who are immunocompromised. This finding has led some experts to recommend doing multiple tests, usually a TST and IGRA, to increase the sensitivity before offering anti-TNF therapy.[41,42] The risks and benefits of this approach have never been formally evaluated. Testing individuals before immunosuppression is recommended when feasible.[24]

Children are an important group for diagnosing and treating LTBI but one in which data on new tests often lag. Early studies showed that IGRAs have similar sensitivity compared with TST in children greater than or equal to 5 years old.[51] Concerns in children less than 5 years of age included the technical challenges of drawing blood in young children and higher rates of indeterminate results. Data in this group were slow to accumulate but recently the American Academy of Pediatrics issued updated recommendations supporting the use of IGRAs in children as young as 2 years of age.[52] However, very few data exist regarding the sensitivity and specificity of IGRAs in children less than 2 years of age. One study of IGRAs in infants showed correlation with TB infection risk factors in a high-burden setting.[53] In low-burden settings, growing clinical evidence of IGRAs in children less than 2 years of age shows a low proportion of indeterminate results, but additional data are needed.[54]

PREDICTING PROGRESSION TO ACTIVE TUBERCULOSIS

The primary rationale for diagnosing LTBI is to be able to offer treatment that will prevent future disease. The TST and IGRAs have high negative predictive values and therefore are effective at identifying individuals who are at low risk for developing active TB, including people living with HIV who are not severely immunocompromised. A meta-analysis of isoniazid preventive therapy trials found that people living with HIV who were TST positive benefitted from therapy compared with TST-negative individuals.[55]

However, the positive predictive value for TST and IGRAs is only modest and probably best in patients with recent infection.[56–58] Among children and adolescents evaluated from a setting with higher TB burden, IGRA conversion was associated with an 8-fold increased risk of progressing to active TB.[59] In a review of 28 studies, the pooled positive predictive value for IGRAs was slightly better than for TST at 2.7% versus 1.5% for TST, which was statistically significant.[56] Another meta-analysis of 15 studies totaling 26,680 patients found similar results for the risk of TB after a median of 4 years among those with a positive test result compared with a negative.[57] A large prospective study in the United Kingdom compared TST, QFT-GIT, and T-SPOT.TB in close contacts and migrants from high-TB-burden countries.[58] Among 9610 participants followed for a median of 2.9 years, 97 (1%) developed active TB. The annual TB incidence was very low in people who were negative, regardless of the test. The annual incidence was similar in participants who were positive by T-SPOT.TB, QFT-GIT, or TST using a 15-mm cutoff.

MONITORING RESPONSE TO THERAPY

One major challenge with managing LTBI is determining when infection has been eradicated or when a new infection has occurred. TSTs were never routinely repeated after a documented positive because of concerns for severe reactions. Studies using IGRAs have found inconsistent treatment responses, defined as reversion from positive to negative.[60,61] Therefore, it is currently not recommended to check an IGRA after treatment of latent TB.

FUTURE DIAGNOSTIC TESTS

C-Tb (Statens Serum Institute, Copenhagen, Denmark) is a newer-generation skin test that uses ESAT-6 and CFP-10 instead of PPD. The test is meant to combine the operational advantages of the TST with the performance characteristics of an IGRA. A phase 3, double-blind, randomized trial compared C-Tb, PPD-based TST, and QFT-GIT in people with no TB risk, occasional contact, close contact, and active TB.[62] Using a 5-mm cutoff, C-Tb positivity correlated with exposure risk, performed better than TST in BCG-vaccinated people, and had a high concordance with QFT-GIT.[62] A recent trial in South Africa that included children less than 5 years of age and people living with HIV found that C-Tb was safe and the positivity rate was similar to TST and QFT-GIT.[63] Whether C-Tb will become commercially available and prove cost-effective is unknown.

Recent studies have identified potential biomarkers that can better predict risk of TB progression.[64–66] These studies analyzed whole-blood RNA sequencing data from large cohorts to identify gene expression combinations that correlate with risk for developing TB. Some combinations of gene signatures show a good correlation with risk for progression to active TB in 6 to 12 months. Further validation studies and the development of a point-of-care platform are needed before these could be used in clinical practice.

SUMMARY

TB is the leading cause of death from an infectious disease globally and is often preventable.[1] Despite their limitations, the TST and IGRAs remain valuable tools for diagnosing LTBI and identifying people most likely to benefit from treatment. They are not sensitive or specific enough in all populations to be used indiscriminately. LTBI testing should target those with clinical or epidemiologic risk for TB. Newer tests may become available but, until then, clinicians need to maximize the use of the current tools, which will continue to require clinical judgment when deciding who to test and whether to recommend treatment.

REFERENCES

1. World Health Organization. Global tuberculosis report 2017. Geneva (Switzerland): World Health Organization; 2017.
2. Salinas JL, Mindra G, Haddad MB, et al. Leveling of tuberculosis incidence - United States, 2013-2015. MMWR Morb Mortality Wkly Rep 2016;65(11):273–8.
3. Stewart RJ, Tsang CA, Pratt RH, et al. Tuberculosis - United States, 2017. MMWR Morb Mortality Wkly Rep 2018;67(11):317–23.
4. Yuen CM, Kammerer JS, Marks K, et al. Recent transmission of tuberculosis - United States, 2011-2014. PLoS One 2016;11(4):e0153728.
5. Houben RM, Dodd PJ. The global burden of latent tuberculosis infection: a re-estimation using mathematical modelling. PLoS Med 2016;13(10): e1002152.
6. Mancuso JD, Diffenderfer JM, Ghassemieh BJ, et al. The prevalence of latent tuberculosis infection in the United States. Am J Respir Crit Care Med 2016; 194(4):501–9.
7. Miramontes R, Hill AN, Yelk Woodruff RS, et al. Tuberculosis infection in the United States: prevalence estimates from the national health and nutrition examination survey, 2011-2012. PLoS One 2015; 10(11):e0140881.
8. Dye C, Glaziou P, Floyd K, et al. Prospects for tuberculosis elimination. Annu Rev Public Health 2013;34: 271–86.
9. Uplekar M, Weil D, Lonnroth K, et al. WHO's new end TB strategy. Lancet 2015;385(9979):1799–801.
10. LoBue PA, Mermin JH. Latent tuberculosis infection: the final frontier of tuberculosis elimination in the USA. Lancet Infect Dis 2017;17(10):e327–33.
11. Kranzer K, Houben RM, Glynn JR, et al. Yield of HIV-associated tuberculosis during intensified case finding in resource-limited settings: a systematic review and meta-analysis. Lancet Infect Dis 2010; 10(2):93–102.
12. Barry CE 3rd, Boshoff HI, Dartois V, et al. The spectrum of latent tuberculosis: rethinking the biology and intervention strategies. Nat Rev Microbiol 2009;7(12):845–55.
13. Von Pirquet C. Frequency of tuberculosis in childhood. J Am Med Assoc 1909;LII(9):675–8.
14. Shulman ST. Clemens von Pirquet: a remarkable life and career. J Pediatric Infect Dis Soc 2017;6(4):376–9.
15. Lee E, Holzman RS. Evolution and current use of the tuberculin test. Clin Infect Dis 2002;34(3):365–70.
16. Menzies D, Gardiner G, Farhat M, et al. Thinking in three dimensions: a web-based algorithm to aid the interpretation of tuberculin skin test results. Int J Tuberc Lung Dis 2008;12(5):498–505.
17. American Thoracic Society and Centers for Disease Control and Prevention. Targeted testing and treatment of latent tuberculosis infection. Am J Respir Crit Care Med 2000;161:S221–47.
18. Farhat M, Greenaway C, Pai M, et al. False-positive tuberculin skin tests: what is the absolute effect of BCG and non-tuberculous mycobacteria? Int J Tuberc Lung Dis 2006;10(11):1192–204.
19. Huebner RE, Schein MF, Hall CA, et al. Delayed-type hypersensitivity anergy in human immunodeficiency virus-infected persons screened for infection with Mycobacterium tuberculosis. Clin Infect Dis 1994; 19(1):26–32.
20. Graham NM, Nelson KE, Solomon L, et al. Prevalence of tuberculin positivity and skin test anergy in HIV-1-seropositive and -seronegative intravenous drug users. JAMA 1992;267(3):369–73.

21. Bartalesi F, Vicidomini S, Goletti D, et al. Quanti-FERON-TB gold and the TST are both useful for latent tuberculosis infection screening in autoimmune diseases. Eur Respir J 2009;33(3):586–93.

22. Ponce de Leon D, Acevedo-Vasquez E, Alvizuri S, et al. Comparison of an interferon-gamma assay with tuberculin skin testing for detection of tuberculosis (TB) infection in patients with rheumatoid arthritis in a TB-endemic population. J Rheumatol 2008;35(5):776–81.

23. Gogus F, Gunendi Z, Karakus R, et al. Comparison of tuberculin skin test and QuantiFERON-TB gold in tube test in patients with chronic inflammatory diseases living in a tuberculosis endemic population. Clin Exp Med 2010;10(3):173–7.

24. Epstein DJ, Subramanian AK. Prevention and management of tuberculosis in solid organ transplant recipients. Infect Dis Clin North Am 2018;32(3):703–18.

25. Lewinsohn DM, Leonard MK, LoBue PA, et al. Official American Thoracic Society/infectious diseases Society of America/Centers for disease control and prevention clinical practice guidelines: diagnosis of tuberculosis in adults and children. Clin Infect Dis 2017;64(2):111–5.

26. Bass JA Jr, Serio RA. The use of repeat skin tests to eliminate the booster phenomenon in serial tuberculin testing. Am Rev Respir Dis 1981;123(4 Pt 1):394–6.

27. Menzies D. Interpretation of repeated tuberculin tests. Boosting, conversion, and reversion. Am J Respir Crit Care Med 1999;159(1):15–21.

28. Eilers PH, Borgdorff MW. Modeling and correction of digit preference in tuberculin surveys. Int J Tuberc Lung Dis 2004;8(2):232–9.

29. Pai M, Riley LW, Colford JM Jr. Interferon-gamma assays in the immunodiagnosis of tuberculosis: a systematic review. Lancet Infect Dis 2004;4(12):761–76.

30. Andersen P, Munk ME, Pollock JM, et al. Specific immune-based diagnosis of tuberculosis. Lancet 2000;356(9235):1099–104.

31. Geluk A, van Meijgaarden KE, Franken KL, et al. Identification and characterization of the ESAT-6 homologue of Mycobacterium leprae and T-cell cross-reactivity with Mycobacterium tuberculosis. Infect Immun 2002;70(5):2544–8.

32. Pai M, Denkinger CM, Kik SV, et al. Gamma interferon release assays for detection of mycobacterium tuberculosis infection. Clin Microbiol Rev 2014;27(1):3–20.

33. Banaei N, Gaur RL, Pai M. Interferon gamma release assays for latent tuberculosis: what are the sources of variability? J Clin Microbiol 2016;54(4):845–50.

34. Theel ES, Hilgart H, Breen-Lyles M, et al. Comparison of the QuantiFERON-TB gold plus and QuantiFERON-TB gold in-tube interferon gamma release assays in patients at risk for tuberculosis and in health care workers. J Clin Microbiol 2018;56(7) [pii:e00614-18].

35. Ryu MR, Park MS, Cho EH, et al. Comparative evaluation of QuantiFERON-TB gold in-tube and QuantiFERON-TB gold plus in diagnosis of latent tuberculosis infection in immunocompromised patients. J Clin Microbiol 2018;56(11) [pii: e00438-18].

36. Barcellini L, Borroni E, Brown J, et al. First evaluation of QuantiFERON-TB Gold Plus performance in contact screening. Eur Respir J 2016;48(5):1411–9.

37. Hogan CA, Tien S, Pai M, et al. Higher positivity rate with fourth-generation QuantiFERON-TB gold plus assay in low-risk U.S. health care workers. J Clin Microbiol 2019;57(1) [pii:e01688-18].

38. Pai M, Zwerling A, Menzies D. Systematic review: T-cell-based assays for the diagnosis of latent tuberculosis infection: an update. Ann Intern Med 2008;149(3):177–84.

39. Cattamanchi A, Smith R, Steingart KR, et al. Interferon-gamma release assays for the diagnosis of latent tuberculosis infection in HIV-infected individuals: a systematic review and meta-analysis. J Acquir Immune Defic Syndr 2011;56(3):230–8.

40. Santin M, Munoz L, Rigau D. Interferon-gamma release assays for the diagnosis of tuberculosis and tuberculosis infection in HIV-infected adults: a systematic review and meta-analysis. PLoS One 2012;7(3):e32482.

41. Smith R, Cattamanchi A, Steingart KR, et al. Interferon-gamma release assays for diagnosis of latent tuberculosis infection: evidence in immune-mediated inflammatory disorders. Curr Opin Rheumatol 2011;23(4):377–84.

42. Winthrop KL, Weinblatt ME, Daley CL. You can't always get what you want, but if you try sometimes (with two tests–TST and IGRA–for tuberculosis) you get what you need. Ann Rheum Dis 2012;71(11):1757–60.

43. Shahidi N, Fu YT, Qian H, et al. Performance of interferon-gamma release assays in patients with inflammatory bowel disease: a systematic review and meta-analysis. Inflamm Bowel Dis 2012;18(11):2034–42.

44. Dorman SE, Belknap R, Graviss EA, et al. Interferon-gamma release assays and tuberculin skin testing for diagnosis of latent tuberculosis infection in healthcare workers in the United States. Am J Respir Crit Care Med 2014;189(1):77–87.

45. Schablon A, Harling M, Diel R, et al. Serial testing with an interferon-gamma release assay in German healthcare workers. GMS Krankenhhyg Interdiszip 2010;5(2):1–8.

46. Stout JE, Belknap R, Wu YJ, et al. Paradox of serial interferon-gamma release assays: variability width more important than specificity size. Int J Tuberc Lung Dis 2018;22(5):518–23.

47. Moon HW, Gaur RL, Tien SS, et al. Evaluation of QuantiFERON-TB gold-plus in health care workers in a low-incidence setting. J Clin Microbiol 2017; 55(6):1650–7.

48. Telisinghe L, Amofa-Sekyi M, Maluzi K, et al. The sensitivity of the QuantiFERON((R))-TB Gold Plus assay in Zambian adults with active tuberculosis. Int J Tuberc Lung Dis 2017;21(6):690–6.

49. Konig Walles J, Tesfaye F, Jansson M, et al. Performance of QuantiFERON-TB Gold Plus for detection of latent tuberculosis infection in pregnant women living in a tuberculosis- and HIV-endemic setting. PLoS One 2018;13(4):e0193589.

50. Guidelines for the prevention and treatment of opportunistic infections in HIV-infected adults and adolescents 2017. 2019. Available at: https://www.aidsinfo.nih.gov/guidelines/html/4/adult-and-adolescent-opportunistic-infection/325/tb. Accessed February 3, 2019.

51. Mandalakas AM, Detjen AK, Hesseling AC, et al. Interferon-gamma release assays and childhood tuberculosis: systematic review and meta-analysis. Int J Tuberc Lung Dis 2011;15(8):1018–32.

52. Kimberlin DW. Red Book: report of the Committee on Infectious Diseases, 2018-2021, 31st Edition. Elk Grove Village (IL): American Academy of Pediatrics; 2018.

53. Andrews JR, Nemes E, Tameris M, et al. Serial QuantiFERON testing and tuberculosis disease risk among young children: an observational cohort study. Lancet Respir Med 2017;5(4):282–90.

54. Gaensbauer J, Gonzales B, Belknap R, et al. Interferon-gamma release assay-based screening for pediatric latent tuberculosis infection in an urban primary care network. J Pediatr 2018;200:202–9.

55. Ayele HT, Mourik MS, Debray TP, et al. Isoniazid prophylactic therapy for the prevention of tuberculosis in HIV infected adults: a systematic review and meta-analysis of randomized trials. PLoS One 2015;10(11):e0142290.

56. Diel R, Loddenkemper R, Nienhaus A. Predictive value of interferon-gamma release assays and tuberculin skin testing for progression from latent TB infection to disease state: a meta-analysis. Chest 2012;142(1):63–75.

57. Rangaka MX, Wilkinson KA, Glynn JR, et al. Predictive value of interferon-gamma release assays for incident active tuberculosis: a systematic review and meta-analysis. Lancet Infect Dis 2012;12(1):45–55.

58. Abubakar I, Drobniewski F, Southern J, et al. Prognostic value of interferon-gamma release assays and tuberculin skin test in predicting the development of active tuberculosis (UK PREDICT TB): a prospective cohort study. Lancet Infect Dis 2018; 18(10):1077–87.

59. Machingaidze S, Verver S, Mulenga H, et al. Predictive value of recent QuantiFERON conversion for tuberculosis disease in adolescents. Am J Respir Crit Care Med 2012;186(10):1051–6.

60. Chiappini E, Fossi F, Bonsignori F, et al. Utility of interferon-gamma release assay results to monitor anti-tubercular treatment in adults and children. Clin Ther 2012;34(5):1041–8.

61. Adetifa IM, Ota MO, Jeffries DJ, et al. Interferon-gamma ELISPOT as a biomarker of treatment efficacy in latent tuberculosis infection: a clinical trial. Am J Respir Crit Care Med 2013;187(4):439–45.

62. Ruhwald M, Aggerbeck H, Gallardo RV, et al. Safety and efficacy of the C-Tb skin test to diagnose Mycobacterium tuberculosis infection, compared with an interferon gamma release assay and the tuberculin skin test: a phase 3, double-blind, randomised, controlled trial. Lancet Respir Med 2017;5(4): 259–68.

63. Aggerbeck H, Ruhwald M, Hoff ST, et al. C-Tb skin test to diagnose Mycobacterium tuberculosis infection in children and HIV-infected adults: a phase 3 trial. PLoS One 2018;13(9):e0204554.

64. Zak DE, Penn-Nicholson A, Scriba TJ, et al. A blood RNA signature for tuberculosis disease risk: a prospective cohort study. Lancet 2016;387(10035): 2312–22.

65. Suliman S, Thompson E, Sutherland J, et al. Four-gene Pan-African blood signature predicts progression to tuberculosis. Am J Respir Crit Care Med 2018;197(9):1198–208.

66. Warsinske HC, Rao AM, Moreira FMF, et al. Assessment of validity of a blood-based 3-gene signature score for progression and diagnosis of tuberculosis, disease severity, and treatment response. JAMA Netw Open 2018;1(6):e183779.

Treatment of Latent Tuberculosis Infection—An Update

Moises A. Huaman, MD, MSc[a,b,c],*, Timothy R. Sterling, MD[c,d]

KEYWORDS

- Latent tuberculosis infection • Treatment • Tuberculosis • Prevention and control • Isoniazid
- Rifampin • Rifapentine • Review

KEY POINTS

- Treatment of latent tuberculosis infection is an important component of tuberculosis control and elimination.
- Treatment regimens for latent tuberculosis infection include once-weekly isoniazid plus rifapentine for 3 months, daily rifampin for 4 months, daily isoniazid plus rifampin for 3 months to 4 months, and daily isoniazid for 6 months to 9 months.
- Isoniazid monotherapy is efficacious in preventing tuberculosis, but the rifampin-containing and rifapentine-containing regimens are shorter and have similar efficacy, adequate safety, and higher treatment completion rates.

INTRODUCTION

Latent tuberculosis infection (LTBI) is defined by the presence of detectable immune responses to *Mycobacterium tuberculosis* antigens with no clinical evidence of active TB disease.[1] It has been estimated that one-quarter of the world population has LTBI; however, there are wide variations in the rates of LTBI across regions.[2] In high-income countries, the incidence of active TB disease has continued to decline over the recent decades,[3,4] but the prevalence of LTBI has remained stable. For example, in the United States, 4% to 5% of the population was estimated to have LTBI in 2011 to 2012,[5] similar to prevalence rates reported in 1999 to 2000.[6] This indicates a persistent reservoir of *M tuberculosis* infection even in countries where active disease is less frequent. Because a majority of new TB cases in these settings are a result of reactivation of remote LTBI rather than recent infection,[7–9] intensification of LTBI screening and treatment strategies is recognized as a crucial component of TB elimination in low TB prevalence settings.[3,10,11] Modeling studies also show the significant contribution of LTBI

Disclosure Statement: The authors have no potential conflicts to disclose.
Financial Support: This work was supported in part by the National Center for Advancing Translational Sciences (KL2 TR001426 to M.A. Huaman). The content is solely the responsibility of the authors and does not represent the official views of the National Institutes of Health or the institutions with which the authors are affiliated.
[a] Department of Internal Medicine, Division of Infectious Diseases, University of Cincinnati College of Medicine, University of Cincinnati, 200 Albert Sabin Way, Room 3112, Cincinnati, OH 45267, USA; [b] Hamilton County Public Health Tuberculosis Control Program, 184 McMillan Street, Cincinnati, OH 45219, USA; [c] Vanderbilt Tuberculosis Center, Vanderbilt University School of Medicine, 1161 21st Avenue South, A-2200 Medical Center North, Nashville, TN 37232, USA; [d] Department of Medicine, Division of Infectious Diseases, Vanderbilt University School of Medicine, Vanderbilt University, 1161 21st Avenue South, A-2209 MCN, Nashville, TN 37232, USA
* Corresponding author. Department of Internal Medicine, Division of Infectious Diseases, University of Cincinnati, 200 Albert Sabin Way, Room 3112, Cincinnati, OH 45267.
E-mail address: moises.huaman@uc.edu

chestmed.theclinics.com

treatment in controlling the TB epidemic in high burden settings.[4,12] Ongoing efforts to target LTBI are challenged by limitations of current diagnostic tests to identify LTBI and persons at highest risk for progression to TB disease, potential toxicities of available LTBI therapies, suboptimal treatment adherence rates, and limited resources of TB control programs.[13–15]

This article reviews current LTBI treatment regimens. The primary focus is on LTBI treatment in low TB prevalence settings, such as the United States and Canada. Sections of LTBI management in special populations (ie, HIV-positive individuals, transplant patients, pregnant women, children, and contacts of multidrug-resistant TB) and considerations for LTBI treatment in high TB prevalence settings are included.

INDICATIONS FOR LATENT TUBERCULOSIS INFECTION SCREENING AND TREATMENT

LTBI screening is indicated in populations with a high risk of progression to TB disease and populations with increased risk for LTBI (**Box 1**).[1,16,17] Persons at increased risk of progression to TB disease include household contacts of confirmed pulmonary TB cases (in particular, children <5 years of age), persons living with human immunodeficiency virus (HIV)/AIDS (PLWHA), patients initiating anti–tumor necrosis factor (TNF)-α therapy, candidates

> **Box 1**
> **Populations at risk of latent tuberculosis infection and tuberculosis disease**
>
> - Contact of pulmonary TB cases
> - Immigrants from high-burden TB areas
> - Persons with HIV infection
> - Transplant candidates
> - Patients receiving hemodialysis
> - Patients starting TNF-α inhibitors
> - Patients with silicosis
> - Homeless individuals
> - Correctional facilities
> - Health care workers
> - Injection drug users
>
> Other agencies include additional populations at risk, such as persons receiving immunosuppression other than anti-TNF treatment.[17,34] Recent LTBI test convertors are at highest risk of TB progression within the first 2 years after infection.
> *Data from* World Health Organization. Latent tuberculosis infection: updated and consolidated guidelines for programmatic management. Geneva, Switzerland. 2018.

for hematologic or solid organ transplant, patients receiving dialysis, and patients with silicosis.[1] In low TB prevalence settings, populations at increased risk for LTBI may include immigrants from countries with high TB prevalence, health care workers, persons who live in high-risk congregate settings such as homeless shelters or correctional facilities, and users of illicit drugs.[1,16,17] Recently, diabetes mellitus has been identified as a risk factor for LTBI and progression to TB disease[18,19]; however, routine LTBI screening in diabetic patients is not recommended by current World Health Organization guidelines.[1]

Screening tests for LTBI include the tuberculin skin test (TST) and interferon-gamma release assays (IGRAs).[20] Readers can refer to Michelle K. Haas and Robert W. Belknap's article, "Diagnostic Tests for Latent Tuberculosis Infection," in this issue for a discussion on LTBI diagnosis and testing modalities.

LATENT TUBERCULOSIS INFECTION TREATMENT REGIMENS

Four main antimicrobial regimens are currently available for LTBI treatment: isoniazid monotherapy, rifampin monotherapy, isoniazid plus rifampin in combination, and isoniazid plus rifapentine in combination (**Table 1**). Isoniazid monotherapy for 6 months to 12 months has been used for decades, and its efficacy in preventing progression to TB disease is approximately 90%.[21] Its overall effectiveness, however, has been hindered by low adherence and completion rates due to its prolonged duration and hepatotoxicity risk.[22,23] Shorter rifamycin-based regimens have similar efficacy and are increasingly used. These regimens are associated with improved completion rates as well as reduced risk of hepatotoxicity compared with isoniazid monotherapy.[24] Importantly, studies have not shown an increased risk of developing isoniazid-resistant or rifamycin-resistant TB disease after receiving LTBI treatment regimens that contain these drugs.[25,26]

Isoniazid Daily for 6 Months to 12 Months

Isoniazid inhibits the synthesis of mycolic acids, which are essential components of the mycobacterial cell wall.[27] Isoniazid monotherapy has been considered standard of care for LTBI treatment for several decades.[28,29] Multiple studies have demonstrated the TB preventive efficacy of this drug. Isoniazid is administered at a dose of 5 mg/kg/d (conventional adult dose, 300 mg daily).[30] A meta-analysis of randomized controlled trials showed that the odds ratios of TB disease in persons with LTBI treated with 6 months

Table 1
Latent tuberculosis infection treatment regimens

Regimen	Duration	Dose	Frequency	Total Doses
Isoniazid plus rifapentine	3 mo	Isoniazid, 900 mg (15 mg/kg) Rifapentine, 750 mg if 32–50 kg; 900 mg if >50 kg	Once weekly[a]	12
Rifampin	4 mo	600 mg (10 mg/kg)	Daily	120
Isoniazid plus rifampin	3–4 mo	Isoniazid, 300 mg (5 mg/kg) Rifampin, 600 mg (10 mg/kg)	Daily	90–120
Isoniazid	6–9 mo	300 mg (5 mg/kg) 900 mg (15 mg/kg)	Daily Twice-weekly[b]	180–270 52–76

[a] Isoniazid and rifapentine weekly can be given as SAT or DOT.[52]
[b] Isoniazid twice-weekly regimens must be provided by DOT.[34]

and greater than or equal to 12 months of isoniazid were 0.65 (95% credible interval, 0.50–0.83) and 0.50 (95% credible interval, 0.41–0.62), respectively, compared with placebo.[31] In a trial of 28,000 HIV-negative persons with fibrotic pulmonary lesions, 12 months of isoniazid achieved a 75% reduction on the incidence of TB disease compared with a 65% reduction in the group receiving 6 months of isoniazid.[32] A re-analysis of US Public Health Service trials data suggested, however, that the maximal benefit from isoniazid monotherapy was achieved by 9 months.[33] Therefore, the recommended duration of isoniazid monotherapy for LTBI has been 6 months to 9 months.[1,34] Isoniazid has been used as the main standard of care comparator regimen in recent clinical trials of LTBI. Pyridoxine should be administered concomitantly with isoniazid.

Side effects from isoniazid may include hepatitis (fatigue, decreased appetite, abdominal discomfort, nausea, and jaundice) and peripheral neuropathy (**Table 2**).[34] A survey of 13,838 persons who received isoniazid found a rate of probable and possible isoniazid-related hepatitis of 1.3%.[23] The risk of hepatitis increases with age and alcohol consumption. Preexisting liver conditions, such as chronic hepatitis C infection, also are associated with higher risk of hepatotoxicity; therefore, closer follow-up is advised in these patients.[34,35] Isoniazid may interact with some drugs, such as phenytoin, carbamazepine, valproate, acetaminophen, warfarin, and monoamine oxidase inhibitors.[36]

Rifampin Daily for 3 Months to 4 Months

Rifampin inhibits RNA synthesis by binding to the mycobacterial RNA polymerase.[37] Rifampin monotherapy for LTBI has been associated with similar efficacy and lower hepatotoxicity rates compared with isoniazid.[1,38,39] Rifampin is administered at a dose of 10 mg/kg/d (conventional adult dose, 600 mg daily) for 3 months to 4 months. In a recent multicenter trial, 6063 adults with LTBI were randomized to receive 4 months of daily rifampin or 9 months of daily isoniazid.[38] Participants

Table 2
Potential adverse events of drugs used for latent tuberculosis infection treatment

Drug	Potential Adverse Effects	Comments
Isoniazid	Elevation of aminotransferases Symptomatic hepatitis Peripheral neuropathy	Close follow-up and caution in patients with baseline liver disease

Rifamycins (includes rifampin, rifapentine, and rifabutin)	Cutaneous rash
	Hematologic abnormalities
	Flulike illness
	Elevation of aminotransferases
	Symptomatic hepatitis
	Orange discoloration of body
	  fluids
		Consider multiple potential drug-drug
		  interactions (ie, warfarin,
		  anticonvulsants, opioids, and
		  antiretrovirals)
		Isoniazid-rifapentine not recommended in
		  pregnant women or women expecting
		  to be pregnant during treatment
		Isoniazid-rifapentine not recommended
		  for children <2 y of age

were followed-up to 28 months for the development of active TB. The rates of confirmed and clinically diagnosed TB disease were similar between the study groups and thus rifampin was determined to be noninferior to isoniazid for TB prevention. Rifampin was associated with higher treatment completion rates than isoniazid (78.8% vs 63.2%). As shown in a prior smaller trial,[40] rifampin had a more favorable safety profile, including lower frequency of grade 3 to grade 4 hepatotoxicity events that required permanent drug discontinuation compared with isoniazid (0.3% vs 1.8%).[38]

Rifampin may cause gastrointestinal symptoms (ie, abdominal pain and nausea), dermatologic reactions, hypersensitivity reactions, hematological side effects, and hepatotoxicity. Urine and other body fluids may develop an orange discoloration, which can lead to staining of soft contact lenses and dentures.[34] Rifampin is a potent CYP3A inducer and may affect the metabolism of several drugs, including antiretrovirals, anticonvulsants, warfarin, azole antifungals, methadone, cyclosporine, and other immunosuppressants.[21,36] Therefore, checking for potential drug-drug interactions is advised when considering rifampin for LTBI.

Isoniazid and Rifampin Daily for 3 Months to 4 Months

A meta-analysis showed that the odds ratio of TB disease in persons with LTBI treated with daily isoniazid plus rifampin for 3 months to 4 months was 0.53 (95% credible interval, 0.36–0.78) compared with placebo.[31] Randomized trials have compared 3 months to 4 months of daily isoniazid plus rifampin to 6 months to 12 months of daily isoniazid monotherapy in HIV-positive and HIV-negative persons.[41–45] Overall, similar TB prevention efficacy rates and safety profiles have been reported for the isoniazid plus rifampin combination regimen compared with standard isoniazid monotherapy.[46]

Isoniazid and Rifapentine Once Weekly for 3 Months

Rifapentine is a rifamycin derivative with a longer half-life and increased potency compared with rifampin.[47,48] In the Tuberculosis Trials Consortium Study 26/AIDS Clinical Trials Group 5259 (PREVENT TB), 7731 high-risk individuals with positive TST (contacts of pulmonary TB cases, recent TST convertors, PLWHA, and presence of fibrosis on chest radiograph) were randomized to receive 3 months of directly observed isoniazid, 900 mg, and rifapentine, 900 mg, once weekly, or 9 months of isoniazid, 300 mg, daily monotherapy.[49] Participants were followed for 33 months. The isoniazid-rifapentine combination regimen was noninferior to isoniazid in preventing TB disease. The risk of hepatotoxicity was lower in the isoniazid-rifapentine combination group compared with isoniazid (0.4% vs 2.7%). Treatment completion rates were higher with the isoniazid-rifapentine combination than with isoniazid (82.1% vs 69%). Similar completion rates have been reported among patients receiving the 3-month isoniazid-rifapentine regimen for LTBI in US TB control programs after its implementation in routine practice.[50] Based on the PREVENT TB trial design, the isoniazid-rifapentine regimen initially was administered only by directly observed therapy (DOT). A recent study, however, compared the isoniazid-rifapentine regimen given by DOT versus self-administered therapy (SAT).[51] Among US sites, once-weekly isoniazid-rifapentine given as SAT achieved similar treatment completion rates and safety outcomes as DOT; therefore, this regimen is now recommended as SAT by Centers for Disease Control and Prevention (CDC) guidelines.[52] Rifapentine is a potent CYP3A inducer (approximately 85% as potent as rifampin). Rifapentine and rifampin share similar drug-drug interaction and toxicity profiles.[53]

INITIAL ASSESSMENT

Patients found to have LTBI should be evaluated by health care provider teams with experience in managing LTBI to rule out active TB and discuss implications of the diagnosis, risk of TB reactivation, and available treatment options. A detailed history of TB risk factors, presence of comorbidities, and current medications should be obtained. Electronic decision support tools that provide personalized estimates of annual and cumulative risks of progression to TB disease, such as the Online TST/IGRA Interpreter (www.tstin3d.com), are available to assist patients and providers.[54,55] HIV testing is advised in all patients with LTBI. Baseline liver function tests should be considered in patients with baseline liver disease and/or risk factors for hepatotoxicity. Women of childbearing potential should be screened for pregnancy. Patients in whom rifamycin-containing regimens are considered should have their current list of medications analyzed for potential drug-drug interactions. Providers should discuss potential side effects of LTBI therapy and inform patients of signs and symptoms that require medical attention. Resources for educating patients on LTBI and available therapies can be found at the CDC Web site (www.cdc.gov/tb/topic/treatment/ltbi.htm).

For the 3-month isoniazid plus rifapentine regimen, the decision on SAT versus DOT should be based on patient age, medical history, social circumstances, risk factors for TB disease progression, and program resources.[52]

LATENT TUBERCULOSIS INFECTION TREATMENT MONITORING

Patients who initiate LTBI treatment should be routinely monitored for medication adherence and tolerability. The CDC recommends monthly visits to assess medication adherence and signs or symptoms of drug toxicity.[34] No laboratory tests are routinely ordered at follow-up visits, unless there is a clinical indication and/or concern for drug toxicity. In patients with abnormal baseline liver enzymes and/or at risk for hepatotoxicity, periodic laboratory monitoring is recommended.[34] LTBI drugs should be held if a patient is symptomatic and transaminase levels exceed 3 times the upper limit of normal or if asymptomatic and transaminase levels are greater than or equal to 5 times the upper limit of normal. Patients who develop signs or symptoms of active TB disease should be screened with a chest radiograph even if they are receiving LTBI treatment.

SPECIAL POPULATIONS
Persons Living with Human Immunodeficiency Virus/AIDS

HIV/AIDS carries a significant risk of progression to TB disease. It is estimated that in the absence of antiretroviral therapy (ART) as many as 10% of PLWHA with LTBI coinfection may develop TB disease each year.[56,57] The risk of progression to active TB among PLWHA on ART and optimal virologic response remains higher than the general population.[58] ART and treatment of LTBI both decrease the risk of TB among PLWHA[59–62]; thus, both are indicated.[63] Isoniazid monotherapy has been the preferred LTBI treatment regimen for PLWHA given its proved efficacy.[34,63] A meta-analysis showed that isoniazid decreased the incidence of TB disease in 64% among PLWHA with a positive TST.[64] The 3-month once-weekly isoniazid plus rifapentine regimen is noninferior to isoniazid monotherapy in PLWHA who have not yet started ART[65] and can be used in PLWHA taking compatible ART, such as efavirenz-containing or raltegravir-containing regimens.[66,67] Additional investigation is needed to determine the safety of once-weekly isoniazid plus rifapentine in PLWHA receiving dolutegravir-containing ART, because a severe flulike syndrome occurred in 2 of 4 healthy volunteers.[68] A recent trial (AIDS Clinical Trials Group 5279) showed that an ultrashort course of 1 month of daily isoniazid, 300 mg, and rifapentine, 300 mg to 600 mg, was noninferior to 9 months of isoniazid for TB prevention in PLWHA (most of the study participants were living in high TB burden settings and were TST-negative).[69] The 1-month daily isoniazid-rifapentine regimen had fewer adverse events and higher treatment completion rates than 9 months of isoniazid.

In PLWHA in settings with high TB prevalence, 36 months of isoniazid has been associated with a greater reduction in the risk of incident TB disease than 6 months of isoniazid[70]; however, the potential toxicities and adherence difficulties of such prolonged TB preventive therapy have made its implementation challenging.

Transplant Candidates and Persons Receiving Tumor Necrosis Factor–α Inhibitors

Transplant candidates found to have LTBI should receive one of the recommended LTBI treatment regimens, ideally prior to transplantation.[71] If transplantation occurs prior to LTBI treatment completion, treatment should be resumed after transplant as soon as medically feasible to complete the originally planned duration. Most of the clinical experience in transplant candidates with LTBI has been with isoniazid monotherapy. Case series of kidney, liver, and heart transplant candidates receiving the 3-month isoniazid-rifapentine regimen suggest adequate completion rates and tolerability in selected patients.[72–74] Close follow-up is required in transplant candidates who initiate LTBI treatment to monitor for side effects and treatment adherence.

Persons initiating TNF-α inhibitors should be systematically tested and treated for LTBI.[1] The American College of Rheumatology recommends completing at least 1 month of LTBI treatment prior to starting or resuming TNF-α inhibitors and other biologic agents in patients with rheumatoid arthritis.[75]

Pregnant Women

Current CDC guidelines recommend considering LTBI treatment in pregnant women who are HIV positive or recent TB contacts.[34] In pregnant women not at high risk of progression to TB, LTBI treatment may be delayed until 2 months to 3 months postpartum. Isoniazid has been the preferred regimen for LTBI treatment during pregnancy.[1,34] Rifampin is an alternative option. Both isoniazid and rifampin are considered category C drugs during pregnancy. Whether to initiate or delay LTBI treatment during pregnancy should be a joint decision with each individual patient, considering a patient's risks factors for TB reactivation and potential side effects from LTBI treatment. A recent randomized trial showed that HIV-positive pregnant women living in high TB burden settings (most of whom did not have evidence of LTBI) who initiated isoniazid therapy during pregnancy had higher rates of adverse pregnancy outcomes compared with women who deferred LTBI treatment until 12 weeks postpartum.[76] Therefore, the recommendation for LTBI treatment during pregnancy in HIV-positive pregnant women is being re-evaluated. A subanalysis of the PREVENT TB and iAdhere trials assessed the outcomes of 125 pregnant women who received some isoniazid-rifapentine or isoniazid monotherapy.[77] No unexpected fetal loss or congenital abnormalities were reported in these women, providing some reassurance that these drugs may be used in pregnancy or women of childbearing potential when deemed clinically necessary.

Children

Children with LTBI are at increased risk for progression to TB disease, particularly in the setting of HIV coinfection.[78] In the United States, isoniazid monotherapy for 9 months remains the preferred recommended regimen for children and adolescents.[34] Daily rifampin for 6 months is recommended by the American Academy of Pediatrics when the case source is known to be isoniazid resistant and rifampin susceptible.[79] Four months of rifampin is safe and effective in children.[80] Isoniazid plus rifampin for 3 months to 4 months seems safe and effective in the pediatric population.[81,82] The CDC now recommends the use of the 3-month isoniazid-rifapentine regimen in adolescents and children aged 2 or older.[52]

Multidrug-Resistant Tuberculosis Contacts

Studies have confirmed that contacts of multidrug-resistant (MDR) TB patients are at increased risk of developing MDR TB disease.[83] There are no standardized recommendations for MDR TB contacts due to lack of randomized clinical trials of TB preventive therapy in this population. Consultation with an expert in MDR TB is generally advised to assist with monitoring and therapy decisions.[34] If preventive treatment is considered, the drug(s) should be selected based on the drug susceptibility profile of the source patient.[1] Although there is no consensus on whether periodic screening versus preventive therapy is better for LTBI management in MDR TB contacts, observational studies suggest a benefit of preventive therapy. A study showed that none of 104 MDR TB

contacts who started a fluoroquinolone-based LTBI regimen developed MDR TB after 36 months of follow-up, whereas 3 of 15 (20%) contacts who refused LTBI treatment developed MDR TB.[84] A recent meta-analysis of 21 observational studies found that LTBI treatment reduced MDR TB incidence by 90% (9%–99%), with greatest cost-effectiveness using fluoroquinolone plus ethambutol in combination.[85] Thus, many programs have adopted the use of fluoroquinolone-based regimens for MDR TB contacts with LTBI based on growing clinical experience and expert opinion.[24,86,87] Randomized trials are urgently needed in this population, however. In the ongoing V-QUIN trial, household contacts of MDR TB cases are randomized to 6 months of levofloxacin or placebo. The PHOENIx MDR-TB trial (NCT03568383) will randomize household contacts of MDR TB cases to 6 months of delamanid or isoniazid therapy.

TREATMENT OF LATENT TUBERCULOSIS INFECTION IN HIGH TUBERCULOSIS PREVALENCE SETTINGS

LTBI screening and preventive therapy in high TB prevalence settings prioritize groups with the highest risk for TB reactivation, such as PLWHA and contacts of pulmonary TB cases, especially children less than 5 years of age.[1] Unfortunately, implementation of LTBI programs has been difficult, because most available resources are utilized to manage active TB cases. Isoniazid given for 6 months to 9 months has been the preferred treatment regimen due to its low cost, availability, and proved efficacy. Studies indicate, however, that the 3-month isoniazid-rifapentine regimen is likely to be cost-effective relative to isoniazid in high TB burden settings.[88]

FUTURE APPROACHES

Shorter and better-tolerated LTBI regimens are under development. The 3-month isoniazid-rifapentine combination regimen represents an important step forward in reducing LTBI treatment duration and improving adherence, thus facilitating large-scale implementation. In an effort to overcome challenges posed by poor treatment adherence and low completion rates of current LTBI therapies, there is ongoing work to develop long-acting formulations suitable for LTBI.[89] For PLWHA in high TB prevalence settings, cyclic administration of LTBI treatment may be an alternative to single rounds of prolonged, continuous TB preventive therapy. Such strategy is being investigated in the WHIP3TB trial

(NCT02980016), which is comparing the 3-month isoniazid-rifapentine regimen given in annual cycles for 2 consecutive years with standard 3-month isoniazid-rifapentine or 6 months of isoniazid given as single cycles. Novel vaccination strategies are under development, because the only licensed TB vaccine available (bacillus Calmette-Guérin) does not provide substantial protection against pulmonary TB disease.[90] A phase 2b trial of an adjuvant subunit vaccine containing 2 *M tuberculosis* antigens showed 54% efficacy in preventing TB disease development among HIV-negative adults with LTBI from endemic areas.[91] Readers can refer to Lisa Stockdale and Helen Fletcher's article, "The Future of Vaccines for Tuberculosis," in this issue for further discussion on the future of vaccines in TB prevention. Targeted host–directed therapies that enhance immune responses to *M tuberculosis* may offer opportunities as future adjuvant and/or primary TB preventive strategies.[92,93]

SUMMARY

Regimens of isoniazid, rifampin, or combinations of isoniazid plus rifampin or rifapentine are available for treating LTBI. Rifamycin-based therapies are shorter and better tolerated than isoniazid monotherapy and thus are important tools to prevent TB disease and contribute to ending the TB epidemic. Novel vaccine strategies, host immunity–directed therapies, and ultrashort antimicrobial regimens for TB prevention are under evaluation.

REFERENCES

1. World Health Organization. Latent tuberculosis infection: updated and consolidated guidelines for programmatic management. Geneva (Switzerland): World Health Organization; 2018.
2. Houben RM, Dodd PJ. The global burden of latent tuberculosis infection: a Re-estimation using mathematical modelling. PLoS Med 2016;13(10):e1002152.
3. Lonnroth K, Migliori GB, Abubakar I, et al. Towards tuberculosis elimination: an action framework for low-incidence countries. Eur Respir J 2015;45(4). 928–52.
4. Dye C, Glaziou P, Floyd K, et al. Prospects for tuberculosis elimination. Annu Rev Public Health 2013;34: 271–86.
5. Mancuso JD, Diffenderfer JM, Ghassemieh BJ, et al. The prevalence of latent tuberculosis infection in the United States. Am J Respir Crit Care Med 2016; 194(4):501–9.
6. Bennett DE, Courval JM, Onorato I, et al. Prevalence of tuberculosis infection in the United States population: the national health and nutrition examination survey, 1999-2000. Am J Respir Crit Care Med 2008;177(3):348–55.
7. Tsang CA, Langer AJ, Navin TR, et al. Tuberculosis among foreign-born persons diagnosed >/=10 years after arrival in the United States, 2010-2015. MMWR Morb Mortal Wkly Rep 2017;66(11):295–8.
8. Yuen CM, Kammerer JS, Marks K, et al. Recent transmission of tuberculosis - United States, 2011-2014. PLoS One 2016;11(4):e0153728.
9. Shea KM, Kammerer JS, Winston CA, et al. Estimated rate of reactivation of latent tuberculosis infection in the United States, overall and by population subgroup. Am J Epidemiol 2014;179(2):216–25.
10. Stewart RJ, Tsang CA, Pratt RH, et al. Tuberculosis - United States, 2017. MMWR Morb Mortal Wkly Rep 2018;67(11):317–23.
11. Bayer R, Castro KG. Tuberculosis elimination in the United States - the need for renewed action. N Engl J Med 2017;377(12):1109–11.
12. Abu-Raddad LJ, Sabatelli L, Achterberg JT, et al. Epidemiological benefits of more-effective tuberculosis vaccines, drugs, and diagnostics. Proc Natl Acad Sci U S A 2009;106(33):13980–5.
13. Tang P, Johnston J. Treatment of latent tuberculosis infection. Curr Treat Options Infect Dis 2017;9(4): 371–9.
14. Rangaka MX, Cavalcante SC, Marais BJ, et al. Controlling the seedbeds of tuberculosis: diagnosis and treatment of tuberculosis infection. Lancet 2015; 386(10010):2344–53.
15. Alsdurf H, Hill PC, Matteelli A, et al. The cascade of care in diagnosis and treatment of latent tuberculosis infection: a systematic review and meta-analysis. Lancet Infect Dis 2016;16(11):1269–78.
16. Getahun H, Matteelli A, Abubakar I, et al. Management of latent Mycobacterium tuberculosis infection: WHO guidelines for low tuberculosis burden countries. Eur Respir J 2015;46(6):1563–76.
17. U.S. Preventive Services Task Force, Bibbins-Domingo K, Grossman DC, Curry SJ, et al. Screening for latent tuberculosis infection in adults: US preventive services task force recommendation statement. JAMA 2016;316(9):962–9.
18. Lee MR, Huang YP, Kuo YT, et al. Diabetes mellitus and latent tuberculosis infection: a systemic review and metaanalysis. Clin Infect Dis 2017;64(6): 719–27.
19. Jeon CY, Murray MB. Diabetes mellitus increases the risk of active tuberculosis: a systematic review of 13 observational studies. PLoS Med 2008;5(7):e152.
20. Turetz ML, Ma KC. Diagnosis and management of latent tuberculosis. Curr Opin Infect Dis 2016; 29(2):205–11.
21. Getahun H, Matteelli A, Chaisson RE, et al. Latent Mycobacterium tuberculosis infection. N Engl J Med 2015;372(22):2127–35.

22. Hirsch-Moverman Y, Daftary A, Franks J, et al. Adherence to treatment for latent tuberculosis infection: systematic review of studies in the US and Canada. Int J Tuberc Lung Dis 2008;12(11):1235–54.

23. Kopanoff DE, Snider DE Jr, Caras GJ. Isoniazid-related hepatitis: a U.S. Public Health Service cooperative surveillance study. Am Rev Respir Dis 1978; 117(6):991–1001.

24. Fox GJ, Dobler CC, Marais BJ, et al. Preventive therapy for latent tuberculosis infection-the promise and the challenges. Int J Infect Dis 2017;56:68–76.

25. Balcells ME, Thomas SL, Godfrey-Faussett P, et al. Isoniazid preventive therapy and risk for resistant tuberculosis. Emerg Infect Dis 2006;12(5):744–51.

26. den Boon S, Matteelli A, Getahun H. Rifampicin resistance after treatment for latent tuberculous infection: a systematic review and meta-analysis. Int J Tuberc Lung Dis 2016;20(8):1065–71.

27. Takayama K, Wang L, David HL. Effect of isoniazid on the in vivo mycolic acid synthesis, cell growth, and viability of Mycobacterium tuberculosis. Antimicrob Agents Chemother 1972;2(1):29–35.

28. Preventive therapy of tuberculous infection. Am Rev Respir Dis 1974;110(3):371–4.

29. Runyon EH. Preventive treatment in tuberculosis: a statement by the Committee on therapy, American Thoracic Society. Am Rev Respir Dis 1965;91:297–8.

30. Ferebee SH, Palmer CE. Prevention of experimental tuberculosis with isoniazid. Am Rev Tuberc 1956; 73(1):1–18.

31. Zenner D, Beer N, Harris RJ, et al. Treatment of latent tuberculosis infection: an updated network meta-analysis. Ann Intern Med 2017;167(4):248–55.

32. Efficacy of various durations of isoniazid preventive therapy for tuberculosis: five years of follow-up in the IUAT trial. International Union against Tuberculosis Committee on Prophylaxis. Bull World Health Organ 1982;60(4):555–64.

33. Comstock GW. How much isoniazid is needed for prevention of tuberculosis among immunocompetent adults? Int J Tuberc Lung Dis 1999;3(10): 847–50.

34. Centers for Disease Control and Prevention. Latent tuberculosis infection: a guide for primary health care providers. Atlanta (GA): Centers for Diseases Control and Prevention; 2013.

35. Bliven-Sizemore EE, Sterling TR, Shang N, et al. Three months of weekly rifapentine plus isoniazid is less hepatotoxic than nine months of daily isoniazid for LTBI. Int J Tuberc Lung Dis 2015;19(9): 1039–44. i-v.

36. Yew WW. Clinically significant interactions with drugs used in the treatment of tuberculosis. Drug Saf 2002;25(2):111–33.

37. Campbell EA, Korzheva N, Mustaev A, et al. Structural mechanism for rifampicin inhibition of bacterial rna polymerase. Cell 2001;104(6):901–12.

38. Menzies D, Adjobimey M, Ruslami R, et al. Four months of rifampin or nine months of isoniazid for latent tuberculosis in adults. N Engl J Med 2018; 379(5):440–53.

39. Chan PC, Yang CH, Chang LY, et al. Latent tuberculosis infection treatment for prison inmates: a randomised controlled trial. Int J Tuberc Lung Dis 2012; 16(5):633–8.

40. Menzies D, Long R, Trajman A, et al. Adverse events with 4 months of rifampin therapy or 9 months of isoniazid therapy for latent tuberculosis infection: a randomized trial. Ann Intern Med 2008;149(10): 689–97.

41. Geijo MP, Herranz CR, Vano D, et al. [Short-course isoniazid and rifampin compared with isoniazid for latent tuberculosis infection: a randomized clinical trial]. Enferm Infecc Microbiol Clin 2007;25(5): 300–4.

42. Whalen CC, Johnson JL, Okwera A, et al. A trial of three regimens to prevent tuberculosis in Ugandan adults infected with the human immunodeficiency virus. Uganda-Case Western Reserve University Research Collaboration. N Engl J Med 1997; 337(12):801–8.

43. Rivero A, Lopez-Cortes L, Castillo R, et al. Randomized clinical trial investigating three chemoprophylaxis regimens for latent tuberculosis infection in HIV-infected patients. Enferm Infecc Microbiol Clin 2007;25(5):305–10 [in Spanish].

44. A double-blind placebo-controlled clinical trial of three antituberculosis chemoprophylaxis regimens in patients with silicosis in Hong Kong. Hong Kong Chest Service/Tuberculosis Research Centre, Madras/British Medical Research Council. Am Rev Respir Dis 1992;145(1):36–41.

45. Martinez Alfaro EM, Cuadra F, Solera J, et al. Evaluation of 2 tuberculosis chemoprophylaxis regimens in patients infected with human immunodeficiency virus. The GECMEI Group. Med Clin (Barc) 2000; 115(5):161–5 [in Spanish].

46. Ena J, Valls V. Short-course therapy with rifampin plus isoniazid, compared with standard therapy with isoniazid, for latent tuberculosis infection: a meta-analysis. Clin Infect Dis 2005;40(5): 670–6.

47. Miyazaki E, Chaisson RE, Bishai WR. Analysis of rifapentine for preventive therapy in the Cornell mouse model of latent tuberculosis. Antimicrob Agents Chemother 1999;43(9):2126–30.

48. Ji B, Truffot-Pernot C, Lacroix C, et al. Effectiveness of rifampin, rifabutin, and rifapentine for preventive therapy of tuberculosis in mice. Am Rev Respir Dis 1993;148(6 Pt 1):1541–6.

49. Sterling TR, Villarino ME, Borisov AS, et al. Three months of rifapentine and isoniazid for latent tuberculosis infection. N Engl J Med 2011;365(23): 2155–66.

50. Sandul AL, Nwana N, Holcombe JM, et al. High rate of treatment completion in program settings with 12-dose weekly isoniazid and rifapentine for latent Mycobacterium tuberculosis infection. Clin Infect Dis 2017;65(7):1085–93.

51. Belknap R, Holland D, Feng PJ, et al. Self-administered versus directly observed once-weekly isoniazid and rifapentine treatment of latent tuberculosis infection: a randomized trial. Ann Intern Med 2017;167(10):689–97.

52. Borisov AS, Bamrah Morris S, Njie GJ, et al. Update of recommendations for use of once-weekly isoniazid-rifapentine regimen to treat latent mycobacterium tuberculosis infection. MMWR Morb Mortal Wkly Rep 2018;67(25):723–6.

53. Mitnick CD, McGee B, Peloquin CA. Tuberculosis pharmacotherapy: strategies to optimize patient care. Expert Opin Pharmacother 2009;10(3):381–401.

54. Scolarici M, Dekitani K, Chen L, et al. A scoring strategy for progression risk and rates of treatment completion in subjects with latent tuberculosis. PLoS One 2018;13(11):e0207582.

55. Menzies D, Gardiner G, Farhat M, et al. Thinking in three dimensions: a web-based algorithm to aid the interpretation of tuberculin skin test results. Int J Tuberc Lung Dis 2008;12(5):498–505.

56. Deffur A, Mulder NJ, Wilkinson RJ. Co-infection with Mycobacterium tuberculosis and human immunodeficiency virus: an overview and motivation for systems approaches. Pathog Dis 2013;69(2):101–13.

57. Selwyn PA, Hartel D, Lewis VA, et al. A prospective study of the risk of tuberculosis among intravenous drug users with human immunodeficiency virus infection. N Engl J Med 1989;320(9):545–50.

58. Gupta A, Wood R, Kaplan R, et al. Tuberculosis incidence rates during 8 years of follow-up of an antiretroviral treatment cohort in South Africa: comparison with rates in the community. PLoS One 2012;7(3):e34156.

59. Rangaka MX, Wilkinson RJ, Boulle A, et al. Isoniazid plus antiretroviral therapy to prevent tuberculosis: a randomised double-blind, placebo-controlled trial. Lancet 2014;384(9944):682–90.

60. TEMPRANO ANRS 12136 Study Group, Danel C, Moh R, et al. A trial of early antiretrovirals and isoniazid preventive therapy in Africa. N Engl J Med 2015;373(9):808–22.

61. Golub JE, Saraceni V, Cavalcante SC, et al. The impact of antiretroviral therapy and isoniazid preventive therapy on tuberculosis incidence in HIV-infected patients in Rio de Janeiro, Brazil. AIDS 2007;21(11):1441–8.

62. Golub JE, Pronyk P, Mohapi L, et al. Isoniazid preventive therapy, HAART and tuberculosis risk in HIV-infected adults in South Africa: a prospective cohort. AIDS 2009;23(5):631–6.

63. Panel on Opportunistic infections in HIV-infected adults and adolescents. Guidelines for the prevention and treatment of opportunistic infections in HIV-infected adults and adolescents: recommendations from the Centers for disease control and prevention, the national Institutes of health, and the HIV medicine association of the infectious diseases Society of America. Available at: http://aidsinfo.nih.gov/contentfiles/lvguidelines/adult_oi.pdf. Accessed December 29, 2018.

64. Akolo C, Adetifa I, Shepperd S, et al. Treatment of latent tuberculosis infection in HIV infected persons. Cochrane Database Syst Rev 2010;(1):CD000171.

65. Sterling TR, Scott NA, Miro JM, et al. Three months of weekly rifapentine and isoniazid for treatment of Mycobacterium tuberculosis infection in HIV-coinfected persons. AIDS 2016;30(10):1607–15.

66. Weiner M, Egelund EF, Engle M, et al. Pharmacokinetic interaction of rifapentine and raltegravir in healthy volunteers. J Antimicrob Chemother 2014;69(4):1079–85.

67. Podany AT, Bao Y, Swindells S, et al. Efavirenz pharmacokinetics and pharmacodynamics in HIV-infected persons receiving rifapentine and isoniazid for tuberculosis prevention. Clin Infect Dis 2015;61(8):1322–7.

68. Brooks KM, George JM, Pau AK, et al. Cytokine-mediated systemic adverse drug reactions in a drug-drug interaction study of dolutegravir with once-weekly isoniazid and rifapentine. Clin Infect Dis 2018;67(2):193–201.

69. Swindells S, Ramchandani R, Gupta A, et al. One month of rifapentine/isoniazid to prevent TB in people with HIV: Brief-TB/A5279. 25th CROI. Boston, MA. 4–7 March 2018. Oral abstract 37LB.

70. Samandari T, Agizew TB, Nyirenda S, et al. 6-month versus 36-month isoniazid preventive treatment for tuberculosis in adults with HIV infection in Botswana: a randomised, double-blind, placebo-controlled trial. Lancet 2011;377(9777):1588–98.

71. Subramanian AK, Morris MI, AST Infectious Diseases Community of Practice. Mycobacterium tuberculosis infections in solid organ transplantation. Am J Transplant 2013;13(Suppl 4):68–76.

72. Simkins J, Abbo LM, Camargo JF, et al. Twelve-week rifapentine plus isoniazid versus 9-month isoniazid for the treatment of latent tuberculosis in renal transplant candidates. Transplantation 2017;101(6):1468–72.

73. Knoll BM, Nog R, Wu Y, et al. Three months of weekly rifapentine plus isoniazid for latent tuberculosis treatment in solid organ transplant candidates. Infection 2017;45(3):335–9.

74. de Castilla DL, Rakita RM, Spitters CE, et al. Short-course isoniazid plus rifapentine directly observed therapy for latent tuberculosis in solid-organ transplant candidates. Transplantation 2014;97(2):206–11.

75. Singh JA, Saag KG, Bridges SL Jr, et al. 2015 American College of Rheumatology guideline for the treatment of rheumatoid arthritis. Arthritis Rheumatol 2016;68(1):1–26.

76. Gupta A, Montepiedra G, Aaron L, et al. Randomised trial of safety of isoniazid preventive therapy during or after pregnancy. 25th CROI. Boston, MA. 4–7 March 2018. Oral abstract 142LB.

77. Moro RN, Scott NA, Vernon A, et al. Exposure to latent tuberculosis treatment during pregnancy. The PREVENT TB and the iAdhere trials. Ann Am Thorac Soc 2018;15(5):570–80.

78. Perez-Velez CM, Marais BJ. Tuberculosis in children. N Engl J Med 2012;367(4):348–61.

79. Targeted tuberculin skin testing and treatment of latent tuberculosis infection in children and adolescents. Pediatrics 2004;114(Supplement 4):1175–201.

80. Diallo T, Adjobimey M, Ruslami R, et al. Safety and side effects of rifampin versus isoniazid in children. N Engl J Med 2018;379(5):454–63.

81. Spyridis NP, Spyridis PG, Gelesme A, et al. The effectiveness of a 9-month regimen of isoniazid alone versus 3- and 4-month regimens of isoniazid plus rifampin for treatment of latent tuberculosis infection in children: results of an 11-year randomized study. Clin Infect Dis 2007;45(6):715–22.

82. Bright-Thomas R, Nandwani S, Smith J, et al. Effectiveness of 3 months of rifampicin and isoniazid chemoprophylaxis for the treatment of latent tuberculosis infection in children. Arch Dis Child 2010; 95(8):600–2.

83. Becerra MC, Appleton SC, Franke MF, et al. Tuberculosis burden in households of patients with multidrug-resistant and extensively drug-resistant tuberculosis: a retrospective cohort study. Lancet 2011;377(9760):147–52.

84. Bamrah S, Brostrom R, Dorina F, et al. Treatment for LTBI in contacts of MDR-TB patients, Federated States of Micronesia, 2009-2012. Int J Tuberc Lung Dis 2014;18(8):912–8.

85. Marks SM, Mase SR, Morris SB. Systematic review, meta-analysis, and cost-effectiveness of treatment of latent tuberculosis to reduce progression to multidrug-resistant tuberculosis. Clin Infect Dis 2017;64(12):1670–7.

86. Curry International Tuberculosis Center, California Department of Public Health. Drug-resistant tuberculosis: a survival guide for clinicians. 3rd edition. Oakland (CA): Curry International TB Center; 2016.

87. Public Health Agency of Canada. Canadian tuberculosis standards. 7th edition. Canada: Centre for Communicable Diseases and Infection Control, Public Health Agency of Canada; 2013. Available at: https://www.canada.ca/en/public-health/services/infectious-diseases/canadian-tuberculosis-standards-7th-edition/edition-22.html.

88. Johnson KT, Churchyard GJ, Sohn H, et al. Cost-effectiveness of preventive therapy for tuberculosis with isoniazid and rifapentine versus isoniazid alone in high-burden settings. Clin Infect Dis 2018;67(7): 1072–8.

89. Swindells S, Siccardi M, Barrett SE, et al. Long-acting formulations for the treatment of latent tuberculous infection: opportunities and challenges. Int J Tuberc Lung Dis 2018;22(2):125–32.

90. Mangtani P, Abubakar I, Ariti C, et al. Protection by BCG vaccine against tuberculosis: a systematic review of randomized controlled trials. Clin Infect Dis 2014;58(4):470–80.

91. Van Der Meeren O, Hatherill M, Nduba V, et al. Phase 2b controlled trial of M72/AS01E vaccine to prevent tuberculosis. N Engl J Med 2018;379(17): 1621–34.

92. Kolloli A, Subbian S. Host-directed therapeutic strategies for tuberculosis. Front Med (Lausanne) 2017; 4:171.

93. Tiberi S, du Plessis N, Walzl G, et al. Tuberculosis: progress and advances in development of new drugs, treatment regimens, and host-directed therapies. Lancet Infect Dis 2018;18(7):e183–98.

The Future of Vaccines for Tuberculosis

Lisa Stockdale, BSc, MPH, PhD[a,b], Helen Fletcher, BSc, PhD[c],*

KEYWORDS

- TB • Vaccines • BCG

KEY POINTS

- Intense international collaborative efforts have resulted in a TB vaccine pipeline comprising 20 candidates at various stages of preclinical and clinical development.
- Efficacy results from 2 clinical vaccine trials published in 2018 offer hope that effective TB vaccines may be on the horizon.
- Guidance from licensing agencies takes into consideration ethical and logistical constraints surrounding large and expensive vaccine efficacy studies. Early contact with agencies should help developers prepare for success.

INTRODUCTION

Tuberculosis (TB) is now the leading cause of death from a single infectious agent (*Mycobacterium tuberculosis*; *M.tb*), ranking above HIV/AIDS.[1] In 2017, 10 million people were ill with TB, and the disease caused an estimated 1.3 million deaths.[1] Bacillus Calmette-Guérin (BCG), a live-attenuated strain of *Mycobacterium bovis*, is the only licensed vaccine against TB, and one of the most widely used vaccines globally. BCG provides variable protection against pulmonary forms of TB,[2] and efficacy is affected by previous infection with *M.tb* or sensitization with environmental mycobacteria.[3] Although duration of protection is variable, protection has been shown to last for up to 10 years,[4] and recent global shortages of BCG point toward a possible underappreciation of the benefit of neonatal vaccination in areas of high incidence,[5] including nonspecific beneficial effects.[6]

In 2013, the World Health Organization (WHO) published a roadmap of how to reduce TB deaths by 95% by 2035.[7] The overall aim being to achieve TB elimination by 2050: to reduce annual incidence to less than 1 case per million population.[8] Central to WHO strategy is the development of effective preexposure and postexposure vaccines, this being especially important given the increasing threat of drug-resistant strains of TB.[9]

As of mid-2018, the TB vaccine pipeline comprised 20 potential candidates. These include subunit vaccines, virally vectored vaccines, and live-attenuated or whole-cell-inactivated *Mycobacteria* (**Table 1**), and are the result of highly collaborative research and development activities[a]. Aside from the biochemical attributes of vaccines, these candidates can also be categorized into the host infection status targeted by vaccination (uninfected, latently infected, or people with active TB), and the desired effect of the vaccine (prevention of

Disclosure Statement: This work was supported by a UK Medical Research Council studentship for LS (MR/J003999/1). HF received support from EC HORIZON2020 TBVAC2020 (grant ref MR/K012126/1).

[a] Department of Paediatrics, University of Oxford, Oxford, UK; [b] NIHR Oxford Biomedical Research Centre and Oxford University Hospitals NHS Foundation Trust, Oxford, UK; [c] Department of Immunology and Infection, London School of Hygiene and Tropical Medicine, Keppel Street, London WC1E 7HT, UK
* Corresponding author.
E-mail address: helen.fletcher@lshtm.ac.uk
twitter: @LisaStockdale (L.S.); @FletcherHelen (H.F.)

[a]https://www.tbvi.eu/what-we-do/pipeline-of-vaccines/.

Clin Chest Med 40 (2019) 849–856
https://doi.org/10.1016/j.ccm.2019.07.009
0272-5231/19/© 2019 Elsevier Inc. All rights reserved.

Table 1
TB vaccines in preclinical and clinical development

Vaccine Name (Recent Publication)	Phase of Development	Developer	Description and Link to Clinical Trial Details (If Available)
Subunit vaccines			
H64:CAF01	Preclin	SII, TBVI	Fusion protein of 6 antigens. Developed as a supplement to BCG with CAF01 adjuvant
CsyVac2/Advax[33]	Preclin	Univ. Sydney. TBVI	Fusion protein of virulence factor CysD and Ag85B with the polysaccharide adjuvant Advax
GamTBVac	1	MoH Russia	
ID93/GLA-SE[34]	2a	IDRI, Wellcome Trust	Rv2608 PPE family member, Rv3619 and Rv3620 virulence factors, and Rv1813 dormancy antigen with GLA-SE oil-in-water emulsion/TLR4 agonist adjuvant (NCT02465216)
H4:IC31[21]	2	Sanofi Pasteur, Aeras	Ag85B and TB10.4 with the adjuvant IC31. Developed as a POI BCG boost (NCT02075203)
M72 AS01$_E$[19]	2b	GSK, Aeras	Rv1196 PPE family member and Rv0125 peptidase with AS01$_E$ liposome/TLR4 agonist adjuvant. *POD* (NCT01755598)
H56:IC31[35]	2b	SII, Valneva, Aeras	H1 and Rv2660c dormancy antigens with IC31 cationic peptide/TLR9 agonist adjuvant. POR (NCT03512249)
Virally vectored vaccines			
ChAdOx/MVA PPE15-85A	Preclin	Univ. Oxford, TBVI	Replication-deficient chimpanzee adenovirus and modified vaccinia virus-vectored PPE and Ag85A
CMV-6Ag[22]	Preclin	Aeras, Vir Biotech, OHSU	Replication-deficient cytomegalovirus-vectored ESAT-6, Ag85A, Ag85B, Rv3407, Rv1733, Rv2626, Rpf A, Rpf C, and Rpf D
MVA multiphasic vac[36]	Preclin	Transgene, TBVI	Up to 14 antigens representative of the 3 phases of TB infection (active, latent, and resuscitation) with a modified vaccinia virus vector
ChAdOx1. 85A MVA 85A	1	Univ. Oxford, TBVI	Chimpanzee adenovirus-vectored Ag85A prime and modified vaccinia virus-vectored Ag85A boost. Aerosol/IM administration (NCT03681860)
Ad5 Ag85A	1	McMaster, CanSino	Replication-deficient human adenovirus 5-vectored Ag85A (NCT02337270)
TB/FLU04L	2a	RIBSP	Replication-deficient influenza virus (H1N1) vectored Ag85A (NCT02501421)
Live Vaccines			
BCG-ZMPI	Preclin	Univ. Zurich, TBVI	Recombinant BCG lacking *zmp1* gene. Developed as a POI BCG replacement in newborns

(*continued on next page*)

Table 1
(continued)

Vaccine Name (Recent Publication)	Phase of Development	Developer	Description and Link to Clinical Trial Details (If Available)
MTBVAC[37]	2a	Biofabri, Univ. Zaragosa, TBVI	Live-attenuated *Mycobacterium tuberculosis* with specific deletion of the virulence factor, *erp*. Developed as a POI BCG replacement (NCT02013245)
VPM1002[38]	3	SII, Max Planck, VPM, TBVI	Live attenuated recombinant BCG with deletion of a range of genes, including the antiapoptotic factor *nuoG*. Developed as a POI BCG replacement and POD after successful antituberculosis drug therapy (NCT03152903)
Inactivated Whole-Cell Mycobacterial Vaccines			
RUTI	2a	Archivel Pharma	Inactivated *Mycobacterium tuberculosis*. Developed as an immunotherapeutic vaccine to be used alongside antibiotic treatment (NCT02711735)
DAR-901[39]	2b	Univ. Dartmouth, Aeras	Inactivated nontuberculous *Mycobacterium obuense*. Developed as a boost to BCG POI (NCT02712424)
MIP	3	Indian department of biotechnology, Cadila Pharma	*Mycobacterium indicus pranii*
M.Vaccae[40]	3	Anhui Zhifei Longcom	Inactivated *Mycobacterium vaccae* (NCT01979900)

Abbreviations: Ag85A, antigen85A (mycolyl transferase); POD, prevention of disease; POI, prevention of infection; POR, prevention of recurrence; PPE, proline, proline, glutamate residues.

infection [POI], prevention of disease [POD] or prevention of recurrence [POR]). Some vaccines are being developed to replace BCG, some as boosters to BCG, and some as therapeutic vaccines to be given with or without concomitant drug treatment. Host infection status, as well as relative efficacy and duration of protection, will have significant impact on decisions on the optimal age for vaccination. These considerations will also be important in the operational roll-out when we have a suitable vaccine.

In this review, we provide an overview of the current TB vaccine pipeline, highlighting exciting recent findings, describe important work relating to epidemiologic impact of vaccines, and discuss the possible future of TB vaccine development.

BIOMARKER RESEARCH

On exposure to *M.tb* bacilli, it is estimated that 70% of individuals remain uninfected. Of the 30% that do become infected, over 90% of

individuals are able to contain the bacilli in a granuloma; leading to latent infection.[10] Although HIV and other forms of immunosuppression increase the likelihood of developing disease, increase the severity of symptoms, and decrease the time to progression,[11,12] the reasons why most individuals exposed to *M.tb* do not develop TB are not known.

An essential part of vaccine development is the ability to determine if a vaccine has been successful. For most licensed vaccines, this has been a direct observation of protection against disease in humans. This situation is rather more complicated in the case of TB, in which disease can occur years after initial infection. Vaccine trials that measure disease as their endpoint are, by necessity, very large, very costly, and require years of follow-up.

Recently, vaccines against the invasive bacterial infection, *Neisseria meningitidis*, have been licensed for human use based on measurement of humoral immune responses.[13] A direct relationship between serum bactericidal activity and protection against disease was shown by Goldschneider and colleagues[14,15] in 1969. It is these more easily measurable immune responses, either being functionally responsible for protection (correlate of protection), or simply associated with protection (surrogate of protection),[16] that can provide early readouts from clinical efficacy studies, which would otherwise require years of follow-up to reach statistical clinical disease endpoints.[17] Despite international collaborative efforts[b,c] and intense research, correlates or surrogates of protection against TB remain elusive.[18]

TUBERCULOSIS VACCINE PIPELINE

Table 1 shows the current TB vaccine pipeline candidates. A major objective of international collaborative research funding has been the identification of novel antigens for use in subunit and virally vectored vaccines. The overall aim is to identify immunogenic proteins and lipoproteins derived from *M.tb*-infected macrophages that will induce polyfunctional effector T cell subsets, and, more recently, a focus on induction of antibody-mediated protection, to protect against infection and, ultimately, disease. The subunit vaccines rely on adjuvants. The role of adjuvants is to help to activate the immune system, thereby assisting the antigens to induce long-term, protective immunity. Here, we highlight some of the most recent advances from the pipeline.

Subunit Vaccines

There are currently 7 subunit vaccine candidates in the TB vaccine pipeline (see **Table 1**). Results from a phase 2b POD trial among adults already infected with *M.tb* of the GSK subunit vaccine M72/AS01$_E$ in Kenya, South Africa, and Zambia were reported in late 2018. In HIV-negative adults with latent TB infection, as determined by QuantiFERON (QFT), the group reported a per protocol vaccine efficacy of 54% (95% CI 3–78) in 3283 individuals followed-up for a mean of 2.3 years against confirmed pulmonary TB disease.[19] In prespecified subgroup analyses, the group found a higher vaccine efficacy among men (75.2% vs 27.4% for women), and among individuals aged 25 years or younger (84.4% vs 10.2% for those aged over 25 years). The authors do note a sex imbalance in terms of

numbers of participants in the younger age group, which likely confounds the age and sex effects seen but, nonetheless, these are exciting findings given that an estimated quarter of the world's population is latently infected with TB.[20] Crucially, samples were stored for analysis of immune correlates of vaccine efficacy. Results from further investigations should help to shed light on mechanisms of protective effect.

Another subunit vaccine trial that reported results in 2018 is the H4:IC31 vaccine.[21] Intended as a BCG boost, this POI study among QFT-negative individuals enrolled adolescents in South Africa between the ages of 12 and 17 years and had 3 arms: neonatal BCG vaccination followed by H4:IC31, or BCG revaccination, or a saline placebo. All 989 participants were HIV-negative and had no evidence of latent TB infection (by QFT). The endpoint for this study was sustained QFT conversion, which the authors propose likely represents sustained *M.tb* infection and a higher risk of progression to TB. Whereas neither H4:IC31 nor BCG revaccination prevented initial QFT conversion, the group reported that BCG revaccination reduced the rate of sustained QFT conversion (efficacy 45%, 95% CI 6–68) compared with H4:IC31 vaccine (efficacy 31%, 95% CI 16–58). Although the clinical implications of sustained QFT conversion are unknown, this study has renewed interest in BCG revaccination.

Virally Vectored Vaccines

There are 6 virally vectored vaccines in development (see **Table 1**). Four of these use either modified vaccinia Ankara, a highly attenuated, replication-deficient poxvirus, or an adenoviral vector specific to either human or chimpanzee. Adenoviral vectors can be replication competent or deficient; however, those in the current pipeline are all replication deficient. One candidate in preclinical development uses a replication-competent herpes virus; cytomegalovirus, and one in clinical development uses a replication-deficient H1N1 influenza virus as the vector.

Results of a preclinical trial in the highly susceptible rhesus macaque were reported in 2018. Vaccination with cytomegalovirus-vectored vaccine containing either 6 or 9 TB antigens showed 41% protective efficacy against

---

[b]https://www.ctvd.co/Pages/default.aspx.

[c]https://www.validate-network.org/.

experimental infection with pathogenic Erdman strain of *M.tb* 1 year after vaccination (14/34 vaccinated macaques showed no TB compared with 0/17 unvaccinated animals).[22] In addition, 10/14 protected macaques were *M.tb* culture-negative for all tissues, indicating sterilizing immunity. The mechanism of protective efficacy has yet to be determined.[23]

Live-Attenuated Vaccines

Of the 3 candidates in development, VPM1002 is the most advanced. Designed both as a replacement for BCG, and as an immunotherapeutic to be given following successful antitubercular treatment, a phase III study was recruiting participants at the time of writing and is due to complete at the end of 2019 (NCT03152903).

Whole-Cell-Inactivated Vaccines

DAR-901 is a whole-cell booster vaccine (based on the *Mycobacterium obuense* construct) to prevent TB infection. A phase 2 placebo-controlled 3-dose trial in adolescents primed with BCG in Tanzania is planned but not yet recruiting (NCT02712424). This study will study the effect of vaccination on POI in 650 13–15 year olds with no evidence of *M.tb* infection.

Bacillus Calmette-Guérin Revaccination

As discussed above, unexpected results from the BCG revaccination arm of the Nemes and colleagues[21] H4:IC31 subunit vaccine POI trial showed that BCG revaccination reduced the rate of sustained QFT conversion. Previous research from Finland,[24] Brazil,[25] Malawi,[26] and Hong Kong[27] failed to show any benefit of revaccination on TB incidence. Whereas these recent data have rekindled interest in the use of BCG in adolescents, it is important to take into consideration the contraindication of BCG among HIV-positive individuals, people on immunosuppressive treatment, and pregnant women.[d] However, the low cost, excellent safety profile, and availability of BCG place BCG revaccination as a leading strategy for control of the global TB epidemic. Key questions to be answered in future trials include: (1) Can the prevention of TB infection result seen by Nemes and colleagues be repeated in an independent study? (2) Does prevention of TB infection translate to prevention of TB disease? (3) Would this strategy be safe and effective on those living with HIV with viral loads controlled by antiretroviral therapy? Although the first question can be answered within a few years, with less than 1000 individuals, the second and third questions would require much longer, larger, and more complex studies.

Modeling of Epidemiologic Impact of Tuberculosis Vaccines

In the absence of an efficacious TB vaccine, epidemiologists have used mathematical models to explore the anticipated population impact, assuming various vaccine profiles. A systematic review by Harris and colleagues[28] included 23 evaluations that varied in characteristics such as their predicted efficacy, duration of protection, host infection status (and therefore the POI/POD/POR effect of the vaccine), and age at vaccination. Economic evaluations of all modeled scenarios were overwhelmingly cost-effective, and results proved agnostic to whether the vaccine functioned preinfection or postinfection. Vaccine usage will need to be tailored to the epidemiology of the intended population. In the systematic review, the most rapid global epidemiologic impact was found to be associated with effective vaccination of adolescents or adults as opposed to neonates.[28] In the case of China, where an aging population means that most TB cases are a result of reactivation of prior *M.tb* infection, evidence suggests that vaccination of adults aged over 60 years would be the most effective way to reduce incidence of TB.[29]

Changes in the Regulatory Landscape

Regulatory agencies in the United States and Europe have recognized that, for some pathogens, it is not possible to perform vaccine efficacy trials because the number of disease endpoints is too low and the time required and costs of conducting clinical efficacy trials too high. Where efficacy trials cannot be performed, an immune correlate of protection can be used as a surrogate for vaccine efficacy, and these data can be accepted by regulatory agencies to obtain vaccine licensure. A phase III TB vaccine efficacy trial with a disease endpoint is possible, but the scale and costs of such trials are so high they verge on unfeasible. For this reason, there would be a legitimate argument for using an immune correlate of TB vaccine efficacy as a surrogate for a disease endpoint for TB vaccine licensure. However, because we have not been able to identify an immune correlate that could be used in such a trial, this route is not open for the licensure of new TB vaccines.

TB is not the only pathogen for which it is difficult to perform vaccine efficacy trials, and for which an immune correlate is unavailable. This is particularly the case for emerging or outbreak pathogens. Significant investment and activity in the development of vaccines for outbreak pathogens is driving change across the whole of the vaccine development landscape. Regulators are working closely with academic communities and industry to find new ways to accelerate vaccine development and licensure.

In 2015, the US Food and Drug Administration (FDA) finalized guidance 21 CFR 601.91(a) to "provide information and recommendations on drug and biological product development when human efficacy studies are not ethical or feasible."[30] Thus far, only 1 vaccine has been licensed using the animal rule; a postexposure vaccine against *Bacillus anthracis*.[31] In a situation in which traditional efficacy trials involving exposure to the disease-causing agent are impractical, this guidance states that the FDA may grant approval of a product based on "adequate and well-controlled animal efficacy studies when the results of those studies establish that the drug is reasonably likely to produce clinical benefit in humans."[30]

The European Medicines Agency (EMA) also has a draft guideline on clinical evaluation of vaccines (EMEA/CHMP/VWP/164653/05 Rev. 1).[32] This document provides guidance when a vaccine efficacy trail is not feasible, and where an immune correlate of protection has not been identified. Efficacy studies may not be needed if "vaccine efficacy can be inferred by demonstrating noninferior immune responses between the candidate vaccine and a licensed vaccine for which efficacy and/or effectiveness has been estimated."[32]

If it is not possible to compare immune responses between a candidate vaccine and a licensed vaccine the EMA suggest 2 alternatives for measuring vaccine efficacy; human challenge studies and animal challenge studies. The EMA caution that if vaccine licensure is based on human or animal challenge studies, a condition should be that an estimate of vaccine efficacy is obtained postlicensure.

Given the acknowledgment by international agencies of the ethical and logistical constraints surrounding vaccine efficacy testing for diseases such as TB, it will be crucial that vaccine developers initiate contact with licensing agencies early in clinical development.

Future of Tuberculosis Vaccines

With the M72 trial and the BCG revaccination study it has been shown that we can protect adolescents against TB. With modeling we have a much better understanding of the impact even a partially effective TB vaccine could have on the global epidemic. With a more flexible regulatory environment it may be possible to progress to the licensure of a new TB vaccine more rapidly than we could have anticipated just a few years ago. Whereas human and animal challenge models cannot substitute for a rigorously performed vaccine efficacy trial with a disease endpoint, the possibility of licensure through more rapid routes including human and animal challenge, and POI studies will act as a much-needed stimulant to the TB vaccine development pipeline.

SUMMARY

Despite a $1.2B funding shortfall needed to reach ambitious goals set by WHO,[e] this year has seen exciting advances in TB vaccine development. These recent advances are the result of intense international and cross-discipline co-operation, which will be critical in future studies. As with the 2 human efficacy studies published in 2018,[19,21] which have stored samples to identify correlates, or surrogates, of protection; resource and forethought will be needed in future studies to make adequate provision for the biobanking of clinical samples.

A changing regulatory landscape, offering more flexibility for obtaining vaccine licensure, will act as a stimulant to the TB vaccine development pipeline and places the licensure of a new TB vaccine within reach.

This is an exciting time to be working in TB vaccine development. Previously disparate fields such as basic immunology, epidemiology, and mathematical modeling have come together, and learned lessons from other disease areas can be applied to TB research. The results of recent studies, and the pending further analyses from these and others, offer hope that effective TB vaccines may be on the horizon.

---

[e]https://www.nature.com/articles/d41586-018-07708-z.

REFERENCES

1. World Health Organization. Global tuberculosis report 2018. Geneva (Switzerland): WHO; 2018. Available at: https://apps.who.int/iris/handle/10665/274453. License: CC BY-NC-SA 3.0 IGO.
2. Fine P. Variation in protection by BCG: implications of and for heterologous immunity. Lancet 1995;346:1339–45.
3. Mangtani P, Abubakar I, Ariti C, et al. Protection by BCG against tuberculosis: a systematic review of randomised controlled trials. Clin Infect Dis 2014;58:470–80.
4. Abubakar I, Pimpin L, Ariti C, et al. Systematic review and meta-analysis of the current evidence on the duration of protection by bacillus Calmette-Guérin vaccination against tuberculosis. Health Technol Assess (Rockv) 2013;17:1–4.
5. du Preez K, Seddon JA, Schaaf HS, et al. Global shortages of BCG vaccine and tuberculous meningitis in children. Lancet Glob Health 2019;7:e28–9.
6. Higgins JPT, Soares-Weiser K, López-López JA, et al. Association of BCG, DTP, and measles containing vaccines with childhood mortality: systematic review. BMJ 2016;355:i5170.
7. Uplekar M, Weil D, Lonnroth K, et al. WHO's new end TB strategy. Lancet 2015;385:1799–801.
8. Dye C, Glaziou P, Floyd K, et al. Prospects for tuberculosis elimination. Annu Rev Public Health 2013;34:271–86.
9. Zignol M, Dean AS, Falzon D, et al. Twenty years of global surveillance of antituberculosis-drug resistance. N Engl J Med 2016;375:1081–9.
10. Shaler CR, Horvath C, Lai R, et al. Understanding delayed T-cell priming, lung recruitment, and airway luminal T-cell responses in host defense against pulmonary tuberculosis. Clin Dev Immunol 2012;2012:628293.
11. Jagirdar J, ZagZag D. Pathology and insights into pathogenesis of tuberculosis. In: Rom N, Garay S, editors. Tuberculosis. Boston: Brown and Co.; 1996. p. 467–91.
12. Smith I. Mycobacterium tuberculosis pathogenesis and molecular determinants of virulence. Clin Microbiol Rev 2003;16:463–96.
13. Andrews SM, Pollard AJ. A vaccine against serogroup B Neisseria meningitidis: dealing with uncertainty. Lancet Infect Dis 2014;14:426–34.
14. Goldschneider I, Gotschlich EC, Artenstein MS. Human immunity to the meningococcus I. The role of humoral antibodies. J Exp Med 1969;129:1307–26.
15. Goldschneider I, Gotschlich EC, Artenstein MS. Human immunity to the meningococcus II. Development of natural immunity. J Exp Med 1969;129:1327–48.
16. Plotkin SA. Correlates of protection induced by vaccination. Clin Vaccine Immunol 2010;17:1055–65.
17. Kaufmann SHE, Weiner JR, Maertzdorf J. Accelerating tuberculosis vaccine trials with diagnostic and prognostic biomarkers. Expert Rev Vaccines 2017;16:845–53.
18. Bhatt K, Verma S, Ellner JJ, et al. Quest for correlates of protection against tuberculosis. Clin Vaccine Immunol 2015;22:258–66.
19. Van Der Meeren O, Hatherill M, Nduba V, et al. Phase 2b controlled trial of M72/AS01 E vaccine to prevent tuberculosis. N Engl J Med 2018;379:1621–34.
20. Houben R, Dodd PJ. The global burden of latent tuberculosis infection: a re-estimation using mathematical modelling. PLoS Med 2016;13:e1002152.
21. Nemes E, Geldenhuys H, Rozot V, et al. Prevention of M. tuberculosis infection with H4:IC31 vaccine or BCG revaccination. N Engl J Med 2018;379:138–49.
22. Hansen SG, Zak DE, Xu G, et al. Prevention of tuberculosis in rhesus macaques by a cytomegalovirus-based vaccine. Nat Med 2018;24:130–43.
23. Carpenter SM, Behar SM. A new vaccine for tuberculosis in rhesus macaques. Nat Med 2018;24:124–6.
24. Tala-Heikkilä MM, Tuominen JE, Tala EOJ. Bacillus Calmette-Guérin revaccination questionable with low tuberculosis incidence. Am J Respir Crit Care Med 1998;157:1324–7.
25. Rodrigues LC, Pereira SM, Cunha SS, et al. Effect of BCG revaccination on incidence of tuberculosis in school-aged children in Brazil: the BCG-REVAC cluster-randomised trial. Lancet 2005;366:1290–5.
26. Karonga Prevention Trial Group. Randomised controlled trial of single BCG, repeated BCG, or combined BCG and killed Mycobacterium leprae vaccine for prevention of leprosy and tuberculosis in Malawi. Karonga Prevention Trial Group. Lancet 1996;348:17–24.
27. Leung CC, Tam CM, Chan SL, et al. Efficacy of the BCG revaccination programme in a cohort given BCG vaccination at birth in Hong Kong. Int J Tuberc Lung Dis 2001;5:717–23.
28. Harris RC, Sumner T, Knight GM, et al. Systematic review of mathematical models exploring the epidemiological impact of future TB vaccines. Hum Vaccin Immunother 2016;12:2813–32.
29. Harris RC, Sumner T, Knight GM, et al. Age-targeted tuberculosis vaccination in China and implications for vaccine development: a modelling study. Lancet Glob Health 2019;7:e209–18.
30. US Department of Health and Human Services, Food and Drug Administration. Product development under the animal rule guidance for industry 2015. Available at: https://www.fda.gov/media/88625/download.

31. Beasley DWC, Brasel TL, Comer JE. First vaccine approval under the FDA animal rule. NPJ Vaccines 2016;1:5–7.

32. European Medicines Agency. Committee on human medicinal products (CHMP) guideline on clinical evaluation of vaccines. (EMEA/CHMP/VWP/164653/05) 2018. Available at: https://www.ema.europa.eu/en/documents/scientific-guideline/draft-guideline-clinical-evaluation-vaccines-revision-1_en.pdf.

33. Counoupas C, Pinto R, Nagalingam G, et al. *Mycobacterium tuberculosis* components expressed during chronic infection of the lung contribute to long-term control of pulmonary tuberculosis in mice. NPJ Vaccines 2016;1:16012.

34. Penn-Nicholson A, Tameris M, Smit E, et al. Safety and immunogenicity of the novel tuberculosis vaccine ID93 + GLA-SE in BCG-vaccinated healthy adults in South Africa: a randomised, double-blind, placebo-controlled phase 1 trial. Lancet Respir Med 2018;6:287–98.

35. Suliman S, Kany A, Luabeya K, et al. Dose optimization of H56: IC31 vaccine for TB endemic populations: a double-blind, placebo-controlled, dose-selection trial. Am J Respir Crit Care Med 2019;199(2):220–31.

36. Leung-Theung-Long S, Gouanvic M, Coupet CA, et al. A novel MVA-based multiphasic vaccine for prevention or treatment of tuberculosis induces broad and multifunctional cell-mediated immunity in mice and primates. PLoS One 2015;10:1–19.

37. Gonzalo-Asensio J, Marinova D, Martin C, et al. MTBVAC: attenuating the human pathogen of tuberculosis (TB) toward a promising vaccine against the TB epidemic. Front Immunol 2017;8:1–8.

38. Nieuwenhuizen NE, Kulkarni PS, Shaligram U, et al. The recombinant Bacille Calmette-Guérin vaccine VPM1002: ready for clinical efficacy testing. Front Immunol 2017;8:1–9.

39. Lahey T, Laddy D, Hill K, et al. Immunogenicity and protective efficacy of the DAR-901 booster vaccine in a murine model of tuberculosis. PLoS One 2016;11:1–12.

40. von Reyn CF, Mtei L, Arbeit RD, et al. Prevention of tuberculosis in Bacille Calmette-Guérin-primed, HIV-infected adults boosted with an inactivated whole-cell mycobacterial vaccine. AIDS 2010;24:675–85.

Preventing Transmission of *Mycobacterium Tuberculosis*—A Refocused Approach

Edward A. Nardell, MD

KEYWORDS

- TB transmission • TB infection control • TB prevention • Respiratory isolation • Screening
- Ultraviolet • Ventilation • Respirators

KEY POINTS

- Traditional tuberculosis (TB) infection control focuses on known patients with tuberculosis already on therapy, whereas most transmission is from patients with unsuspected TB or unsuspected drug resistance, not on effective therapy.
- For high-burden settings, a refocused, intensified, administrative control strategy, FAST (Find cases Actively, Separate temporarily, and Treat effectively based on molecular diagnostics), attempts to shorten the time from entry to a health care facility and the start of effective treatment.
- For low-burden settings, unsuspected TB also poses the greatest transmission risk, but this is better addressed by increased awareness through education.
- Because not every infectious case will be detected and promptly treated, air disinfection is important in high-risk settings. Environmental controls such as ventilation and germicidal air disinfection reduce risk. Increasing use of air conditioning in warming climates require air supplemental disinfection as windows are closed.
- Germicidal ultraviolet air disinfection is underused, but after natural ventilation, it is the most cost-effective and sustainable technology.

INTRODUCTION

Awareness of how *Mycobacterium tuberculosis* (*Mtb*) is spread, and precautions to prevent it, came long after Robert Koch's 1882 discovery of the causative bacillus.[1] In Thomas Mann's 1924 novel set in prewar Europe, for example, Hans Castorp visits his cousin, a tuberculosis patient in an alpine tuberculosis sanatorium, completely oblivious of any risk from sharing a room with his cousin for weeks and taking every meal in a dining hall filled with untreated, coughing patients with TB.[2] Little did he know that he already had the disease. Sanitoria were a form of treatment in the prechemotherapy era, not isolation facilities. Although long suspected as airborne, and the subject of numerous earlier transmission experiments, it was not until mid-twentieth century that Riley and colleagues[3] unequivocally proved the point by demonstrating human-to-guinea pig transmission when the only contact was shared air.[4] Further, Riley showed that all transmission stopped if the ward exhaust air was disinfected with ultraviolet light, and

Funding for the author's research underlying this review was provided primarily by NIOSH (CDC/NIOSH: 1RO1 OH009050) and NIH (1D43TW009379).

Division of Global Health Equity, Harvard Medical School, Brigham & Women's Hospital, 75 Francis Street, Boston, MA 02115, USA

E-mail address: enardell@BWH.harvard.edu

Clin Chest Med 40 (2019) 857–869
https://doi.org/10.1016/j.ccm.2019.07.010
0272-5231/19/© 2019 Published by Elsevier Inc.

chestmed.theclinics.com

most importantly, transmission stopped almost immediately with the start of effective treatment, as shown in **Table 1**.[4]

THE RAPID IMPACT ON TRANSMISSION OF EFFECTIVE *M TUBERCULOSIS* TREATMENT

Table 1 shows the results of Riley's second, 2-year experiment, where patients with sputum smear- and culture-positive TB were admitted to the 6-bed Baltimore Veterans' Administration Hospital ward and either treated immediately or had their treatment delayed so that the impact of treatment could be quantified.[3] Treated patients, based on comparable person-time on the ward, were 98% less infectious that untreated patients. This was at a time when the only drugs available for treating TB were isoniazid (INH), para-aminosalicylic acid, and streptomycin, a relatively weak regimen by today's standards. Patients whose *Mtb* isolates were drug resistant, most often to INH, also became less infectious when treated with the remaining drugs, but the numbers were too few to be sure, according to Riley. An often-overlooked finding of this study was the rapidity of the impact of treatment on transmission. Patients began treatment at the same time that they entered the ward, not 2 weeks or even 2 days earlier. The powerful impact of effective chemotherapy on transmission was essentially *immediate* or as long as it took to reach therapeutic levels in tissues. So important and underappreciated is this observation that it deserves to be expressed in Riley's own words:[4]

> The treated patients were admitted to the ward at the time treatment was initiated and were generally removed before the sputum became completely negative. Hence the decrease in infectiousness preceded the elimination of the organisms from the sputum, indicating that the effect was prompt as well as striking. ...Drug therapy appeared to be effective in reducing the infectivity of patients with drug resistant organisms, but the data do not permit detailed analysis of the problem.[4]

Independent of these landmark human-to-guinea pig experimental results, the rapid impact of effective treatment was also studied epidemiologically in the 1960s and 70s with several household contact investigations summarized by a review paper by Rouillion and colleagues.[5] Beginning with a controlled trial of ambulatory and hospital treatment in Madras, India, several observational studies in the United Studies showed that household contacts of newly diagnosed pulmonary TB cases that were tuberculin skin test (TST) negative after the index case started treatment were no more likely to convert their TST than noncontacts in the general population.[5,6] These studies were used as evidence in favor of the ambulatory treatment of TB, suggesting that patients on therapy rapidly became noninfectious, well before sputum smear and culture conversion, which occurs, on average, at about 2 months into treatment. But exactly how much therapy was needed was not discernible from epidemiologic observations, and Riley's human-to-animal data appear not to have been considered in formulating transmission control policies at that time. Instead, by consensus, Rouillion and colleagues[5] made first reference to "*less than 2 weeks*" as the amount of treatment that renders patients noninfectious, regardless of sputum smear or culture status, assuming a clinical

---

Table 1
Outcome of human-to-guinea pig *Mycobacterium tuberculosis* transmission studies, showing the rapid impact of effective treatment on transmission among drug-susceptible and drug-resistant patients

Patients with Susceptible *Mtb*	Numbers of GPs Infected	Relative Infectiousness[a]
Untreated	29	100%
Treated	1	2%
Patients with drug-resistant *Mtb*		
Untreated	14	28%
Treated	6	5%

Note that the only available drugs at the time were isoniazid (INH), streptomycin, and para-aminosalicylic acid, so drug-resistant patients, usually INH resistant at least, had very few treatment options.[4]

Abbreviation: GP, guinea pig.

[a] All smear-positive patients, relative to the amount of time spent on the ward.

From Riley RL, Mills CC, O'grady F, et al. Infectiousness of air from a tuberculosis ward. Ultraviolet irradiation of infected air: comparative infectiousness of different patients. Am Rev Respir Dis 1962;85:511–25; with permission.

response to treatment evident by decreasing cough, an increasing sense of well-being, and usually, less positive sputum smears.

> There is an ever-increasing amount of evidence in support of the idea that abolition of the patient's infectiousness – a different matter from 'cure,' which takes months, and from negative results of bacteriological examinations, direct and culture, which may take weeks – is very probably obtained after less than 2 weeks of treatment....These facts seem to indicate very rapid and powerful action by the drugs on infectivity...[5]

Although the *"2-week rule"* and the epidemiologic evidence on which it was based have been criticized as potentially biased, it has never been rigorously tested clinically.[7] Such a trial would be challenging to design and conduct in high- or low-risk settings. Instead, in recent years it is still common to see the assertion that patients responding to effective therapy who remain sputum smear- or culture-positive on effective treatment should be considered still infectious.[8] Because sputum smear positivity in untreated patients is appropriately used as one of several indicators of probable infectiousness, the grounds for confusion are clear. But as a result of this confusion, sputum smear conversion is still commonly used as a criterion for ending TB isolation or discharge from hospitals in low-prevalence settings despite the acceptance of entirely ambulatory TB treatment for more than 50 years. Another factor is that hospital infection control polices tend to be conservative at the expense of overisolation of patients rather than risking exposing health care workers or other patients. Finally, during the 1985 to 1992 resurgence of multidrug-resistant (MDR) TB in the United States and other countries, patients with *unsuspected* MDR-TB remained infectious after 2 weeks of what turned out to be *ineffective* therapy, but nevertheless tarnishing the dogma that patients could no longer transmit after 2 weeks treatment.[9] In an era of rapid molecular drug susceptibly testing, unsuspected drug-resistant TB is less likely in many parts of the world, but not everywhere.

THE IMPACT OF EFFECTIVE TREATMENT ON DRUG-RESISTANT TUBERCULOSIS TRANSMISSION

As noted, Riley's human-to-guinea pig studies, conducted in an era before MDR-TB and extensively drug-resistant (XDR) TB, left the issue of the impact of effective treatment for drug-resistant TB unresolved.[4] Given the 1985 to 1992 experience of MDR-TB transmission on treatment,

albeit *infective* treatment, and the higher morbidity, mortality, and difficulty treating MDR-TB, health departments and hospitals adopted more rigorous transmission isolation policies, largely based on sputum smear, and sometimes culture conversion. Those policies largely remain in place today. Although conversion times have shortened with some of the newer treatment regimens for highly resistant TB, they are still measurable in months. But because it has been long known that transmission ceases well before sputum smear and culture conversion, it can be safely assumed that isolation under such policies is unnecessarily long but an understandable caution in the absence of transmission data for MDR-TB on treatment. Two other revivals of the Riley human-to-guinea pig transmission experimental model are relevant to the impact of treatment on transmission.[10–12]

In 2008, Escombe and colleagues[10,11] reported results from the first human-to-guinea pig (H-GP) transmission experiments since Riley's 50 years earlier. Escombe exposed 292 guinea pigs to the exhaust air from a TB-human immunodeficiency virus (HIV) ward in Peru. Over 505 days, 97 patients with HIV-TB infected 125 general practitioners (GPs), 98% were due to 9 patients with unsuspected MDR-TB, being treated for drug-susceptible (DS) TB. Three DS patients infected 1 GP each, but 2 of the patients had delayed treatment and 1 had had treatment stopped. This study confirmed Riley's earlier findings that effective treatment of DS *Mtb* nearly completely suppresses transmission, with transmission predominantly from unsuspected patients with MDR-TB not being effectively treated.[11] But what of MDR-TB treatment?

In 2005, Nardell and colleagues[12] also established an H-GP transmission facility in South Africa (Airborne Infection Research Facility [AIR]), specifically to study MDR-TB transmission, in part because DS patients on therapy do not infect GPs. The purpose was to study the dynamics of transmission and to test transmission interventions, such as germicidal ultraviolet air disinfection and masks on patients (to be discussed later), and also to examine the impact of treatment.[8,13,14] The assumption was that patients with MDR-TB just started on therapy would remain infectious long enough to infect guinea pigs. In the authors' first (pilot) study 26 DR patients infected 74% of 362 exposed GPs.[12] But in the next 4 experiments, a total of 109 patients selected by the same criteria (mostly sputum smear positive, cavitary chest x-ray, coughing, and just started on MDR-TB therapy) had highly variable results, in order, infecting 10% over 3 months, 53% over 2 months, 1% over

3 months, and 77% over 3 months exposure. The reason for this variability was not apparent until fingerprinting results of *Mtb* isolates from GPs infected in the pilot study came back, showing 8 different spoligotypes, but only 2 that transmitted to GPs, both associated with cases of unsuspected XDR-TB. XDR-TB existed but had not yet been described at the time of the AIR pilot study.[8] Although the standard South African MDR treatment regimen rapidly stopped MDR-transmission, it did not stop the transmission from unsuspected XDR-TB. In the fourth H-GP study, importantly, 27 patients with DR-TB exposed 90 GPs over 3 months, but only 1 GP was infected. Fortuitously, none of the 27 patients had XDR by conventional drug susceptibility testing or line probe assay. Effective MDR-TB treatment promptly suppressed all but one instance of MDR-TB H-GP transmission over 3 months.[8] But does specific XDR-TB treatment suppress XDR-TB transmission?

Recently, 2 as yet unpublished studies from the AIR facility address that question. Five patients with MDR-TB failing standard treatment were eligible to receive both bedaquiline and linezolid under South African policy. The patients entered the AIR facility and were studied for 8 days before (exhaust air to 90 GPs in chamber A) and for 11 days after starting therapy (exhaust air from the last 8 days to GPs in chamber B).[15] For the first 72 hours of treatment exhaust air did not expose GPs, to allow some time for drugs to act. There was no difference in the GP infection rate before and after the onset of drugs to which their *Mtb* was susceptible. Using a similar protocol, the highly curative "NIX-TB" regimen (bedaquiline, high-dose linezolid, and pretomanid) was then tested for its ability to rapidly suppress transmission to GPs. Patient-day exposure time of GPs before and after

the start of treatment was the same and was the same as for the first study. Again, 72 hours treatment time was excluded to allow the drugs to reach tissues. This regimen completely suppressed transmission of patients with XDR/MDR-TB who qualified for the regimen.[16]

In summary, effective treatment of DS and MDR-TB seems to rapidly stop transmission, but for more highly resistant *Mtb*, the effect on transmission may depend on the specific drugs used, their pharmacokinetics/pharmacodynamics, and their effects on as yet unknown microbial mechanisms required for airborne transport and reestablishing infection in a new host. More research in this area in needed, including drugs delivered via the airways that might have selective effect on transmission.

UNSUSPECTED TUBERCULOSIS AND UNSUSPECTED DRUG RESISTANCE—THE PRINCIPAL SOURCES OF *M TUBERCULOSIS* TRANSMISSION

TB transmission control as currently practiced is *wrongly focused on patients with TB* and needs to be refocused. This seems to be true in both high- and low-burden setting, but for different reasons. If it is true that effective treatment renders patients with TB rapidly noninfectious, the logical corollary is that the greater risk in health care and other congregate settings is from persons with pulmonary TB not on effective therapy either because they are unsuspected and undiagnosed or because they have unsuspected drug resistance. There have been remarkably few studies quantifying the rate of undiagnosed TB in congregate settings where the most effective transmission is likely to occur.[17,18] **Fig. 1** conceptualizes risk of transmission as progressing slowly from

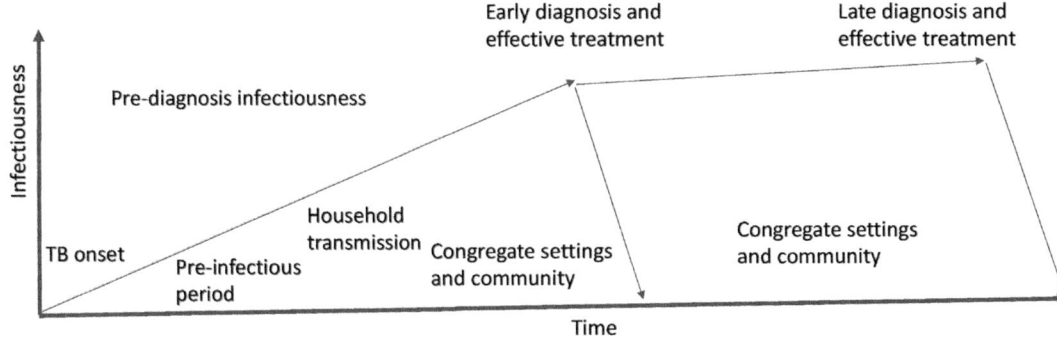

Fig. 1. Progressive TB infectiousness until diagnosis and effective treatment. *Reprinted* with permission of the American Thoracic Society. Copyright © 2019 American Thoracic Society. Riley RL, Mills CC, O'Grady F, et al. Infectiousness of air from a tuberculosis ward. Ultraviolet irradiation of infected air: comparative infectiousness of different patients. Am Rev Respir Dis 1962;85:511-25. The American Journal of Respiratory and Critical Care Medicine is an official journal of the American Thoracic Society.

the time of clinical onset, increasing with the cough, lung cavitation, and sputum smear positivity, to first infect household members sharing common air. But compared with congregate settings and the community, the number of susceptible persons in the household is limited and decreases as the most vulnerable are infected.[19] Despite less individual contact time in the community and nonresidential indoor congregate settings, increasing infectiousness and number of susceptible contacts results in greater spread outside of households, according to some analyses.[19] But as previously emphasized, transmission stops almost immediately with diagnosis and effective treatment of the index case. Active case finding and prompt effective treatment is increasingly recognized as the principal goal for controlling transmission-driven epidemics in high-burden settings. In low-burden settings where reactivation of latent infection predominates, not suspecting TB becomes the norm, and unsuspected cases continue to be the cause of focal outbreaks, for example, in intensive care units, dialysis units, and other clinical settings, as well as homeless shelters, and occasional nursing homes.

FIND CASES ACTIVELY, SEPARATE TEMPORARILY, AND TREAT EFFECTIVELY: A REFOCUSED, INTENSIFIED, ADMINISTRATIVE APPROACH TO TUBERCULOSIS TRANSMISSION CONTROL IN HIGH-BURDEN SETTINGS

If effective treatment renders most cases of TB quickly noninfectious, and most transmission in high-burden settings occurs from patients with unsuspected TB, or unsuspected drug resistance, not on effective treatment, it follows that one administrative approach to transmission control might be active case finding followed by rapid diagnosis and prompt effective treatment based on rapid molecular drug susceptibility testing.[20] This approach, packaged as F-A-S-T (Find cases Actively, Separate temporarily, and Treat effectively), has been piloted in many countries, and some early reports have been published.[21] So far, results indicate that liberally applying rapid molecular diagnostics in a chest hospital in Bangladesh, for example, resulted in the detection of many patients with otherwise unsuspected TB, especially among patients with a past history of TB. Most remarkably, so far, are results from a study of 2 TB hospitals in Russia.[22]

In Voronezh and Petrozavodsk, Russia, for example, investigators implemented a targeted form of F-A-S-T in 2 TBs hospitals to reduce transmission from patients with unsuspected MDR-TB.

Hospitalization was prolonged before and after implementation—an average of 20.7 weeks before and 20.0 weeks after implementation.[22] Universal Xpert testing was initiated on all admissions to both the 800-bed and 120-bed facilities, followed by prompt (less than 48 hours) Xpert-directed treatment of DS and rifampin-resistant TB. Before implementation of universal Xpert testing it took an average of 76.5 days before MDR-TB was diagnosed and patients started on effective treatment. They compared the subsequent rate of MDR-TB generation associated with hospitalization to the baseline rate, pre-FAST. Of a total of 450 patients HR sensitive on admission before implementation, 12.2% were diagnosed with MDR-TB within 12 months of finishing treatment. Of the 259 patients isonizid and rifampin (HR) sensitive after implementation of universal molecular testing and prompt, effective treatment, only 3.1% were subsequently diagnosed with MDR-TB within 12 months of finishing treatment—a 78% odds reduction in MDR acquisition through the interruption of transmission by prompt, effective treatment of MDR-TB case in hospital.[22]

However, F-A-S-T is not applicable to all settings, for example, where the prevalence of TB is too low or too high. Where TB is an uncommon cause of cough, cough surveillance is sure to be a cost-ineffective screening strategy, as might any other screening test. Most positive results would likely be false positives under low-prevalence conditions. But in a crowded ambulatory clinic in Mumbai, for example, where transmission from unsuspected cases is occurring in waiting rooms and corridors, there is currently no inexpensive point-of-care test for TB disease that is sensitive, specific, and fast enough to allow routine detection, triage, and prompt treatment. At this time, an achievable strategy might be applying F-A-S-T for all hospital admission in selected high-burden settings, with a goal of promptly detecting and effectively treating otherwise unsuspected TB, and unsuspected drug resistance, thereby eliminating the likely sources of transmission. Measures of success include greater case detection among hospital admissions and a shorter time from entry until the start of effective treatment based on a molecular DST.[20] But even in such settings, questions remain. Asking patients about to be admitted about any cough, or cough for 2 weeks, may be an insensitive and nonspecific screening question in some populations or times of year. A screening chest radiograph with computer-assisted interpretation might detect most transmissible TB in low-HIV settings, such as Peru, but is it affordable and worth the radiation exposure?

OTHER TUBERCULOSIS TRANSMISSION FACTORS AND INTERVENTIONS

TB transmission is complex, involving characteristic of not only the infectious source case but also the organism, the environment, and the host, all of which are important in preventing transmission. **Fig. 2** depicts transmission broadly, listing key variables in each category, and possible interventions that impact transmission.

Source strength. Not all patients with pulmonary TB infect others. Epidemiologic studies have suggested that perhaps only 1 in 3 patients with pulmonary TB infect any contacts. Likewise, Sultan and colleagues[23] found great patient-to-patient variability in infectiousness even when patients were selected for having positive sputum smears and cultures. Likewise, Fennelly was able to detect culturable aerosol in about one-third of smear-positive patients.[24] Sputum smear positivity, cough frequency and strength, sputum viscosity, and ability to generate aerosol have long been considered source strength factors. As discussed, prompt detection and effective treatment (FAST) may be the best way to limit source strength. *Cough hygiene* and its equivalent, wearing *surgical masks*, stops large respiratory droplets from becoming airborne droplet nuclei. Simple surgical face masks worn by patients most of the day reduced transmission to guinea pigs by 56%.[14]

Organisms. Mtb strain virulence is likely a transmission factor but not one that affects transmission control efforts. Organism number and viability are controllable by air disinfection strategies: dilution, extraction, directional airflow, filtration, precipitation, and killing. Although a variety of chemical disinfectants, such as glycol vapors, have been tried in the past, by far the most effective and cost-effective approach to killing airborne pathogens is upper-room germicidal ultraviolet irradiation (GUV), as detailed later.[25,26] Natural ventilation is the most important means of air disinfection, globally, with mechanical ventilation used in more affluent countries.[27,28]

Host resistance. Resistance to TB infection and disease varies by individual innate and adaptive immunity, and through epigenetic influences, but protection is usually incomplete. Exposure to related environmental mycobacteria and leprosy increases resistance. Heavily exposed populations pass on resistance genetically, and possibly epigenetically, so called learned immunity.[29,30] From a transmission control perspective, BCG and a newer vaccine have been shown to convey resistance to infection as well as disease progression, although incomplete.[31] Diabetes, HIV-AIDS, and other illnesses and drugs lower resistance. The growing use of TNF inhibitors is the fastest growing category of therapeutics that often increase risk to TB infection or disease. Of potential practical importance, several host-directed therapies, notably metformin and the statins, may well prevent Mtb infection and progression to disease, and these or similar drugs may serve a protective role in the

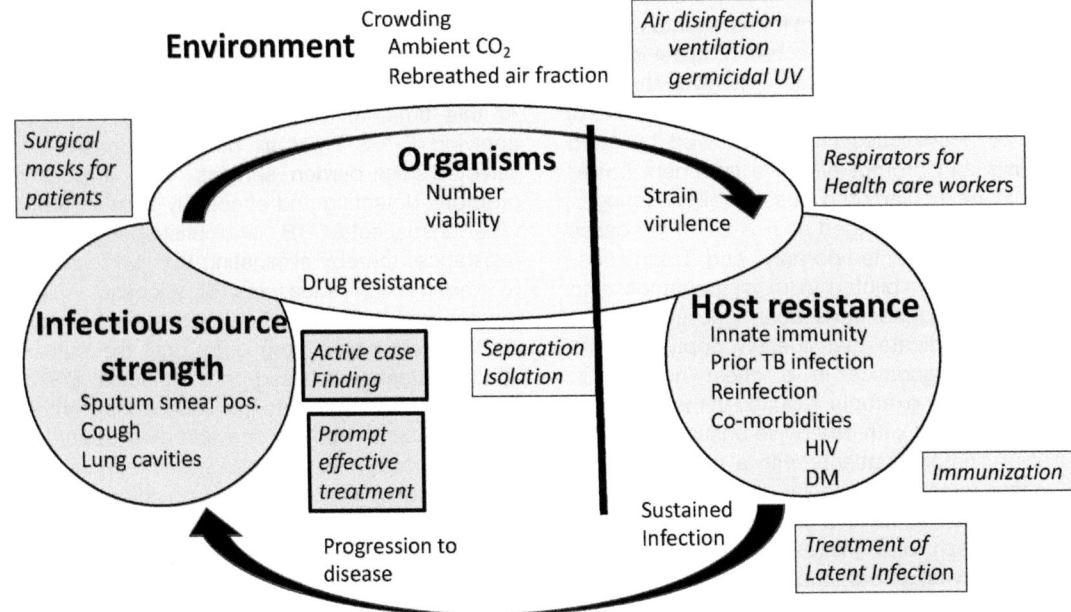

Fig. 2. Transmission factors and potential sites for intervention.

future.[32–34] Treatment of latent infection can prevent progression from infection to disease, but does it reduce the beneficial immunity of infection? There is no direct data, but analogy with BCG immunization suggests that, as hypersensitivity, the estimated 70% protection of previous infection persists long after viable organisms remain.[35]

REDUCING TUBERCULOSIS EXPOSURE FROM UNSUSPECTED SOURCES: THE ROLE OF ENVIRONMENTAL INTERVENTIONS AND RESPIRATORY PROTECTION

As emphasized, persons with infectious pulmonary tuberculosis remain infectious until diagnosed and started on effective therapy. But there are many settings where patients with undiagnosed TB can be anticipated and are not likely to all be promptly diagnosed and started on effective therapy, such as busy emergency rooms and crowded ambulatory waiting areas and corridors. Environmental controls are important in these and other areas.

Natural ventilation. In much of the world where TB is common, natural ventilation is the main form of air disinfection and can be highly effective, but there are many caveats, and there is the new threat of climate change—closed windows because more and more clinical areas are air conditioned and also to keep out polluted air.[36] With a building designed for cross-ventilation, in a warm or temperate climate, and with favorable outside conditions, it is hard to beat the effectiveness, low cost, and sustainability of natural ventilation (**Fig. 3**). Where climate permits, outdoor waiting areas are ideal and largely independent of building design. But many buildings are poorly designed for natural ventilation, with deep interior spaces where air exchange is limited. A common scenario in ambulatory setting are doctor's offices

on both sides of a corridor, windows only in the offices, with cross-ventilation that depends on open transom windows above doors when doors are closed, while the corridors themselves becoming crowded waiting areas, as shown in **Fig. 4**. Windows are often closed because of cool night air or for security. Natural ventilation has long been limited to air infiltration in very cold climates, together with prolonged hospitalization and delayed diagnosis, accounting for the hypertransmission of MDR-TB in recent decades in Eastern Europe, Russia, FSU countries, and Central Asia. With global warming, however, similar conditions are becoming commonplace in hot countries, as windows are closed to allow for effective and efficient cooling with ductless air conditioners.[37] In an office occupied by 5 people in South Africa we recently demonstrated the effect of closing an open window and turning on a ductless air conditioner (AC) unit. Within an hour of closing the window ambient CO_2 measurements increased 4-fold with no plateau in sight, indicating comparable increase in risk of an airborne infection, given an infectious source in the room.[38] What are the options when natural ventilation is limited by building design or outside conditions?

In theory, there are 3 alternatives to natural ventilation. *Mechanical ventilation systems* are the norm in most resource rich countries, especially in large

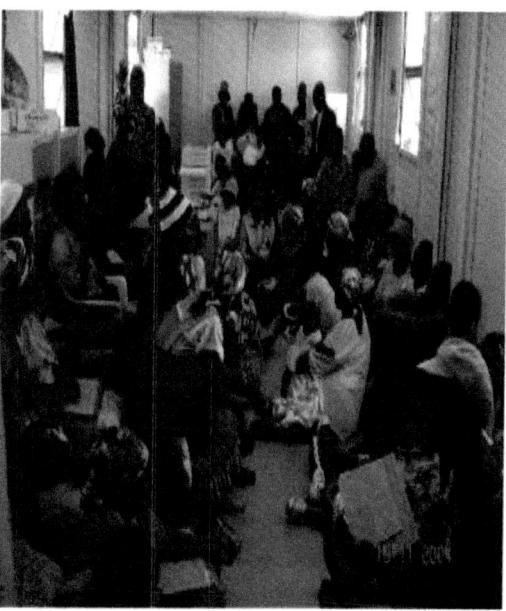

Fig. 4. MDR-TB Clinic, Karachi, Pakistan; Tariq Alexander Qaiser, architect. Note the wind scoop design in the main building and a covered outdoor waiting area, both taking full advantage of natural ventilation.

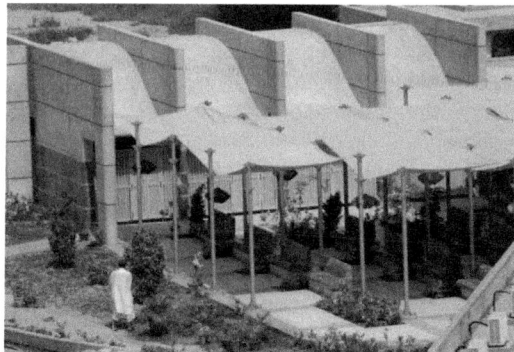

Fig. 3. Crowded waiting area typical of ambulatory clinics in high-burden settings.

buildings such as hospitals. In poor countries where TB is prevalent, mechanical ventilation is uncommon in public buildings. It is expensive to install in new construction, difficult to retrofit, and expensive to operate and maintain, especially when outdoor air must be heated or cooled. Unless specifically designed for airborne infection control, and maintained, air exchange rates of outdoor air rarely reach the recommended 6-12 room air changes per hour (ACH). When operating optimally, however, mechanical ventilation assures that indoor conditions remain predictable day and night, season to season, independent of outside conditions.[39] Basic mechanical ventilation technology is well understood by trained mechanical engineers, despite often poor maintenance in practice due to administrative neglect.

An alternative air disinfection approach, heavily marketed around the world, is *room air cleaner technology*. Room air cleaners move room air through a filter or alternative germicidal technology (ultraviolet, plasma, etc) designed to remove or kill pathogens.[40] Sales presentations commonly show data proving that contaminated air is nearly completely disinfected when it exits in the device, thanks to their unique technology. What they rarely mention is the actual clean air delivery rate—the flow rate of decontaminated air produced by the device—and how many equivalent ACH that equates to in a given room. Moreover, there is a tendency for room air cleaners, with intake and outlet located near each other, to recapture just decontaminated air (short-circuiting), reducing the *effective* equivalent ACH produced. These devices vary greatly from one to another, but many produce no more than 1 to 2 equivalent ACH in average size rooms. It is a difficult engineering task to move all room air through a single device without unacceptable noise and drafts. In theory, room air cleaners should work, but in practice they tend to be suitable for small rooms where alternative technologies cannot be used.

Another air disinfection technology, highly effective but underused for more than 70 years, is GUV (**Fig. 5**). There are now 2 controlled studies showing 70% to 80% efficacy in reducing *Mtb* transmission under real hospital conditions.[41,42] Application guidelines are now scientifically based, and the technology is recommended in the new WHO TB Infection Control Guidelines.[43] Compared with room air cleaners that try to move room air through a disinfecting device, upper-room GUV disinfects large volumes of room air continuously, relying on air mixing between the upper and lower room to protect room occupants.[44,45] Air mixing can be assured by commonly available low-velocity mixing fans,

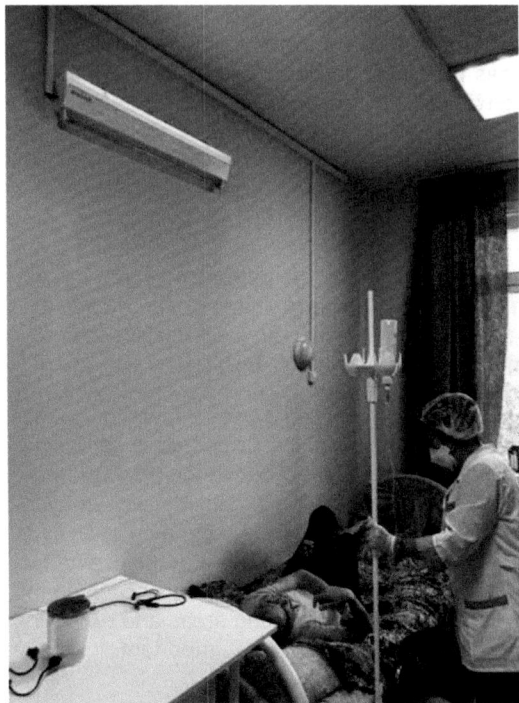

Fig. 5. Upper-room GUV fixture in use in a Russian hospital.

rated to produce at least 20 ACH between the upper and lower room. Properly used, GUV technology is safe. Fixtures are designed to deliver GUV to the upper room, blocking spill and reflection into the lower room. The major risk is eye irritation, almost always the result of poor installation, poor fixtures, or accidental direct exposure of workers to GUV in the upper room, such as painting or cleaning.

A major GUV application development is the requirement that fixture manufacturers have their devices independently tested in a lighting laboratory for total GUV output.[42,46] This is required to allow design engineers to dose rooms at approximately 12 mW/m^3 total volume, based on the published and subsequent experiments preventing transmission in a South African hospital. A disadvantage of GUV, compared with mechanical ventilation systems, is that engineers have generally not been trained in its use. Maintenance is not difficult but is necessary to assure sustained function. A manual on GUV maintenance is available in the literature and online in English, Spanish, and Russian: (http://www.stoptb.org/wg/ett/assets/documents/MaintenanceManual.pdf).

GUV is highly cost-effective compared with mechanical ventilation and room air cleaners. Volchenkov and Jensen used a bacterial aerosol to test the air disinfection effectiveness of mechanical ventilation, 3 different room air cleaners, and GUV in a hospital in Vladimir, Russia, finding that GUV was more than 9 times more cost-effective compared with mechanical ventilation or room air cleaners per equivalent air change.[47] Barriers to the more effective use of GUV as the logical alternative to natural ventilation in high-burden settings include lack of familiarity with the technology, fear (unfounded) of radiation injury, lack of technical expertise to plan installations, lack of locally made high-quality fixtures, unreliable electrical power, and cost of installation and maintenance. A plan for sustainable implementation has been developed for India using an international service company that may solve many of these logistical barriers.[48,49] The rapid development of LED GUV, although years from commercial availability, will enable the use of solar power and battery back-up, addressing the power issue. As global warming leads to greater use of highly efficient cooling through ductless AC, the pairing of upper-room GUV fixtures and wall AC units that also provide excellent air mixing may further stimulate the development of high-quality, lower-cost GUV products.

RESPIRATORY ISOLATION

Respiratory isolation, as defined by the CDC, refers to a combination of administrative policies and environmental controls designed to prevent the spread of infectious droplet nuclei from patient known or suspected to have symptomatic, infectious pulmonary or extrapulmonary TB. Respiratory isolation is expensive to achieve in modern mechanically ventilated buildings because it means controlling and monitoring the pressure differences between rooms and corridors that drive directional airflow, assuring that flow is always entering the isolation room. For that reason, several respiratory isolation rooms are routinely found in hospitals in resource-rich settings, where they are used for a variety of potentially contagious respiratory infections, including patients thought to have TB. Respiratory isolation rooms are rarely found in resource-poor settings not only because of cost and technical limitations but also because of the number of patients who would require isolation if it were available. Instead, cohorting of like patients is the norm in many high-risk settings. For example, in Haiti, a naturally ventilated ward is used for sputum smear-positive patients assumed to have drug-susceptible TB for the initial days or weeks of treatment. For relapse patients in whom MDR-TB is more likely, a simple single-bed room is used, with doors and windows closed and an exhaust fan producing negative pressure

(resulting in airflow into the room under the door). Air disinfection is enhanced by an upper-room GUV fixture and mixing fan. With the growing availability of rapid diagnostics and DST, the use of respiratory isolation in hospitals can and should be limited to just a few days as effective treatment is initiated and patients respond clinically.

In low-risk settings for TB, *hospital isolation is often overused*. Because TB has become uncommon and unfamiliar to health care workers and public health departments, it generates greater fear and fear of liability. Low-risk persons with upper lobe infiltrates are often isolated, but if they have no sputum, they remain in isolation based on strict smear-based discharge criteria. Because TB patients need *not* be admitted to hospital to start treatment, and household members have already been exposed, the threshold for discharge home for patients with DS TB once therapy starts should usually be low and not dependent on sputum smear conversion, as emphasized earlier. Smear-positive patients on effective therapy who are responding to therapy can and should be sent home after a few days, if hospitalized at all. Household members will be tested and started on preventive treatment if indicated. Homeless patients and other special situations require individualized treatment and isolation plans. Likewise, public health home quarantine guidelines need to be revised. Although patients with TB responding to effective therapy ought not immediately return to work in day care or a neonatal unit, for example, a few days of treatment is adequate, if they are responding to treatment, coughing less, and feeling better to return to most jobs based on available evidence. TB is a serious infection with systemic symptoms that often justifies time off for recovery but not for transmission control per se.

RESPIRATORS AND SURGICAL MASKS

Air disinfection only works in specific areas where it is applied and is not applied in every high-risk situation, transporting an unsuspected or untreated patient in an elevator or in the back of an ambulance, for example, Respiratory protection is considered the last category of interventions to prevent *Mtb* transmission because they only work when applied, which assumes awareness of risk.[50] Ironically, for that reason, they are most often used by health care workers in the presence of patients on effective therapy who are incorrectly assumed to be still infectious. They are more appropriate for health care workers in the emergency room or ambulatory setting seeing new patients with undiagnosed respiratory symptoms who may be at risk of pulmonary TB. They are especially important for workers present at cough-generating procedures such as bronchoscopy and sputum induction in both high- and low-burden settings.

The distinction between *respirators* and *surgical masks* is important.[50] *Respirators* are designed to protect the wearer by excluding airborne particles, whereas *surgical masks* are designed to protect a surgical field or others in the room by reducing the production of airborne particles by the wearer. When recommended as an influenza precaution, surgical masks primarily serve as a barrier to touching contaminated surfaces and then touching your own nose or mouth. Although surgical masks block some (probably fewer than 50% depending on the mask) inhaled airborne particles, they are not a substitute for a "fit-tested" disposable or reusable N95 or equivalent respiratory, the filtration material that excludes virtually all airborne particles, allowing particles only around the imperfect face seal.[51] Face seal leak from most disposable respirators ranges from 10% to 20% and much lower if respirators have been qualitatively fit tested and a selection of sizes and models to fit a variety of face shapes is available. Beards make proper fit of ordinary respirators impossible. Persons with facial hair need to use a positive-pressure air-purifying respirator where fit testing is unnecessary, as all leakage is out. Such respirators offer maximum respiratory protection for a variety of applications, including exposure to known highly drug-resistant patients or their laboratory specimens or cultures.

Surgical masks are sometimes used temporarily on patients with known or suspected TB as a form of cough hygiene. Surgical masks are stigmatizing and should be used selectively for short periods *before*, but *not after* effective treatment starts. In human-to-guinea pig transmission experiments, simple over-the-ear surgical masks were 56% effective in preventing transmission when worn most of the day—that is, removed for eating, teeth brushing, etc.[14] Appropriate short-term use of surgical masks includes coughing patients in a waiting room or during transport before diagnosis and treatment or longer if drug resistance is suspected while awaiting laboratory results. Discharging patients on effective therapy with a box of face masks to be worn at home or at work is unnecessary and stigmatizing.

TESTING AND TREATING HEALTH CARE WORKERS FOR TUBERCULOSIS INFECTION AND DISEASE

The details of latent TB infection (LTBI) testing and treatment are discussed elsewhere in this issue. Its relevance to transmission control is mentioned here.

In low-burden settings, testing and treating health care workers for latent infection had long been the norm based on studies of nurses and doctors showing risks 2 or more times that of the general population. But just before the 1985 resurgence of TB, the necessity of ongoing screening was questioned, as conversion rates approached that of the community. With the 1985 to 1992 TB resurgence, worker testing was again emphasized, although Centers for Disease Control published criteria for institutions where testing is not required.[50] Now again, as TB rates in this country are far lower than 1985 rates, the value of ongoing testing for many workers should be reassessed. It is well known that under low-risk conditions, many positive results, TST or Interferon Gamma Release Assay (IGRA), will be false positives. Many 10 mm TST reactions and borderline positive IGRA tests are unlikely to represent TB infection, much less a risk of reactivation. Most "convertors" from just less than to just greater than the positive threshold under low-risk conditions are unlikely to have been recently TB infected—an event that normally cause a much greater immunologic response in an otherwise healthy host. Testing often results in unnecessary radiographs and treatment. Stopping testing, of course, risks missing some true health care worker infections, sometimes the only clue to recent exposure to a patient with unsuspected, untreated TB.

In high-burden settings, testing and treating LTBI, even among health care workers, is rarely done for a variety of reasons: limited resources for testing and treatment, stigma, and a different understanding of TB infection risk among them. Confounding by BCG vaccination makes tuberculin testing difficult to interpret. Although IGRA testing was developed to avoid BCG cross-reactivity, the high cost of IGRA testing and the difficulty of interpreting variable responses, likely representing ongoing exposure, combined with reluctance to accept treatment, has limited implementation. Still, as the ultrasound and other low-burden settings decades ago, health care workers are being exposed, infected, and becoming sick with TB at rates well greater than the general population. The prevention strategies outlined in this article should be implemented. In addition, efforts to develop targeted IGRA testing programs for high-risk workers, evidence-based interpretation algorithms, and practical treatment strategies accompanied by worker education still seem justified. New preventative treatments for drug-resistant infection are needed, possibly including host-directed therapies in the near future.

MORE COMPREHENSIVE, WORLD HEALTH ORGANIZATION EVIDENCE-BASED GUIDELINES

A revised WHO TB transmission control policy has recently been issued, and an accompanying implementation guide is being developed.[43] The policy document is limited by recommendations based on (scarce) hard evidence supplemented by expert opinion, whereas the implementation guide is less constrained, based on experience, with additional practical application advice.

SUMMARY

The focus of traditional TB transmission control needs to change from the patient known to have TB who is believed to be on effective therapy and who is responding to treatment, to interventions to prevent transmission from patients unsuspected of having TB or of having drug-resistant TB, who are not on effective treatment. In high-burden settings, by definition, any patient with new or prolonged cough, or other TB symptoms, should be rapidly "ruled out" for TB. How best to cost-effectively rule out TB with currently available diagnostics is unclear at this time. WHO has defined the properties of an effective "rule-out" test for TB, which is different (highly sensitive, but less specific) than a confirmatory "rule-in" test for the disease. For HIV, rapid tests have served both functions for years. In low-burden settings, most patients with typical but nonspecific TB symptoms will not have the disease, so the challenge for sensitive, but reasonably specific rule-out tests is even greater. The newest molecular diagnostics discussed elsewhere in this issue are both highly sensitive and highly specific, also providing rapid drug susceptibility results to guide initial therapy—but require a sputum specimen—a barrier at the TB screening stage.

As emphasized, effective treatment rapidly stops transmission of drug susceptible and MDR-TB. The "NIX-TB" oral regimen, still at the investigative stage" seem to also rapidly stop XDR-TR transmission in preliminary, as yet unpublished H-GP studies. Once on effective therapy, with evidence of a clinical response, further transmission control interventions are probably not needed, although warranted in settings (hospitals, congregate settings) where vulnerable populations could be exposed, should treatment prove ineffective.

Environmental controls, ventilation and GUV, are an important intervention where unsuspected, untreated, or inadequately treated TB poses a risk. Natural ventilation is the main mode of air disinfection where climate permits, but even in warm countries, its effectiveness is threatened by increasing use of air conditioning, requiring closed windows. The most effective, affordable, and sustainable companion technology (or substitute where natural ventilation is not possible) is GUV, properly planned, installed (using high-quality fixtures and air mixing), commissioned, and maintained according to readily available guidelines. Finally, respiratory protection should refocus limited use of quality, fit-tested respiratory protection for encounters with symptomatic persons at risk for pulmonary TB who are not likely on effective treatment. Surgical masks should be reserved for short-term use before effective treatment starts.

REFERENCES

1. Riley R, O'Grady F, editors. Airborne infection. New York: The Macmillan Company; 1961.
2. Mann T, editor. The magic moutain. New York: Alfred A. Knopf; 1924.
3. Riley RL, Mills CC, O'grady F, et al. Infectiousness of air from a tuberculosis ward. Ultraviolet irradiation of infected air: comparative infectiousness of different patients. Am Rev Respir Dis 1962;85:511–25.
4. Donald PR, Diacon AH, Lange C, et al. Droplets, dust and Guinea pigs: an historical review of tuberculosis transmission research, 1878-1940. Int J Tuberc Lung Dis 2018;22:972–82.
5. Rouillion A, Perdrizet S, Parrot R. Transmission of tubercle bacilli: the effects of chemotherapy. Tubercle 1976;57:275–99.
6. Andrews RH, Devadatta S, Fox W, et al. Prevalence of tuberculosis among close family contacts of tuberculous patients in South India, and influence of segregation of the patient on early attack rate. Bull World Health Organ 1960;23:463–510.
7. Menzies D. Effect of treatment on contagiousness of patients with active pulmonary tuberculosis. Infect Control Hosp Epidemiol 1997;18:582–6.
8. Dharmadhikari AS, Mphahlele M, Venter K, et al. Rapid impact of effective treatment on transmission of multidrug-resistant tuberculosis. Int J Tuberc Lung Dis 2014;18:1019–25.
9. Frieden TR, Sherman LF, Maw KL, et al. A multi-institutional outbreak of highly drug-resistant tuberculosis: epidemiology and clinical outcomes. JAMA 1996;276:1229–35.
10. Escombe AR, Oeser C, Gilman RH, et al. The detection of airborne transmission of tuberculosis from HIV-infected patients, using an in vivo air sampling model. Clin Infect Dis 2007;44:1349–57.
11. Escombe AR, Moore DA, Gilman RH, et al. The infectiousness of tuberculosis patients coinfected with HIV. PLoS Med 2008;5:e188.

12. Dharmadhikari AS, Basaraba RJ, Van Der Walt ML, et al. Natural infection of Guinea pigs exposed to patients with highly drug-resistant tuberculosis. Tuberculosis (Edinb) 2011;91(4):329–38.

13. Mphaphlele M, Dharmadhikari AS, Jensen PA, et al. Institutional Tuberculosis Transmission: controlled trial of upper room ultraviolet air disinfection - A basis for new dosing guidelines. Am J Resp Crit Care Med 2015;192(4):477–84.

14. Dharmadhikari AS, Mphahlele M, Stoltz A, et al. Surgical face masks worn by patients with multidrug-resistant tuberculosis: impact on infectivity of air on a hospital ward. Am J Respir Crit Care Med 2012; 185:1104–9.

15. Stoltz A, de Kock E, Nathavitharana RR, et al. Multidrug resistant TB treatment regimen, including bedaquiline and linezolid, failed to reduce transmission over 11 days. International Scientific Meeting of the American Thoracic Society. Washington, DC, May 19-24, 2019: ATS: abstact 2017.

16. Nardell E, de Kock E, Nathavitharana RR, et al. Measuring the early impact on transmission of new treatment regimens for drug resistant tuberculosis. Annual Scientific Meeting of the American Thoracic Society; 2019 May, 2019; Dallas, Texas.

17. Willingham FF, Schmitz TL, Contreras M, et al. Hospital control and multidrug-resistant pulmonary tuberculosis in female patients, Lima, Peru. Emerg Infect Dis 2001;7:123–7.

18. Bates M, O'Grady J, Mwaba P, et al. Evaluation of the burden of unsuspected pulmonary tuberculosis and co-morbidity with non-communicable diseases in sputum producing adult inpatients. PLoS One 2012;7:e40774.

19. Yates TA, Khan PY, Knight GM, et al. The transmission of Mycobacterium tuberculosis in high burden settings. Lancet Infect Dis 2016;16:227–38.

20. Barrera E, Livchits V, Nardell E. F-A-S-T: a refocused, intensified, administrative tuberculosis transmission control strategy. Int J Tuberc Lung Dis 2015; 19:381–4.

21. Nathavitharana RR, Daru P, Barrera AE, et al. FAST implementation in Bangladesh: high frequency of unsuspected tuberculosis justifies challenges of scale-up. Int J Tuberc Lung Dis 2017; 21:1020–5.

22. Miller AC, Livchits V, Ahmad Khan F, et al. Turning off the tap: using the FAST approach to stop the spread of drug-resistant tuberculosis in the Russian Federation. J Infect Dis 2018;218:654–8.

23. Sultan L, Nyka C, Mills C, et al. Tuberculosis disseminators - a study of variability of aerial infectivity of tuberculosis patients. Am Rev Respir Dis 1960;82: 358–69.

24. Fennelly KP, Martyny JW, Fulton KE, et al. Cough-generated aerosols of Mycobacterium tuberculosis: a new method to study infectiousness. Am J Respir Crit Care Med 2004;169:604–9.

25. Robertson OH. Disinfection of the air with triethylene glycol vapor. Am J Med 1949;7:293–6.

26. Riley RL, Nardell EA. Clearing the air. The theory and application of ultraviolet air disinfection. Am Rev Respir Dis 1989;139:1286–94.

27. Escombe AR, Oeser CC, Gilman RH, et al. Natural ventilation for the prevention of airborne contagion. PLoS Med 2007;4:e68.

28. Richardson ET, Morrow CD, Kalil DB, et al. Shared air: a renewed focus on ventilation for the prevention of tuberculosis transmission. PLoS One 2014;9: e96334.

29. Stead WW, Senner JW, Reddick WT, et al. Racial differences in susceptibility to infection by Mycobacterium tuberculosis [see comments]. N Engl J Med 1990;322:422–7.

30. Lerner TR, Borel S, Gutierrez MG. The innate immune response in human tuberculosis. Cell Microbiol 2015;17:1277–85.

31. Nemes E, Geldenhuys H, Rozot V, et al. Prevention of M. tuberculosis infection with H4:IC31 vaccine or BCG revaccination. N Engl J Med 2018;379:138–49.

32. Tseng CH. Metformin decreases risk of tuberculosis infection in type 2 diabetes patients. J Clin Med 2018;7 [pii:E264].

33. Magee MJ, Salindri AD, Kornfeld H, et al. Reduced prevalence of latent tuberculosis infection in diabetes patients using metformin and statins. Eur Respir J 2019;53 [pii:1801695].

34. Su VY, Su WJ, Yen YF, et al. Statin use is associated with a lower risk of tuberculosis. Chest 2017;152(3): 598–606.

35. Aronson NE, Santosham M, Comstock GW, et al. Long-term efficacy of BCG vaccine in American Indians and Alaska Natives: a 60-year follow-up study. JAMA 2004;291:2086–91.

36. Davis LW, Gertler PJ. Contribution of air conditioning adoption to future energy use under global warming. Proc Natl Acad Sci U S A 2015;112:5962–7.

37. Nardell EA, Lederer P, Mishra H, et al. Cool but dangerous: how climate change is increasing the risk of airborne infections. Indoor Air, in press.

38. Rudnick SN, Milton DK. Risk of indoor airborne infection transmission estimated from carbon dioxide concentration. Indoor Air 2003;13:237–45.

39. Nardell EA, Keegan J, Cheney SA, et al. Airborne infection. Theoretical limits of protection achievable by building ventilation. Am Rev Respir Dis 1991; 144:302–6.

40. Miller-Leiden S, Lobascio C, Nazaroff WW, et al. Effectiveness of in-room air filtration and dilution ventilation for tuberculosis infection control. J Air Waste Manag Assoc 1996;46:869–82.

41. Escombe AR, Moore DA, Gilman RH, et al. Upper-room ultraviolet light and negative air ionization to

prevent tuberculosis transmission. PLoS Med 2009; 6:e43.

42. Mphaphlele M, Dharmadhikari AS, Jensen PA, et al. Institutional tuberculosis transmission. Controlled trial of upper room ultraviolet air disinfection: a basis for new dosing guidelines. Am J Respir Crit Care Med 2015;192:477–84.

43. World Health Organization. WHO guidelines on tuberculosis infection prevention and control: 2019 update. Geneva (Switzerland): WHO; 2019.

44. Rudnick SN, First MW. Fundamental factors affecting upper-room ultraviolet germicidal irradiation - part II. Predicting effectiveness. J Occup Environ Hyg 2007;4:352–62.

45. First M, Rudnick SN, Banahan KF, et al. Fundamental factors affecting upper-room ultraviolet germicidal irradiation - part I. Experimental. J Occup Environ Hyg 2007;4:321–31.

46. Rudnick SN. Predicting the ultraviolet radiation distribution in a room with multilouvered germicidal fixtures. AIHAJ 2001;62:434–45.

47. Holmes KK, Bertozzi S, Bloom BR, et al. Major infectious diseases. 3rd edition. Washington, DC: World Bank Group; 2017.

48. Nardell E, Vincent R, Sliney DH. Upper-room ultraviolet germicidal irradiation (UVGI) for air disinfection: a symposium in print. Photochem Photobiol 2013;89: 764–9.

49. Nardell EA, Bucher SJ, Brickner PW, et al. Safety of upper-room ultraviolet germicidal air disinfection for room occupants: results from the Tuberculosis Ultraviolet Shelter Study. Public Health Rep 2008;123: 52–60.

50. Jensen PA, Lambert LA, Iademarco MF, et al. Guidelines for preventing the transmission of Mycobacterium tuberculosis in health-care settings, 2005. MMWR Recomm Rep 2005;54: 1–141.

51. Coffey CC, Lawrence RB, Campbell DL, et al. Fitting characteristics of eighteen N95 filtering-facepiece respirators. J Occup Environ Hyg 2004;1:262–71.

UNITED STATES POSTAL SERVICE ®

Statement of Ownership, Management, and Circulation
(All Periodicals Publications Except Requester Publications)

1. Publication Title	2. Publication Number	3. Filing Date
CLINICS IN CHEST MEDICINE	000 - 706	9/18/2019

4. Issue Frequency	5. Number of Issues Published Annually	6. Annual Subscription Price
MAR, JUN, SEP, DE_	4	$377.00

7. Complete Mailing Address of Known Office of Publication (Not printer) (Street, city, county, state, and ZIP+4®)

ELSEVIER INC.
230 Park Avenue, Suite 800
New York, NY 10159

Contact Person
STEPHEN R. BUSHING

Telephone (Include area code)
215-239-3688

8. Complete Mailing Address of Headquarters or General Business Office of Publisher (Not printer)

ELSEVIER INC.
230 Park Avenue, Suite 800
New York, NY 10169

9. Full Names and Complete Mailing Addresses of Publisher, Editor, and Managing Editor (Do not leave blank)

Publisher (Name and complete mailing address)

TAYLOR BALL, ELSEVIER INC.
1600 JOHN F KENNEDY BLVD. SUITE 1800
PHILADELPHIA, FA 19103-2899

Editor (Name and complete mailing address)

COLLEEN DIETZLER, ELSEVIER INC.
1600 JOHN F KENNEDY BLVD. SUITE 1800
PHILADELPHIA, PA 19103-2899

Managing Editor (Name and complete mailing address)

PATRICK MANLEY, ELSEVIER INC.
1600 JOHN F KENNEDY BLVD. SUITE 1800
PHILADELPHIA, PA 19103-2899

10. Owner (Do not leave blank. If the publication is owned by a corporation, give the name and address of the corporation immediately followed by the names and addresses of all stockholders owning or holding 1 percent or more of the total amount of stock. If not owned by a corporation, give the names and addresses of the individual owners. If owned by a partnership or other unincorporated firm, give its name and address as well as those of each individual owner. If the publication is published by a nonprofit organization, give its name and address.)

Full Name	Complete Mailing Address
WHOLLY OWNED SUBSIDIARY OF REED/ELSEVIER, US HOLDINGS	1600 JOHN F KENNEDY BLVD. SUITE 1800 PHILADELPHIA, PA 19103-2899

11. Known Bondholders, Mortgagees, and Other Security Holders Owning or Holding 1 Percent or More of Total Amount of Bonds, Mortgages, or Other Securities. If none, check box ▶ ☐ None

Full Name	Complete Mailing Address
N/A	

12. Tax Status (For completion by nonprofit organizations authorized to mail at nonprofit rates) (Check one)
The purpose, function, and nonprofit status of this organization and the exempt status for federal income tax purposes:
☒ Has Not Changed During Preceding 12 Months
☐ Has Changed During Preceding 12 Months (Publisher must submit explanation of change with this statement)

PS Form **3526**, July 2014 [Page 1 of 4 (see instructions page 4)] PSN: 7530-01-000-9931   PRIVACY NOTICE: See our privacy policy on www.usps.com.

13. Publication Title		14. Issue Date for Circulation Data Below
CLINICS IN CHEST MEDICINE		JUNE 2019

15. Extent and Nature of Circulation			Average No. Copies Each Issue During Preceding 12 Months	No. Copies of Single Issue Published Nearest to Filing Date
a. Total Number of Copies (Net press run)			376	393
b. Paid Circulation (By Mail and Outside the Mail)	(1)	Mailed Outside-County Paid Subscriptions Stated on PS Form 3541 (Include paid distribution above nominal rate, advertiser's proof copies, and exchange copies)	205	229
	(2)	Mailed In-County Paid Subscriptions Stated on PS Form 3541 (Include paid distribution above nominal rate, advertiser's proof copies, and exchange copies)	0	0
	(3)	Paid Distribution Outside the Mails Including Sales Through Dealers and Carriers, Street Vendors, Counter Sales, and Other Paid Distribution Outside USPS®	106	129
	(4)	Paid Distribution by Other Classes of Mail Through the USPS (e.g. First-Class Mail®)	0	0
c. Total Paid Distribution (Sum of 15b (1), (2), (3), and (4))		▶	311	358
d. Free or Nominal Rate Distribution (By Mail and Outside the Mail)	(1)	Free or Nominal Rate Outside-County Copies included on PS Form 3541	45	15
	(2)	Free or Nominal Rate In-County Copies Included on PS Form 3541	0	0
	(3)	Free or Nominal Rate Copies Mailed at Other Classes Through the USPS (e.g. First-Class Mail)	0	0
	(4)	Free or Nominal Rate Distribution Outside the Mail (Carriers or other means)	0	0
e. Total Free or Nominal Rate Distribution (Sum of 15d (1), (2), (3) and (4))		▶	45	15
f. Total Distribution (Sum of 15c and 15e)		▶	356	373
g. Copies not Distributed (See Instructions to Publishers #4 (page #3))		▶	20	20
h. Total (Sum of 15f and g)		▶	376	393
i. Percent Paid (15c divided by 15f times 100)		▶	87.36%	95.99%

* If you are claiming electronic copies, go to line 16 on page 3. If you are not claiming electronic copies, skip to line 17 on page 3.

16. Electronic Copy Circulation		Average No. Copies Each Issue During Preceding 12 Months	No. Copies of Single Issue Published Nearest to Filing Date
a. Paid Electronic Copies	▶		
b. Total Paid Print Copies (Line 15c) + Paid Electronic Copies (Line 16a)	▶		
c. Total Print Distribution (Line 15f) + Paid Electronic Copies (Line 16a)	▶		
d. Percent Paid (Both Print & Electronic Copies) (16b divided by 16c × 100)	▶		

☒ I certify that 50% of all my distributed copies (electronic and print) are paid above a nominal price.

17. Publication of Statement of Ownership

☒ If the publication is a general publication, publication of this statement is required. Will be printed ☐ Publication not required in the DECEMBER 2019 issue of this publication.

18. Signature and Title of Editor, Publisher, Business Manager, or Owner

STEPHEN R. BUSHING - INVENTORY DISTRIBUTION CONTROL MANAGER

Date 9/18/2019

I certify that all information furnished on this form is true and complete. I understand that anyone who furnishes false or misleading information on this form or who omits material or information requested on the form may be subject to criminal sanctions (including fines and imprisonment) and/or civil sanctions (including civil penalties).

PS Form **3526**, July 2014 (Page 3 of 4)   PRIVACY NOTICE: See our privacy policy on www.usps.com

Printed and bound by CPI Group (UK) Ltd, Croydon, CR0 4YY

08/05/2025

01864745-0020